Brain Organization and Memory

Brain
Organization
and Memory:
Cells, Systems, and Circuits

Edited by

JAMES L. McGAUGH

NORMAN M. WEINBERGER

GARY LYNCH

New York   Oxford
OXFORD UNIVERSITY PRESS

Oxford University Press

Oxford   New York   Toronto
Delhi   Bombay   Calcutta   Madras   Karachi
Kuala Lumpur   Singapore   Hong Kong   Tokyo
Nairobi   Dar es Salaam   Cape Town
Melbourne   Auckland

and associated companies in
Berlin   Ibadan

Copyright © 1990 by Oxford University Press

First published in 1990 by Oxford University Press, Inc.,
200 Madison Avenue, New York, New York 10016

First issued as an Oxford University Press paperback, 1992

Oxford is a registered trademark of Oxford University Press

Library of Congress Cataloging-in-Publication Data
Brain organization and memory : cells, systems, and circuits /
edited by James L. McGaugh, Norman M. Weinberger, Gary Lynch.
p.   cm.
Based on the Third Conference on the Neurobiology of Learning and Memory
organized by the Center for Neurobiology of Learning and Memory of
the University of California, Irvine, held at Irvine on Oct. 14-17, 1987.
Includes bibliographies and index.
ISBN 0-19-505496-2   ISBN 0-19-507712-1 (Pbk.)
1. Memory—Congresses.   2. Cerebral cortex—Physiology—Congresses.
3. Neural circuitry—Congresses.   I. McGaugh, James L.
II. Weinberger, Norman M.   III. Lynch, Gary.
IV. University of California, Irvine. Center for the Neurobiology of Learning and Memory.
[DNLM: 1. Cerebral Cortex—physiology—congresses.   2. Memory—physiology—congresses.
3. Models, Neurological—congresses.   4. Nervous System—physiology—congresses.
WL 102 B8132 1987]   QP406.B735   1989   153.1'2—dc19
DNLM/DLC for Library of Congress   88-38920

9   8   7   6   5   4   3   2   1
Printed in the United States of America

Preface

This volume is the third in a series. Like its predecessors, *Neurobiology of Learning and Memory* and *Memory Systems of the Brain,* this book is the outgrowth of a conference that was organized by the Center for the Neurobiology of Learning and Memory of the University of California, Irvine. The Third Conference was held at Irvine on October 14–17, 1987. One might ask, as we did, whether a book summarizing work on how the brain encodes and uses memory is needed every two to three years. An examination of the tables of contents of the three books clearly answers this question. Some of the central theoretical and methodological issues addressed in this book are not so much as noted in the indexes of the previous volumes. This attests to the active and expanding interest in research on brain, learning, and memory.

This book focuses on three related topics: forms of memory, regulation of cortical function in memory, and representations. Some of the themes developed in the first two volumes are given further emphasis in this book. Prominent among these are the efforts to relate learning and memory as they are studied in animals to those processes observed in humans. Despite steady experimental and conceptual progress, development of an adequate taxonomy of memory continues to hamper efforts to achieve unification of memory theory. This annoying fact should temper our hopes for a rapid and complete integration of the subtle and surprising phenomena of memory with those of brain cells, systems, and circuits. Nonetheless, it is clear that the rate of progress in understanding the cellular processes underlying memory continues to accelerate. We are beginning to see the emergence of a consensus regarding the physiological and chemical events that translate activity patterns into long-term changes in the strength of connections between brain cells. We are also now seeing behavioral studies of memory using predictions derived from understanding of synaptic plasticity. One can only be impressed at how quickly the world of ions and receptors is being translated into the realm of memory systems and mazes.

Special emphasis is given in this volume to computational and modeling approaches to the study of brain and memory. The development of network models and computer simulations of memory permeates current research. This effort is explicitly recognized in the final section of the book, but the use of network models is seen throughout the book. Experimentalists working on cortex and hippocampus are attempting to link cells to systems with interesting and powerful models. However, the gap between formal mathematically tractable models and the stuff of brains remains clear and provides a continuing challenge for experimentalists and theorists alike.

In all, the leitmotif of this book, like that of its predecessors, is excitement. Excitement about what we have learned as well as what we can now ask. We hope that readers of *Brain Organization and Memory: Cells, Systems, and Circuits* will share our excitement as well as our eagerness to follow this intellectual drama in volumes yet to come.

Irvine, Calif.   J. L. McG.
October 1988   N. M. W.
                                                                     G. L.

Acknowledgments

The conference on which this book is based was planned and organized by the members of the Center for the Neurobiology of Learning and Memory at the University of California, Irvine. The selection of topics and authors grew out of extensive discussions with our colleagues John Ashe, Michel Baudry, Richard Granger, Mary-Louise Kean, Mark Rosenzweig, Gordon Shaw, Larry Squire, and Larry Stein. Funding for the conference was provided by a number of organizations: the UCI Office of Research and Graduate Studies, the Office of Naval Research, the Air Force Office of Scientific Research, the National Science Foundation, the Sloan Foundation, the Irvine Company, Searle Research and Development, Beckman Instruments, and Hoechst-Roussel Pharmaceuticals. We thank Lynn Brown, Nan Collett, and Lori LaSalle for their skilled coordination of all aspects of the conference. Special thanks are also due to Lynn Brown for editorial assistance.

Contents

II Regulation of Cortical Function in Memory

III Representations: Beyond the Single Cell

Contributors

RICHARD A. ANDERSEN
Department of Brain and Cognitive Sciences
Massachusetts Institute of Technology
Cambridge, Massachusetts 02139

MARK F. BEAR
Center for Neural Science
Brown University
Providence, Rhode Island 02912

JAN BUREŠ
Institute of Physiology
Czechoslovak Academy of Sciences
Prague 4, Czechoslovakia

THOMAS J. CAREW
Departments of Psychology and Biology
Yale University
New Haven, Connecticut 06520

LEON N. COOPER
Department of Physics and Center for Neural Science
Brown University
Providence, Rhode Island 02912

ROBERT W. DOTY
Department of Physiology
University of Rochester
Rochester, New York 14642

FORD F. EBNER
Center for Neural Science
Brown University
Providence, Rhode Island 02912

WALTER J. FREEMAN
Department of Physiology–Anatomy
University of California
Berkeley, California 94720

MICHELA GALLAGHER
Department of Psychology
University of North Carolina
Chapel Hill, North Carolina 27514

GEORGE L. GERSTEIN
Department of Physiology
University of Pennsylvania
Philadelphia, Pennsylvania 19104

PATRICIA S. GOLDMAN-RAKIC
Section of Neuroanatomy
Yale University School of Medicine
New Haven, Connecticut 06510

RICHARD GRANGER
Center for the Neurobiology of Learning and Memory
   and Department of Information and Computer Science
University of California
Irvine, California 92717

PETER C. HOLLAND
Psychology Department
Duke University
Durham, North Carolina 27706

MARCIA K. JOHNSON
Department of Psychology
Princeton University
Princeton, New Jersey 08544

HERBERT P. KILLACKEY
Department of Psychobiology
University of California
Irvine, California 92717

TEUVO KOHONEN
Laboratory of Computer and Information Science
Helsinki University of Technology
Espoo, Finland

JOHN LARSON
Center for the Neurobiology of Learning and Memory
University of California
Irvine, California 92717

GARY LYNCH
Center for the Neurobiology of Learning and Memory
and Department of Psychobiology
University of California
Irvine, California 92717

EMILIE A. MARCUS
Department of Psychology
Yale University
New Haven, Connecticut 06520

RICHARD G. M. MORRIS
Department of Pharmacology
University of Edinburgh Medical School
Edinburgh EH8 9JZ
Scotland

DOMINIQUE MULLER
Department of Pharmacology
Centre Medical Universitaire
Geneva 4, Switzerland

THOMAS G. NOLEN
Department of Biology
University of Miami
Coral Gables, Florida 33124

CATHARINE H. RANKIN
Department of Psychology
University of British Columbia
Vancouver, British Columbia, Canada V6T1W5

EDMUND T. ROLLS
Department of Experimental Psychology
University of Oxford
Oxford OX1 3UD
England

MARK R. ROSENZWEIG
Department of Psychology
University of California
Berkeley, California 94720

CHRISTOPHER SCOFIELD
Nestor Inc.
Providence, Rhode Island 02906

TERRENCE J. SEJNOWSKI
The Salk Institute
La Jolla, California 92037

GORDON L. SHAW
Center for the Neurobiology of Learning and Memory
   and Department of Physics
University of California
Irvine, California 92717

ARTHUR P. SHIMAMURA
Veterans Administration Medical Center
San Diego, California 92161

WOLF SINGER
Max-Planck-Institute for Brain Research
Frankfurt 71
Federal Republic of Germany

CHRISTINE A. SKARDA
Department of Physiology–Anatomy
University of California
Berkeley, California 94720

MARK STOPFER
Department of Psychology
Yale University
New Haven, Connecticut 06520

GERALD TESAURO
IBM Thomas J. Watson Research Center
Yorktown Heights, New York 10598

GARY W. VAN HOESEN
Department of Anatomy
University of Iowa
Iowa City, Iowa 52242

CHRISTOPH VON DER MALSBURG
Computer Science Department
University of Southern California
Los Angeles, California 90089

NORMAN M. WEINBERGER
Center for the Neurobiology of Learning and Memory
    and Department of Psychobiology
University of California
Irvine, California 92717

DAVID ZIPSER
Institute for Cognitive Science
University of California, San Diego
La Jolla, California 92093

Brain Organization and Memory

1

Neurobiology of Memory:
The Significance of Anomalous Findings

JAN BUREŠ

The neurobiology of learning and memory is a relatively young discipline with a vague status that lacks a unifying theory. Facts are accumulating at a rate that vastly exceeds our capability to explain them. Research strategies highly valued in physics find little application in neurobiology. The almost obsessive interest of physicists in anomalies, an attitude that has led to the discovery of planets, subatomic particles, big bang, and superconductivity, is not seen in neurobiology, where it is often difficult to distinguish an anomaly from the normal state of affairs, to recognize an anomalous phenomenon against the background variability of the process studied. Even when the oddity of a finding is obvious and proved beyond any doubt, it is easier to consider it an enigmatic exception than to seek an explanation requiring a fundamental revision of the accepted beliefs. I believe that our discipline is mature enough to face embarrassing facts and that the study of anomalies will not undermine the coherence of the field but open the way to more comprehensive cross-level synthesis of cellular, systemic, and behavioral investigations.

ROBUST LEARNING CAN PROCEED WITHOUT AWARENESS

One of the basic tenets of contemporary neurobiology is that associative learning requires not only the specific input of signals to be processed (i.e., CS and US), but also various auxiliary mechanisms—for example, attention, motivation, emotion—that together account for a particular central state characterized as consciousness, awareness, or alertness and expressed by the corresponding level of arousal. In spite of countless examples supporting this belief, it would be a mistake to assert that awareness is a necessary condition of learning. Conditioned taste aversion (CTA) is a dramatic counterexample. The rat's capability to avoid a flavor whose ingestion has been followed by illness (Barker, Best, & Domjan, 1977; Braveman & Bronstien, 1985; Garcia, Kimeldorf, & Koelling,

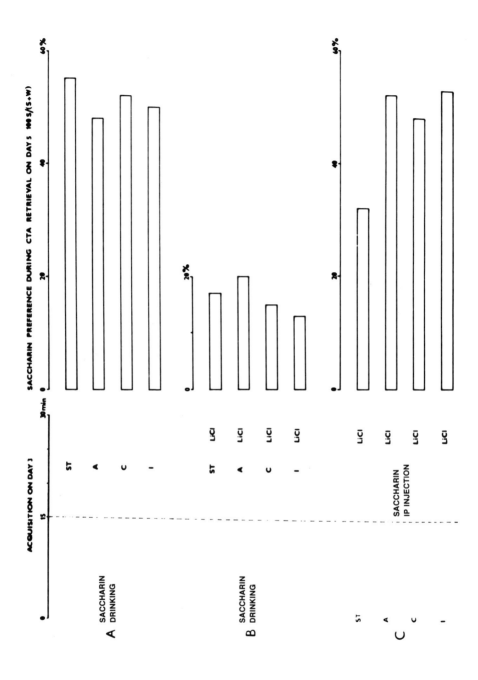

1955) is not diminished when immediately after presentation of the taste stimulus the animal is anesthetized with pentobarbital and maintained under deep anesthesia throughout the duration of the poison-elicited illness (Berger, 1970). The gustatory stimulus has left in the rat's brain a trace that is later associated with the visceral symptoms of intoxication. Anesthesia interferes neither with the persistence of this trace nor with its association with the poison-elicited signals. Similar results were obtained with other comatose states elicited by functional decortication (Burešová & Bureš, 1973), deep (20°C) hypothermia (Ionescu & Burešová, 1977), cerebral ischemia, or prolonged seizures (Bureš & Burešová, 1987). When these states are elicited after presentation of the taste stimulus (Fig. 1.1) they do not induce CTA when applied alone, and they do not prevent CTA acquisition when inserted between the CS and US, that is, when applied before administration of the poison. In fact, we have not yet found any reversible intervention that would disrupt CTA acquisition under the above conditions. This is perhaps not surprising if we take into account the biological significance of CTA, which protects animals against the fatal error of repeated ingestion of lethal poisons.

Accurate memory record of the sensory properties of food whose ingestion has preceded poisoning gives the animal a clear advantage in the struggle for survival. The value of this behavior is greatly increased when the learning is not disrupted by a comatose state that may be a part of the poisoning. Evolution has recognized the vital significance of the taste–poisoning association and has equipped animals with failure-proof brain mechanisms that ensure reliable recording of the relevant information as long as the animal is alive; thus an animal that recovers can profit from the experience and prevent fatal poisoning by avoiding the particular flavor.

The various instances of learning form a continuum ranging from the most universal associative phenomena, allowing combination of any pair of stimuli while requiring prolonged training and activation of auxiliary mechanisms, to dedicated associative processes automatically entering variables of a definite class into highly prepared behavioral schemes. Learning mechanisms supporting food selection are typical examples of the latter questionnaire-type learning. The sensory properties (particularly the taste) of ingested food are automatically

---

←

FIGURE 1.1.   The effect of pentobarbital anesthesia (50 mg/kg, A), picrotoxin convulsions (5 mg/kg, C), cerebral ischemia (5-min occlusion of neck vessels under ether anesthesia, I), or sham treatment (ST) on the acquisition of CTA. The columns indicate mean ($\pm$ SEM, n = 10) saccharin preference during the retention test on day 5. W = water; S = saccharin. The conditions during CTA acquisition on day 3 are schematically shown on the left. (A) Saccharin drinking followed by any of the foregoing experimental treatments alone does not elicit CTA. (B) Saccharin drinking followed by intraperitoneal injection of lithium chloride (0.15 mol/l, 2% body weight) elicits strong CTA, which is not prevented by the foregoing interventions applied after the gustatory CS and before the visceral US. (C) The same interventions (with the exception of ST) prevent CTA acquisition when applied prior to systemic administration of the taste stimulus (2% saccharin, 1% body weight) followed by lithium chloride poisoning.

recorded in a short-term memory file where they wait during several hours for visceral signals generated by the passage of the food through the gastrointestinal tract. Only two outcomes are monitored: (1) the food has no adverse consequences and satisfies hunger or thirst and (2) the food elicits gastrointestinal distress and other signs of sickness. After a time sufficient for food digestion and resorption has elapsed, the neutral input signal is transferred from short-term memory into permanent memory with the label acceptable or aversive. The only intentional part of the process is the initial food intake, which starts an automatic chain of events generating a reliable record of gustatory–visceral contingencies, essential for the future feeding behavior of the animal.

The gustatory trace–poisoning association in anesthetized animals was discovered by Berger (1970) and has since been replicated in a score of studies in different laboratories (Burešová & Bureš, 1977, 1979a, 1979b, 1984; Millner & Palfai, 1975; Rabin & Rabin, 1984; Roll & Smith, 1972). Although these reliable and easily reproducible experiments clearly demonstrate that robust learning can proceed without awareness, the evidence was dismissed as an interesting peculiarity that does not require any fundamental revision of the conventional view. Of course this is not true. A single demonstration of this type shows that the theory is not generally valid and that other, not immediately obvious alternatives must be considered.

CONDITIONED–UNCONDITIONED STIMULUS PAIRING PROCEEDS IN STAGES DIFFERENTIALLY SENSITIVE TO DISRUPTION

Some of the problems involved can again be illustrated through CTA research. Whereas the gustatory trace–poisoning association is not disrupted by the deepest coma, formation of the gustatory trace is a fragile process that can be blocked by mild hypothermia (Burešová & Bureš, 1981), previous paradoxical sleep deprivation (Danguir & Nicolaidis, 1976), or anterograde ECS effects (Burešová & Bureš, 1979a). Interventions that block spontaneous drinking and feeding, for example, functional decortication by cortical spreading depression (CSD) (Burešová & Bureš, 1973) or general anesthesia, prevent formation of the gustatory trace by forcefeeding or by systemic application of the concentrated flavor (e.g., intraperitoneal injection of 2% saccharin, 1% body weight; Bellingham & Lloyd, 1987; Burešová & Bureš, 1977), which is effective in intact animals. Thus the same intervention, for example, anesthesia, disrupts or does not disrupt CTA acquisition according to its timing with respect to the various phases of the learning process (Fig. 1.2). An important advantage of the CTA model is that the long CS–US delay makes it possible to differentially influence CS processing and formation of the gustatory trace, persistence of this trace, and its association with the symptoms of poisoning. This is not likely to occur in other types of learning characterized by CS–US delays of less than a few seconds. Even such instances of conditioning may proceed in several successive stages that are differentially sensitive to disruption but cannot be easily separated from one another.

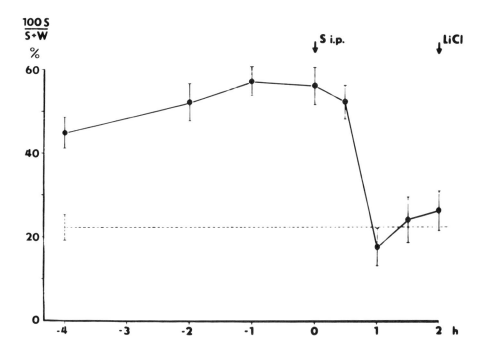

FIGURE 1.2.   The effect of pentobarbital anesthesia (50 mg/kg) on CTA acquisition on day 3. *Ordinate:* Mean saccharin preference ($\pm$ SEM, $n = 10$) during the retention test on day 5. *Abscissa:* Time of pentobarbital injection (50 mg/kg) before ($-$) or after systemic administration of the taste stimulus (2% saccharin, 1% body weight) followed two hours later by lithium chloride poisoning (0.15 mol/l, 2% body weight). Note that CTA is disrupted when the taste stimulus is applied to anesthetized rats or to rats recovering from anesthesia, but that strong CTA develops when the gustatory stimulus precedes the onset of anesthesia.

The successive stages of CTA acquisition are implemented by different brain structures. The finding that formation of the gustatory trace is disrupted by reversible functional decortication suggests that this stage of CTA acquisition requires cortical participation. But the same intervention does not impair persistence of the gustatory trace and/or its association with the visceral symptoms of poisoning because the underlying plastic change takes place at a subcortical level, probably in the lower brain stem. It is important to realize that this differential sensitivity to interference cannot be established by brain lesions, which always affect the most failure-prone link of the process but do not allow recognition of the better protected links. The vast literature on the effects of brain lesions on CTA (Riley & Tuck, 1985) almost exclusively describes the significance of the damaged structures for the formation of the short-term gustatory trace but does not assess their role in the gustatory trace–poisoning association. Papers describing CTA acquisition deficits after ablation of the gustatory cortex (see Kiefer, 1985, for review) do not consider the possibility that the cortex is not necessary for the persistence of the gustatory trace and for its association with poisoning. A more realistic picture of the neural mechanisms involved can be obtained with the use of functional ablation procedures. Thus the finding that CTA acquisition is impaired in amygdalectomized rats was analyzed by Bermudez-Rattoni, Rusiniak, and Garcia (1983), who demonstrated that reversible inactivation of amygdala by novocaine prevents taste-potentiated odor aversion when employed before presentation of the compound odor–taste stimulus. The same intervention applied after the CS but before the visceral US was ineffective. Like the gustatory cortex, amygdala participates in the initial formation of the short-term memory trace but is not indispensable for the poisoning-induced aversive labeling of this trace.

Another deeply ingrained concept represents the association process by direct interaction of the CS- and US-activated circuits. In fact, classical conditioning is best expressed when CS and US overlap in time and deteriorates with increasing CS–US delay in case of trace conditioning. It is possible to surmise that the CTA blockade observed when the gustatory CS has been presented during CSD or anesthesia is due to the failure to form the gustatory trace and to bridge the temporal gap between the CS and US. The gustatory trace might be considered unnecessary when the taste signal overlaps with poisoning and when there is an opportunity for direct convergence of the CS and US volleys on the circuits mediating aversive labeling of the gustatory experience (Fig. 1.3), but experiments show that this is not the case. Whereas forcefeeding saccharin to intact rats poisoned with lithium chloride elicits moderate CTA, no CTA is acquired under the same conditions by rats under bilateral CSD (Bureš & Burešová, 1981). This indicates that CSD or other CTA-disrupting interventions prevent transcription of the gustatory signal into a memory buffer accessible to visceral signals. The purpose of this buffer is not only to cope with the CS–US delay, but also to provide a device for interaction between the temporarily stored neutral signal with other relevant signals and for its eventual transformation into an interpreted, labeled engram stored in permanent memory. It is conceivable that a similar scheme applies to other forms of conditioning that are implemented not by direct interaction between CS- and US-elicited volleys but between representations of the CS and/or US signals. The indispensability of the short-term gustatory trace for CTA formation is thus an important argument in support of the cognitive theories indicating that the multistage organization of the learning process cannot be replaced by a simpler system, corresponding to a verbatim interpretation of the S–R or S–S theories.

MOTOR LEARNING DOES NOT ALWAYS OBEY THE LAW OF EFFECT

Thus far we have discussed the sensory aspects of learning, the processes that store a neutral sensory stimulus and change it into a signal of biologically significant events. In most cases this is sufficient for effective coping behavior, consisting of inhibition of some and activation of other preprogrammed items of

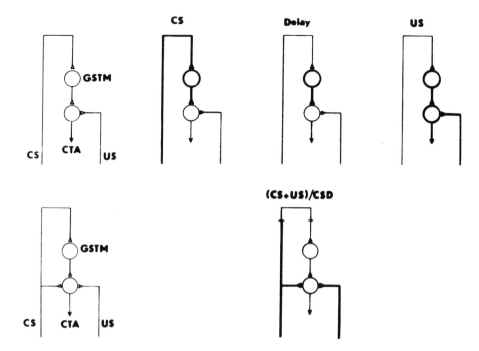

FIGURE 1.3. Schematic representation of the putative stages of CTA acquisition. *Above*: Serial model. *Below*: Serioparallel model. CS = conditioned gustatory stimulus; US = unconditioned visceral stimulus; GSTM = gustatory short-term memory; CTA = aversive labeling of the gustatory stimulus; (CS + US)/CSD = simultaneous presentation of CS and US during bilateral cortical spreading depression. Heavy lines indicate the part of the circuit that is active during the particular stage of the experiment.

the animal's repertoire such as eating, running, and freezing. Sometimes, however, adaptive behavior cannot be achieved by the already available motor programs. In this case, learning consists not only of the detection and interpretation of stimulus contingencies, but also of the modification of the motor response of the animal in the acquisition of new skills.

An obvious advantage of motor learning for brain and behavior research is that the putative plastic change takes place close to the motor output and can therefore be readily observed, localized, and analyzed by electrophysiological methods. The remarkable progress in research into the motor functions (Brooks & Thach, 1981) has significantly advanced our understanding of motor learning, particularly in primates. But the validity of some general principles must be reassessed in light of the physiological analysis of motor learning. The most important of these principles is the "law of effect," formulated almost a century ago by Thorndike (1911), which states that the strength of an operant not followed by reinforcement gradually decreases. This law, borne out by countless experiments, is the theoretical basis of operant conditioning and represents an important tenet of the universalistic concepts asserting that learning can associate any pair of stimuli or establish bonds between any stimulus and any reaction of the organism. Whereas important species-specific constraints described by Breland and Breland (1961) have demonstrated the limited validity of the law of effect in general, analysis of the physiological mechanisms of motor learning shows that the law requires a wider interpretation, taking into account not only the delivery of reinforcement but also the effort required for the necessary reorganization of the existing motor programs. This assertion can be illustrated by experiments attempting to modify rhythmic licking in rats by motor learning.

Licking, like mastication and swallowing, belongs to feeding-related oral behaviors implemented by a central rhythmic generator residing in the lower brain stem (Halpern, 1977; Malmo, Malmo, & Weijnen, 1987; Weijnen & Mendelson, 1977). The generator is switched on and off from higher forebrain centers and is influenced by trigeminal, glossopharyngeal, and vagal inputs. In a thirsty rat, the generator is switched on in the presence of a drinking spout and switched off only some time after the spout has been suddenly removed (Mamedov & Bureš, 1984). The nonrewarded licks emitted in the absence of the spout decrease the overall efficiency of behavior and the law of effect requires that their incidence is maximally reduced. This assumption was tested by training rats to alternate between two retractable drinking spouts accessible through adjacent openings in the wall of the cage (Mamedov, Hernandez-Mesa, & Bureš, 1987). After the first lick at the left spout, this spout was removed by a solenoid out of the reach of the animal's tongue, while the other spout was advanced to the right opening. After the first lick at the right spout, this spout was retracted and the left spout was advanced (Fig. 1.4). The licks at the two spouts were monitored with photoelectric lickometers and their incidence was analyzed with a laboratory computer.

After up to 10 days of training and thousands of spout alternations, the animals continued to emit more than one lick per spout presentation (2.5 licks on average) and this value even grew when the spout separation was increased by introduction of a vertical partition. This apparent violation of the law of effect is not a result of the inability of the rat to emit single licks: if the animal had to alternate between an empty spout and a spout containing water, the additional licks were produced only at the rewarded spout, whereas they were almost absent at the empty spout (Fig. 1.5). It seems that the additional licks reflect the tendency of the animal not to interrupt the activity of the central timing network between spout presentations. Although no overt licks are visible during transition between spouts, the timing network is probably not stopped but only disconnected from the intracycle pattern generator (Lennárd & Hermanson, 1985) and from the motor output. The noninterrupted activity of the pacemaker of licking is indicated by good synchronization of the posttransition licks with the pretransition licking.

The postulate that animals tend to maximize the value of their behavioral output must be based on a complete cost–benefit analysis (Rachlin & Burkhard, 1978), taking into account not only the response–reinforcement ratio but also

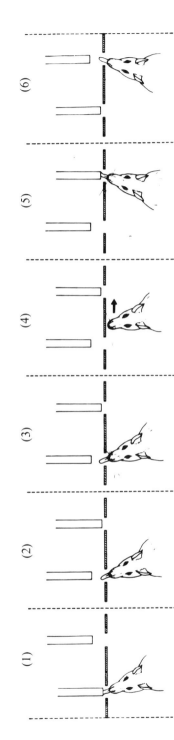

FIGURE 1.4. Forced spout alternation. (1) First lick at the left spout. (2,3) Left spout is retracted and right spout advanced; the rat continues to lick at the left wall opening, although it cannot contact the distant spout. (4) After two nonrewarded licks at the left opening the rat moves to the right opening. (5) First lick at the now available right spout. (6) The right spout is retracted, but the animal continues to lick at the right wall opening.

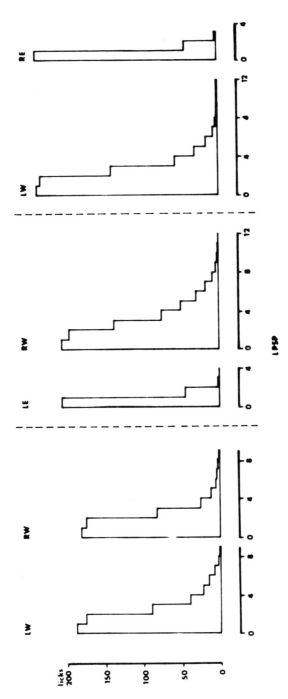

FIGURE 1.5. Cumulative histogram of successive licks emitted during forced spout alternation at the left (L) and right (R) spouts which either contain water (W) or are empty (E). *Ordinate:* Number of licks (vertical bar denotes 100 licks). *Abscissa:* Number of licks per spout presentation (LPSP). Note that the two distributions were symmetric when both spouts contained water, but that LPSP approached 1 at the empty spout while additional licks continued to be emitted at the other water-containing spout.

the difficulties connected with generation of the new response pattern. It seems that rats find it acceptable to get only one reinforced lick out of five if they can avoid in this way the need to switch the central timing network on and off. It is also conceivable that the consummatory licks, resulting in transport of a small amount (about 5 μl) of water into the mouth cavity, require continued licking in vacuo in order to induce swallowing, which usually follows after 3 to 5 licks (Weijnen, Wouters, & Van Hest, 1984). This may explain why the instrumental lick at the dry spout is not followed by additional licks, whereas the consummatory licks at the water-containing spout are.

This simple experiment demonstrates that the law of effect formulated on the basis of behavioral observations exerts only limited control over specific physiological mechanisms and must therefore be applied with great caution for the interpretation of cellular phenomena.

MEMORY READOUT IS NOT IMPAIRED
BY COMPLETE RECONSTITUTION OF SENSORY INPUT

Finally, let us consider yet another anomaly in the neurobiology of memory access, concerned with the problem of central stimulus representation. Although it is not yet clear whether information encoding employs a hierarchical system of neurons converging through progressively more complex feature detectors to the so-called gnostic units (Konorski, 1967), distributed stimulus representation by spatiotemporal patterns of activity in large neuronal populations (Freeman, 1975), or a combination of both principles (Perrett, Mistlin, & Chitty, 1987), orderly mapping of the receptor surface on the appropriate brain centers is a basic prerequisite for each of these alternatives. The fact that neurons are not replaced in the adult brain is usually considered to be an organizational principle supporting the invariance of such mappings. This is the reason why three generations of neurobiologists have been fascinated by Sperry's (1944) demonstration that the regenerating optic nerve axons in frogs and fish can find their respective targets in the tectum and reestablish through appropriate synaptic connections (Jacobson, 1978) apparently normal retinotectal mapping and vision. Recent progress in transplantation of embryonal brain tissue makes it possible to perform analogous experiments in mammals. McLoon and Lund (1980) demonstrated that embryonal retina transplanted close to the superior colliculus of adult rats retains its morphology and light sensitivity and that the axons of the ganglion cells form synaptic contacts with the host tectum. Freed (1983) used light stimulation of the grafted retina through an implanted light-conducting rod to test the possible transmission of CS signals through this ectopic input. Experiments of this type resemble Doty's (1969) analysis of conditioning with the use of electrical stimulation of brain as the CS. There is little doubt that the retinal graft can transmit information about presence or absence of light to the host and allow at least some crude form of brightness discrimination learning.

Whereas the exciting attempts to provide the rat with the additional *Hatteria*-type parietal eye are in their infancy, another mammalian sensory system resembles the optic nerve regeneration in amphibia more closely. Graziadei and Monti-Graziadei (1978) convincingly demonstrated that the sensory neurons of the olfactory epithelium in the nasal cavity are in a permanent state of renewal. After several months they degenerate and are replaced by new neurons developing from the germinative layer of basal cells. Since the olfactory nerve is formed by axons of sensory neurons, all fila olfactoria are completely exchanged within a few months, as are their synaptic connections in the glomerular layer of the olfactory bulb.

The regenerative power of the olfactory epithelium is better expressed after transection of the olfactory nerve: all sensory neurons whose axons were cut degenerate, but the newly formed sensory neurons send their axons through the cribriform bone to the olfactory bulb again. After several months the sense of smell is restored and old olfactory memories are reliably retrieved through new sensory elements, nerve fibers, and synapses. Since the efficiency of this reorganized input is comparable to that observed in case of the optic nerve–tectum reconnection in frogs, olfactory nerve regeneration can serve as a convenient model for the investigation of the molecular mechanisms governing reconnection of millions of axons to their respective targets.

There is an important difference between the two models, however. Whereas in the case of the optic nerve the regenerating axons connect the surviving ganglion cells of retina with tectum, transection of the olfactory nerve leads to initial degeneration and subsequent regeneration of the neuroepithelium so that appropriate connections must be formed between a substantially reduced and reconstituted population of input elements and the original target structure.

Olfactory nerve regeneration makes it possible to go still further: Graziadei and Monti-Graziadei (1986), using rats and mice with olfactory bulbs removed, showed that the olfactory axons can form the characteristic glomeruli and the corresponding synapses in other forebrain structures extending into the bulbectomy-created cavity (frontal lobes, oflactory tract, anterior olfactory nucleus). Whether the synapses between primary olfactory fibers and nonolfactory brain structures or higher olfactory centers are functional is a matter of controversy. Wright and Harding (1982) reported good recovery of smell in bulbectomized mice, but their results were questioned by Butler, Graziadei, Monti-Graziadei, and Slotnick (1984), who found irreversible loss of smell in animals with morphologically verified complete ablation of the olfactory bulb. Amemori, Soukup, Valoušková, and Bureš (1986) confirmed recovery of smell in bulbectomized rats (Fig. 1.6). In most animals the positive results could be explained by reinnervation of small remnants of the olfactory bulb adjacent to the olfactory tract, but several rats succeeded in the olfactory tests in spite of complete bulbectomy. In such cases, intensive glomerulization was seen in the anterior olfactory nucleus and frontal cortex or in embryonal grafts transplanted into the cavity produced by bulbectomy, and units responding to olfactory stimuli were found

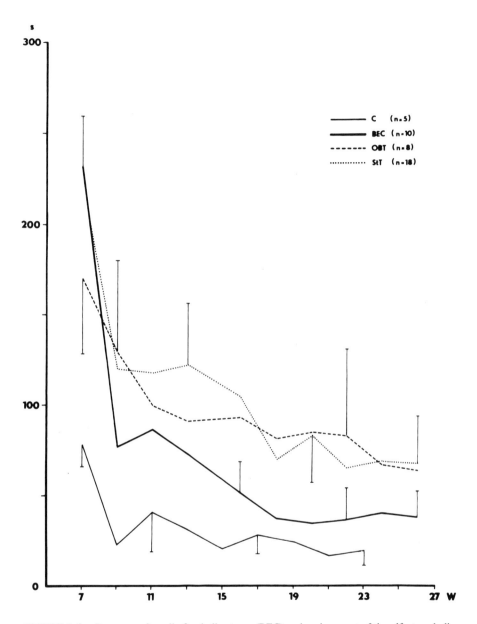

FIGURE 1.6.   Recovery of smell after bulbectomy (BEC) and replacement of the olfactory bulb with grafts of embryonal olfactory bulb (OBT) or neostriatum (StT). *Ordinate:* Average latency (±SEM, *n* = 10) to find a food pellet buried under a 5-cm-deep layer of polystyrene balls. *Abscissa:* Time after bulbectomy in weeks. C = unoperated control animals.

in such nonbulbar brain structures. On the other hand, glomeruli and olfactory responses were absent in the brains of rats failing in the olfactory test.

These results point to the possibility that regenerating olfactory axons can bypass the first relay of the olfactory pathway and transmit olfactory signals to higher olfactory centers. This possibility raises a number of fundamental questions at the molecular level (matching of presynaptic and postsynaptic components of chemical transmission) and system level (relaying the information to appropriate neural circuits), which should be examined by morphological, neurochemical, electrophysiological, and behavioral methods.

CONCLUSION

The preceding examples of experimental evidence incompatible with the conventional view of brain organization and function are certainly not unique. I am sure that others could name even more striking anomalies which show that the accepted explanations are incorrect in a number of specific situations. It is probably more than a coincidence that anomalous findings are encountered more frequently at the system level of investigation than in cellular and behavioral studies. This is understandable because the attempts to find physiological mechanisms for well-established behavioral phenomena led from the days of Pavlov (1927) and Lashley (1929) to construction of conceptual brains whose putative properties approached the properties of real brains at a much later date. The most influential concept of this type, Hebb's (1949) model of neuronal plasticity, decisively influenced present research into cellular and subcellular events mediating simple forms of learning in *Aplysia* (Kandel, 1976) and *Hermissenda* (Farley & Alkon, 1985) as well as long-term potentiation in the hippocampal slice (Dingledine, 1984). We are clearly approaching the moment when at least some instances of plasticity will be described as accurately as have been the generation and conduction of nerve impulse (Woody, 1986).

Achievements at the molecular and cellular levels must not lead to the erroneous conviction that by disclosing the mechanisms of changes occurring at the individual nodes of the neural network we may understand learning in general. It must be stressed that learning is meaningful only at the level of the organism, as an extension of the adaptive phenomena governing the evolution of species to the needs of an individual. Stating that a cell has learned a CS–US contingency, that it recognizes a complex visual stimulus, or that it controls delivery of reward is an unwarranted ascription to a neuron of the properties of a system of which it is a part. Progress at the molecular and cellular levels will not resolve the enigma of learning without commensurate progress at the system level. Unfortunately, the pace of system investigations has been disappointingly slow because the problems encountered here are necessarily much more complex than at the cellular or the behavioral level. Nature has employed similar elements (neurons, synapses) and signals (nerve impulses, transmitters) to assemble and operate the full scale of brain types, from the most primitive invertebrates to humans. And all these brains are used to perform a limited list of essential behavioral programs (e.g., feeding, defense, mating, locomotion), obeying the same fundamental principles.

To use a technical analogy, you can run the same BASIC program on all types of computers and be sure that it is carried out by transmission of electrical impulses through the computer's circuits, but there will be great differences in the architecture of different computers and in the chips employed. Like computers, all brains use similar gates and similar impulses but differ in the density of gates, in their connectivity, and in the overall organization of the system. Hardware-transparent study of behavior, espoused by Skinner (1938), has greatly advanced our knowledge of higher level programming of brain function and is now being supplemented by detailed knowledge of the processes taking place at the individual nodes of the neural networks, but we are still far from understanding how these elementary processes are organized to implement behavior.

In many respects neuroscience faces the same difficulties as the technical disciplines simulating brain functions—artificial intelligence, robotics, computer science—which have only recently discovered that efficient solution of their problems requires not only faster gates, higher density of components, and advanced programming languages, but mainly new principles of computer architecture, characterized by massive parallel processing, reconfigurable setups, and fault-tolerant computation. This is best illustrated by the recent interest in neurocomputers, which should emulate brain function by following biological principles not in the construction of individual gates but in their organization, that is, at the system level. Most needed now is a synthesis of different approaches from molecular and cellular investigations to behavioral experiments and technical simulations, aimed at accelerating the progress of system research.

REFERENCES

Amemori, T., Soukup, T., Valoušková, V., & Bureš, J. (1986). Embryonal brain grafts and recovery of smell in bulbectomized rats. *Physiologia Bohemoslovaca, 35,* 519.

Barker, L. M., Best, M. R., & Domjan, M. (1977). *Learning mechanisms in food selection.* Waco, Tex.: Baylor University Press.

Bellingham, W. P., & Lloyd, D. (1987). Injected flavor as a CS in the conditioned aversion preparation. *Animal Learning and Behavior, 15,* 62–68.

Berger, B. D. (1970). Learning in the anesthetized rat. *Federation Proceedings, 29,* 749.

Bermudez-Rattoni, F., Rusiniak, K. W., & Garcia, J. (1983). Flavor-illness aversions: Potentiation of odor by taste is disrupted by application of novocaine into amygdala. *Behavioral and Neural Biology, 37,* 61–75.

Braveman, N. S., & Brostein, P. (Eds.). (1985). Experimental assessments and clinical applications of conditioned food aversions. *Annals of the New York Academy of Sciences, 443.*

Breland, K., & Breland, M. (1961). The misbehavior of organisms. *American Psychologist, 16,* 681–684.

Brooks, V. B., & Thach, W. T. (1981). Cerebellar control of posture and movement. In V. B. Brooks (Ed.), *Handbook of Physiology: Vol. 2. The Nervous System* (pp. 877–946). Washington, D.C.: American Physiological Society.

Bureš, J., & Burešová, O. (1981). Elementary learning phenomena in food selection. In G. Ádám, I. Mészáros, & É. I. Bányai (Eds.), *Advances in Physiological Science: Vol. 17. Brain and behavior* (pp. 81–94). Budapest: Akadémiai Kiadó.

Bureš, J., & Burešová, O. (1987). Conditioned taste aversion is neither elicited nor prevented by deep anesthesia, anoxia or convulsions. *Neuroscience, 22* (Suppl.), S517.

Burešová, O., & Bureš, J. (1973). Cortical and subcortical components of the conditioned saccharin aversion. *Physiology and Behavior, 11,* 435–439.

Burešová, O., & Bureš, J. (1977). The effect of anaesthesia on acquisition and extinction of conditioned taste aversion. *Behavioral Biology, 20,* 41–50.

Burešová, O., & Bureš, J. (1979a). The anterograde effect of ECS on the acquisition, retrieval and extinction of conditioned taste aversion. *Physiology and Behavior, 22,* 641–645.

Burešová, O., & Bureš, J. (1979b). Extinction of a newly acquired conditioned taste aversion: Effect of gustatory CS administered under anesthesia. *Behavioral Processes, 4,* 329–339.

Burešová, O., & Bureš, J. (1981). Threshold hypothermia disrupting acquisition of conditioned taste aversion and attenuation of neophobia in rats. *Behavioral and Neural Biology, 31,* 274–282.

Burešová, O., & Bureš, J. (1984). Central mediation of the conditioned taste aversion induced in rats by harmaline. *Psychopharmacology, 34,* 384–389.

Butler, A. B., Graziadei, P. P. C., Monti-Graziadei, G. A., & Slotnick, B. M. (1984). Neonatally bulbectomized rats with new olfactory neocortical connection are anosmic. *Neuroscience Letter, 48,* 247–254.

Danguir, J., & Nicolaidis, S. (1976). Impairments of learned aversion acquisition following paradoxical sleep deprivation in the rat. *Physiology and Behavior, 17,* 489–492.

Dingledine, R. (Ed.). (1984). *Brain slices.* New York: Plenum.

Doty, R. W. (1969). Electrical stimulation of the brain in behavioral context. *Annual Review of Psychology, 20,* 299–320.

Farley, J., & Alkon, D. L. (1985). Cellular mechanisms of learning, memory and information storage. *Annual Review of Psychology, 36,* 419–494.

Freed, W. J. (1983). Functional brain tissue transplantation: Reversal of lesion-induced rotation by intraventricular substantia nigra and adrenal medulla grafts. With a note on intracranial retinal grafts. *Biological Psychiatry, 18,* 1205–1267.

Freeman, W. J. (1975). *Mass action in the nervous system.* New York: Academic Press.

Garcia, J., Kimeldorf, D. J., & Koelling, R. A. (1955). A conditioned aversion towards saccharin resulting from exposure to gamma radiation. *Science, 122,* 157–159.

Graziadei, P. P. C., & Monti-Graziadei, G. A. (1978). Continuous nerve cell renewal in the olfactory system. In M. Jacobson (Ed.), *Handbook of sensory physiology* (Vol. 9, pp. 55–83). New York: Springer-Verlag.

Graziadei, P. P. C., & Monti-Graziadei, G. A. (1986). Principles of organization of the vertebrate olfactory glomerulus: An hypothesis. *Neuroscience, 19,* 1025–1035.

Halpern, B. P. (1977). Functional anatomy of the tongue and mouth of mammals. In J. A. W. M. Weijnen & J. Mendelson (Eds.), *Drinking behavior* (pp. 1–92). New York: Plenum.

Hebb, D. O. (1949). *The organization of behavior.* New York: Wiley.

Ionescu, E., & Burešová, O. (1977). Effects of hypothermia on the acquisition of conditioned taste aversion in rats. *Journal of Comparative and Physiological Psychology, 91,* 1297–1307.

Jacobson, M. (1978). *Developmental biology* (2nd ed.). New York: Plenum.

Kandel, E. R. (1976). *Cellular basis of behavior.* San Francisco: Freeman.

Kiefer, S. W. (1985). Neural mediation of conditioned food aversions. In N. S. Braveman & P. Bronstein (Eds.), *Experimental assessments and clinical applications of conditioned food aversions* (pp. 100–109). (Annals of the New York Academy of Sciences, Vol. 443). New York: New York Academy of Sciences.

Konorski, J. (1967). Integrative activity of the brain: An interdisciplinary approach. Chicago: University of Chicago Press.

Lashley, K. S. (1929). *Brain mechanisms and intelligence: A quantitative study of injuries to the brain.* Chicago: University of Chicago Press.

Lennárd, P. R., & Hermanson, J. W. (1985). Central reflex modulation during locomotion. *Trends in Neuroscience, 8,* 483–486.

Malmo, H. P., Malmo, R. B., & Weijnen, J. A. W. M. (1987). Individual consistency and modifiability of lapping rates in rats: A new look at the variance-invariance question. *International Journal of Psychophysiology, 4,* 111–119.

Mamedov, Z., & Bureš, J. (1984). Sensory feedback modulates the central pacemaker of licking in rats. *Neuroscience Letter, 45,* 1–6.

Mamedov, Z., Hernandez-Mesa, N., & Bureš, J. (1987). Inefficient licking during forced spout alternation in rats: Violation of the law of effect? *Physiology and Behavior, 39,* 153–160.

McLoon, S. C., & Lund, R. D. (1980). Specific projections of retina transplanted to rat brain. *Experimental Brain Research, 40,* 273–282.

Millner, J. R., & Palfai, T. (1975). Metrazol impairs conditioned aversion produced by LiCl: A time dependent effect. *Pharmacology Biochemistry and Behavior 3,* 201–204.

Pavlov, I. P. (1927). *Conditioned reflexes.* London: Oxford University Press.

Perrett, D. I., Mistlin, A. J., & Chitty, A. J. (1987). Visual neurons responsive to faces. *Trends in Neuroscience, 10,* 358–364.

Rabin, B. M., & Rabin, J. S. (1984). Acquisition of radiation- and lithium chloride-induced conditioned taste aversions in anesthetized rats. *Animal Learning and Behavior, 12,* 439–441.

Rachlin, H. C., & Burkhard, B. (1978). The temporal triangle: Response substitution in instrumental conditioning. *Psychological Review, 85,* 22–47.

Riley, A. L., & Tuck, D. L. (1985). Conditioned taste aversions: A behavioral index of toxicity. *Annals of the New York Academy of Sciences, 443,* 272–292.

Roll, D. L., & Smith, J. C. (1972). Conditioned taste aversion in anesthetized rats. In M. E. P. Seligman & J. L. Hager (Eds.), *Biological boundaries of learning* (pp. 93–102). New York: Appleton-Century-Crofts.

Skinner, B. F. (1938). *The Behavior of organisms.* New York: Appleton-Century-Crofts.

Sperry, R. W. (1944). Optic nerve regeneration with return of vision in Anurans. *Journal of Neurophysiology, 7,* 57–69.

Thorndike, E. L. (1911). *Animal intelligence. Experimental studies.* New York: Macmillan.

Weijnen, J. A. W. M., & Mendelson, J. (1977). *Drinking behavior.* New York: Plenum.

Weijnen, J. A. W. M., Wouters, J., & Van Hest, J. M. H. H. (1984). Interaction between drinking and swallowing in the drinking rat. *Brain, Behavior and Evolution, 25,* 117–127.

Woody, C. D. (1986). Understanding the cellular basis of memory and learning. *Annual Review of Psychology, 37,* 433–493.

Wright, J. W., & Harding, J. (1982). Recovery of olfactory function after bilateral bulbectomy. *Science, 216,* 322–324.

I
Forms of Memory

Introduction

MICHELA GALLAGHER

> It is not a real contradiction that the most creative scientists are fre-
> quently just those, not only willing to accept the existence of disorder,
> but also positively attracted to it. The evident reason is that the recog-
> nition of disorder is an opportunity, and in fact a necessary preliminary,
> for the creative act of ordering.
>
> G. GAYLORD SIMPSON, *Principles of Animal Taxonomy* (1961)

Memory, defined in general terms, refers to the effects of experience that are manifest at a later time. This capacity permits animals to acquire, retain, and use a great variety of information. Thus memory can be captured by an encompassing definition, but can it be profitably studied as a unitary function? Alternatively, does the phenomenon of memory represent a diversity of systems or mechanisms that have evolved to execute different essential types of memory? In this introduciton it is only fair to acknowledge that there is no general consensus that different forms of memory should be distinguished; dissenting views can be found (e.g., Craik, 1983).

In discussing this question, Tulving (1983)—a proponent of the concept that memory is not unitary—uses an analogy in which he compares the problem of understanding memory with that of understanding locomotion. An encompassing definition of locomotion can be formulated along the lines of a change in the position of an animal from one location to another location. From this point, however, any further attempt to describe, or model, or specify the mechanisms used for locomotion requires identification of some type of this general phenomenon. Indeed, a conspicuous and amazing variety of systems/mechanisms have evolved for the purpose of locomotion. Animals swim, jump, burrow, or fly from one place to another. A study of locomotion that provides an appreciation of the behavioral properties, the neural systems, or the cellular mechanisms involved requires an acknowledgment that locomotion is not a unitary phenomenon with a single set of governing principles and underlying mechanisms. If isolated empirical observations are to increase our understanding of the phenomenon, it is also important to know whether different specific instances of

23

locomotion belong to some larger classes that share common features. However, a general theory of locomotion would not be nourished by many empirical facts that apply overall.

Properties that distinguish different forms of memory are conspicuous to many who study memory. There is a growing vocabulary to describe types of memory. Distinctions are made based on the durability of information that is acquired. Short-term, long-term, and intermediate forms of memory often figure in contemporary discussions of memory. The content of information that is preserved has also been used as a basis for distinguishing different forms of memory; there is, for example, memory for facts, or skills, or spatial information. Other distinctions are based on operational characteristics such as working and reference memory.

Different information about memory—its varieties and organization—comes from studies with a biological focus. In one such line of investigation, different forms of memory are characterized by brain damage, which alters performance on some types of memory tasks while sparing performance on others. It is well known, for example, that relatively circumscribed brain damage in diencephalic and temporal lobe structures in humans is associated with an amnesic syndrome. Perhaps the most striking realization of the last decade or so is that these amnesic patients possess some apparently intact memory capacities: they perform as well as normals in retaining certain motor, perceptual, or cognitive skills and show residual effects of exposure to items such as individual words, a phenomenon known as the repetition priming effect (see Squire, 1987, for recent discussion).

Other work with a neurobiological focus has indicated that mechanisms for memory may be distinguished at a cellular level. The short- and long-term representations of nonassociative memory for sensitization in *Aplysia* are likely to require the engagement of qualitatively different intracellular processes (Montarolo et al., 1986). In addition, it is apparent that changes in synaptic function can be controlled by distinct mechanisms in different neural circuits. From the properties of the circuitry, to the identity of neurotransmitters/neuromodulators that regulate neural plasticity, to the species of conductances or nature of morphological changes that occur, there is at least a hint that the cast of characters used to preserve biological records of experience is highly diverse.

The nature of much thought and many empirical studies on memory at different levels of analysis, both behavioral and neurobiological, indicates an expectation that some taxonomy of memory is likely to emerge. At this point, it is perhaps worthwhile to ask whether the criteria applied in this endeavor are useful and/or valid.

In a recent review of this general topic, Sherry and Schacter (1987) provide some guidance about the defining features of a memory system. They propose that a memory system refers to the acquisition, retention, and retrieval mechanisms for information that are governed by distinctive rules of operation. Multiple forms of memory thus emerge when two or more systems are "characterized by fundamentally different rules of operation." By this definition, the type of information—the content of memory—is not alone a sufficient basis for identification of a distinct form of memory. The handling of information by different bits of neural circuitry or different regions of the brain is likewise an insufficient basis for making critical distinctions between types of memory. Indeed, different operations might well be performed by systems that share at least some neural components.

An emphasis on rules of operation—as distinct from content-based or neuroanatomically sequestered systems of memory—emerges in the chapters that follow. It is also evident from some of these presentations that behavioral and neurobiological data may converge to provide a mutually supportive basis for making distinctions. The opening chapter is a developmental analysis for the emergence of nonassociative learning in an invertebrate in which Carew and colleagues provide behavioral and neurobiological evidence for distinctive processes underlying dishabituation and sensitization, forms of nonassociative learning that had previously been subsumed by a common process. Morris then offers a strong argument for examination of the rules of operation at behavioral and neurobiological levels; in the case of the latter a particular emphasis is placed on the information that is likely to be embedded in the neural architecture used to implement the storage of information. By this view, knowledge of neural circuitry is not only a vehicle for discovering sites of plasticity that can be subjected to cellular analysis, but also places interesting and important constraints on the nature of information that is processed and preserved within it. Later chapters in this volume further discuss processing in cortical circuitry and characteristic algorithms used in computational models of such neural architecture.

The chapters by Holland and Johnson share a common thread in viewing memory as a less segregated psychological/neurobiological function. Johnson's discussion of a multiple-entry modular memory system provides a cognitive framework for examining the operating characteristics for information processing in normal humans and amnesic patients. Holland shows that Pavlovian conditioning provides a powerful framework for examining even representation in memory in laboratory animals. These chapters remind us that neurobiological accounts of memory depend critically on study at a behavioral level. Indeed, with current rapid technical advances in the field of neurobiology, it is possible that progress in understanding the neurobiology of memory will be mainly limited by the rate of developing an appropriate behavioral analysis.

These chapters cover an enormous range of research, from behavioral studies of both laboratory animals and human subjects to studies of circuits and cellular mechanisms in mammals and invertebrates. The problem of developing a taxonomy of memory will provide a challenging agenda for many years to come.

REFERENCES

Craik, F. I. M. (1983). On the transfer of information from temporary to permanaent memory. *Philosophical Transactions of the Royal Society (London) 302,* 341, 359.

Montarolo, P. G., Goelet, P., Castellucci, V. F., Morgan, J., Kandel, E. R., & Schacher, S. (1986). A critical period for macromolecular synthesis in long-term heterosynaptic facilitation in *Aplysia. Science, 234,* 1249–1254.
Sherry, D. F., & Schacter, D. L. (1987). The evolution of multiple memory systems. *Psychological Review, 94,* 439–454
Squire, L. R. (1987). *Memory and brain.* New York: Oxford University Press.
Tulving, E. (1983). *Elements of episodic memory.* New York: Oxford University Press.

2

The Development of Learning and Memory in *Aplysia*

THOMAS J. CAREW
EMILIE A. MARCUS
THOMAS G. NOLEN
CATHARINE H. RANKIN
MARK STOPFER

Few issues have captured the imagination of psychologists more than the fundamental question of how, over a lifetime, animals are able to acquire a vast amount of information, store it in their brains, and retrieve it in one form or another for use at a later time. The depth and complexity of this question are reflected in the many rich and diverse approaches psychologists and neurobiologists have taken in analyzing mechanisms of learning and memory. As exemplified by the contributors to this volume, these approaches range from the analysis of membrane currents and molecular events in individual neurons to the investigation of computational strategies in highly complex neural networks. A unifying theme underlying all these approaches is a fascination with the remarkable capacity of animals to learn and remember.

One powerful approach to the analysis of neuronal mechanisms of learning and memory is the use of simple invertebrate animals whose nervous systems are well suited for detailed cellular and molecular studies (for reviews, see Byrne, 1987; Carew & Sahley, 1986; Hawkins, Clark, & Kandel, 1987; Mpitsos & Lukowiak, 1985). Among these invertebrate preparations, the marine mollusc *Aplysia californica* has proved extremely useful, since the animal exhibits a variety of types of learning that range in complexity from nonassociative forms such as habituation, dishabituation, and sensitization to associative forms such as classical and operant conditioning. Moreover, these various forms of learning can be retained on a time scale from short-term memory (lasting hours) to long-term memory (lasting days and weeks). Finally, it has been possible to specify in some detail the synaptic, biophysical, and molecular events that contribute to the expression of these various forms of learning and memory (Byrne, 1987; Carew, 1987; Hawkins et al., 1987).

In our laboratory in recent years we have extended the analysis of learning and memory in *Aplysia* by combining it with a developmental analysis, aimed at examining the emergence and assembly of different forms of learning and memory during ontogeny. The rationale for this approach is that by examining the assembly of different forms of learning as they sequentially appear during development, it may be possible to obtain unique insights into underlying cellular and molecular mechanisms. In this chapter we will illustrate our approach by showing how a developmental analysis in *Aplysia* has revealed multiple components underlying simple forms of nonassociative learning. These different components can be dissociated by examining their developmental timetables, which turn out to be quite different. This in turn has afforded us the experimental advantage of examining early emerging forms of learning in developmental isolation from later emerging forms. In this way we have not only been able to dissociate different components of learning, but we have also been able to reveal previously unappreciated behavioral and cellular processes. Finally, the developmental dissociation of different components of learning in juvenile *Aplysia* prompted us to examine adult animals, where we found the same clearly dissociable components. Thus an analysis of the ontogenetic assembly of learning can also provide important insights into the final phenotypic expression of learning in the adult.

DEVELOPMENT OF HABITUATION AND DISHABITUATION IN THE SIPHON WITHDRAWAL REFLEX

In adult *Aplysia* the gill and siphon withdrawal reflex exhibits both nonassociative and associative forms of learning (Carew, 1987; Hawkins et al., 1987). The three different forms of nonassociative learning are illustrated in Figure 2.1. *Habituation* refers to a decrease in response amplitude occurring as a function of repeated stimulation; *dishabituation* describes the facilitation of a habituated response by the presentation of a strong or novel stimulus; and *sensitization* refers to the facilitation of a nondecremented response by a similar strong or noxious stimulus.

In our developmental analysis we focused on the juvenile stages of development because it is during the juvenile period that the gill and siphon first emerge (Kriegstein, 1977a; Rankin, Stopfer, Marcus, & Carew, 1987). The juvenile stages we analyzed are shown in Figure 2.2. In the first set of experiments (Rankin & Carew, 1987a) we investigated whether habituation and dishabituation emerge at the same developmental stage or whether there is a difference in their developmental timetables. We found that habituation of siphon withdrawal is present in very early stages of juvenile development. However, it exists in a relatively immature form. In the youngest animals, significant within-session habituation was produced only by very short interstimulus intervals (ISIs). As the animals continued to develop, significant habituation was produced in

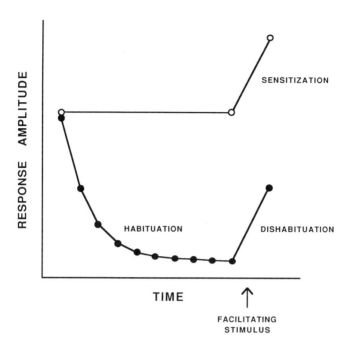

FIGURE 2.1. Three forms of nonassociative learning: habituation, dishabituation, and sensitization.

response to progressively longer ISIs. Thus in stage 9, significant habituation occurred to only a 1-sec ISI, but not to 5- or 10-sec ISIs; in stage 10, to both 1- and 5-sec ISIs but not to a 10-sec ISI; and in stage 11, to all three ISIs. Moreover, even in later juvenile stages, further maturation of habituation was evident. For example, in response to a 30-sec ISI, stage 12 animals show significantly less habituation than do adult animals to this same ISI. Figure 2.3 summarizes the development of habituation: the magnitude of habituation (as an average percentage habituation score) in response to each ISI tested is expressed across juvenile developmental stages. We examined habituation to comparable ISIs across developmental stages and found a clear and significant developmental trend in the magnitude of habituation exhibited to a variety of ISIs (ranging from 1 to 30 sec) throughout most of the juvenile life of *Aplysia.*

Although habituation was present at the earliest stage of development studied, dishabituation was not. Specifically, dishabituation was absent in stage 9, first appearing several days later in stage 10. This can be seen in Figure 2.4, which provides a comparison of habituation (to a 1-sec ISI) and dishabituation (to tail shock) in stages 9, 10, and 11. Whereas dishabituation in response to tail shock was significant in stages 10 and 11, it was completely absent in stage 9. Thus habituation is present in early juvenile development and dishabituation emerges in a distinct later stage (stage 10) approximately one week later.

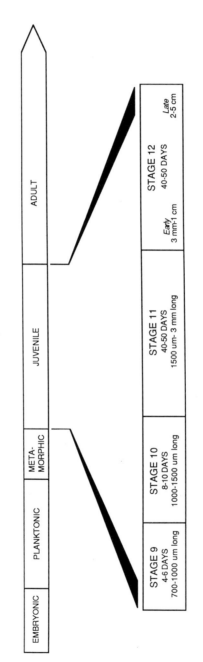

FIGURE 2.2. The *Aplysia* life cycle has been divided into five major phases: embryonic (lasting about 10 days), planktonic (lasting about 30 days), metamorphic (lasting about 3 days), juvenile (lasting about 120 days), and adult. We have focused our attention on the juvenile phase, which can be further subdivided into four stages based on discrete morphological criteria. The approximate duration of each stage (in days) is shown.

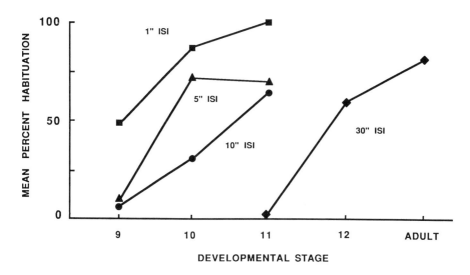

FIGURE 2.3.   The mean percent habituation (100% = complete response decrement) to four different ISIs (1, 5, 10, and 30 sec) as a function of developmental stage. There was a significant increase in habituation (i.e., a positive slope) as a function of age for all four ISIs. Thus progressively older animals were capable of expressing habituation to progressively longer ISIs. (From Rankin and Carew, 1987a)

DEVELOPMENT OF SENSITIZATION IN THE SIPHON WITHDRAWAL REFLEX

Until recently, dishabituation and sensitization had commonly been considered to reflect a single underlying facilitatory process. This view was supported by the general observation that both nondecremented and decremented responses were simultaneously facilitated by the presentation of a single strong or noxious stimulus. The most parsimonious explanation for this kind of result was that a noxious stimulus initiated a general arousal process that was widespread in the nervous system, facilitating habituated and nonhabituated responses alike (Carew, Castellucci, & Kandel, 1971; Groves & Thompson, 1970). Although reasonable, this explanation did not rule out the possibility that dishabituation and sensitization could reflect separate facilitatory processes that are activated in parallel by a strong stimulus. In fact, direct cellular evidence for two separate facilitatory processes has recently been provided by Hochner, Klein, Schacher, and Kandel (1986a, 1986b), who suggested that dishabituation and sensitization in adult *Aplysia* may be produced, at least in part, by different cellular mechanisms.

One way to behaviorally address the question of whether dishabituation and sensitization reflect a unitary process is to determine when they emerge during development. If a single process is involved, both forms of learning should be expressed at the same time ontogenetically. Alternatively, if more than one pro-

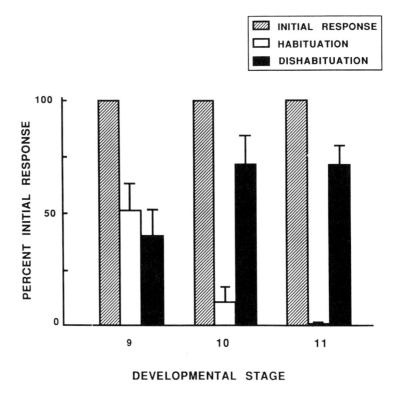

FIGURE 2.4.   Summary of habituation and dishabituation for stages 9, 10, and 11. Summarized data are for a 1-sec ISI. The hatched bar shows the initial response (100%). The clear bar shows habituation (the mean of the last trial for the habituation series). The black bar shows dishabituation (the mean of the first trial following tail shock). Older animals showed greater habituation to a 1-sec ISI than did younger animals. Moreover, there was no dishabituation in stage 9, whereas there was significant dishabituation in stages 10 and 11. (From Rankin and Carew, 1987a)

cess is involved, it might be possible to separate them developmentally. To address this question Rankin and Carew (1988) examined the effects of tail shock on both decremented and nondecremented responses in developmental stages 11, early 12, and late 12. In each stage two groups of animals were examined. One group received dishabituation training (habituation followed by tail shock); the other received sensitization training (several baseline stimuli were delivered at an ISI too long to produce response decrement, followed by a tail shock identical to that of the dishabituation group). Both groups were then tested for response facilitation resulting from tail shock. Our results showed (1) that sensitization emerges between early and late stage 12 of juvenile development and (2) that tail shock actually produces inhibition of the reflex response in young animals prior to the development of sensitization.

Sensitization Emerges in Late Stage 12 of Juvenile Development

The results of dishabituation and sensitization training for each of the stages examined are summarized in Figure 2.5, which shows the mean response amplitudes immediately prior to and immediately following tail shock for each of the three developmental stages studied. During habituation trials, animals at each stage showed significant response decrement as a result of repeated stimulation (not shown). In all stages habituated animals showed significant facilitation of response amplitude following tail shock. Thus, confirming previous results (Rankin & Carew, 1987a), dishabituation was present in each of the developmental stages examined. In contrast, the results for animals that received sensitization training showed a strikingly different pattern: sensitization was completely absent in stage 11 and early stage 12. In these stages the same animals that exhibited dishabituation lacked sensitization. Moreover, sensitization was absent regardless of the intensity of siphon stimulation used to elicit the reflex

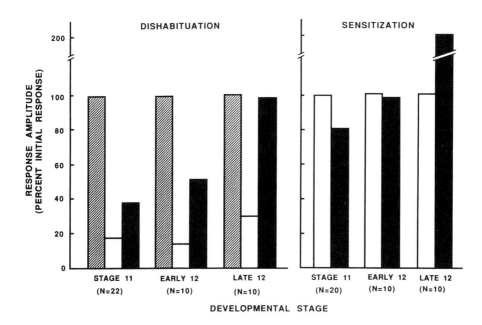

FIGURE 2.5.   Differential emergence of dishabituation and sensitization during juvenile development. *Dishabituation:* Significant habituation is exhibited in all developmental stages: compare initial response (hatched bars) to final habituated responses (clear bars). Moreover, significant dishabituation is also evident in all stages: compare postshock responses (black bars) with habituated responses. Data are expressed as a percentage of initial response. *Sensitization:* In contrast to dishabituation, sensitization is not evident until late stage 12; compare preshock responses (clear bars) to postshock responses (black bars). Significant response facilitation is seen only in late stage 12 animals. Data are expressed as a percentage of mean preshock responses. (From Rankin and Carew, 1988)

or the intensity of tail shock used to attempt to produce sensitization (ranging from weak to very strong). In fact, as we will discuss later, in these early stages in which sensitization was absent, tail shock produced a modest but significant depression in response amplitude. However, in late stage 12, tail shock did indeed produce sensitization of the reflex (Fig. 2.5). Thus these experiments showed that sensitization emerges between early and late stage 12 of juvenile development.

Tail Shock Produces Inhibition of Reflex Responding Before the Emergence of Sensitization

In examining the developmental emergence of sensitization, we assessed the effects of tail shock on nondecremented responses in three juvenile stages: stage 11, early stage 12, and late stage 12. This analysis revealed an unexpected result. In early developmental stages (stage 11 and early stage 12) a modest but reliable inhibitory effect of tail shock was apparent. Then, between early and late stage

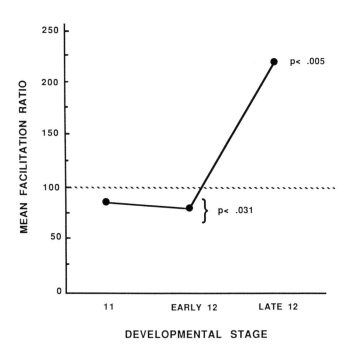

NON-DECREMENTED RESPONSES

FIGURE 2.6.   Developmental transition from inhibition to facilitation of nondecremented responses following tail shock. A composite facilitation ratio was computed for each stage. In stage 11 and early stage 12, tail shock produces significant reflex inhibition. In contrast, in late stage 12, tail shock produces significant facilitation. (From Rankin and Carew, 1988)

12, there was a dramatic transition after which tail shock could produce its facilitatory effect. This transition is illustrated in Figure 2.6, in which the data are
shown as a facilitation ratio for each developmental stage by expressing the first
response following tail shock as a percentage of the average preshock responses.
In any single group of animals the inhibitory effect of tail shock was modest.
However, it was quite consistent: in six out of six different groups of stage 11
and early stage 12 animals the first postshock response was lower than the mean
of the preshock responses. Thus significant response inhibition was seen in early
stages, whereas significant facilitation was seen in the later stage (Rankin &
Carew, 1988). The functional significance of this novel inhibitory process is an
interesting question for further exploration.

Figure 2.7 summarizes the behavioral results for all of the developmental
stages we examined. To permit a comparison of the magnitude of both disha-

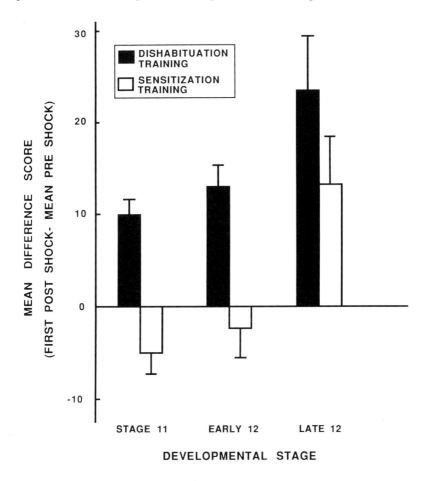

FIGURE 2.7. Summary of the emergence and maturation of dishabituation and sensitization.
Data are expressed in terms of a mean difference score. (From Rankin and Carew, 1988)

bituation and sensitization across different stages, the data are expressed in terms of a mean difference score, which was obtained by computing the differences in amplitude between the first response following tail shock and the mean preshock responses. There was a significant developmental increase in both dishabituation and sensitization. In dishabituation there were no signficant differences between stage 11 and early stage 12; however, there was a significant increase in late stage 12. The same was true for sensitization; there was no significant difference between stage 11 and early stage 12 (sensitization was absent in both), but there was significant facilitation following tail shock in late stage 12, reflecting the expression of sensitization for the first time.

The results shown in Figure 2.7 permit several interesting conclusions. First, although dishabituation is present at all developmental stages examined, sensitization does not emerge until sometime between early and late stage 12 in juvenile development. Second, inspection of the data on the effects of sensitization training shows that the inhibitory effects of tail shock appear to diminish between stage 11 and early stage 12, and in parallel with this reduction of the inhibitory effect there is a concomitant modest increase in the magnitude of dishabituation. It is not clear from these results whether the inhibitory process is truly diminishing during development and/or whether an independent facilitatory process is beginning to emerge in early stage 12, with the net effect of reducing the inhibition expressed at this stage.

Since both the facilitatory process involved in dishabituation and the inhibitory process are produced by tail shock, it is possible that the inhibitory process competes with dishabituation. In fact, evidence has recently been obtained in stage 11 juvenile *Aplysia* (Rankin & Carew, 1987b, 1989) that weak tail shock (which produced no inhibition of nondecremented responses) produces significant dishabituation, whereas strong tail shock (which produced strong inhibition of nondecremented responses) produces no dishabituation, suggesting that the inhibition produced by strong tail shock may directly compete with dishabituation. Moreover, it is striking that at the time in development when the effects of tail shock on nondecremented responses show a transition from inhibition to facilitation (i.e., sensitization emerges), the magnitude of dishabituation also significantly increases. It is likely that this increase is due to the sensitization process adding to dishabituation and/or to the reduction of the inhibitory process.

Our observations during development suggest the hypothesis that the process of dishabituation may be more complex than previously thought (see, e.g., Carew et al., 1971; Carew & Kandel, 1974; Groves & Thompson, 1970). Specifically, the magnitude of dishabituation may ultimately be determined by the interaction of three separate processes: (1) the dishabituation process itself; (2) the inhibitory process that may subtract from dishabituation (see also Marcus, Nolen, Rankin, & Carew, 1987; Rankin & Carew, 1987b); and (3) the sensitization process that may add to dishabituation (see also Hochner et al., 1986a, 1986b). These behavioral results reveal striking differences in the development of dishabituation and sensitization that are not compatible with the notion that dishabituation and sensitization are a single process; rather they suggest that they are, at least in part, separate processes.

THE DEVELOPMENT OF SENSITIZATION IN THE ESCAPE LOCOMOTION SYSTEM

In the work presented thus far, the development of learning has been analyzed in the siphon withdrawal reflex. Having established the timetable for the emergence of sensitization in this reflex system, we then asked if the emergence of sensitization was due to the development of a process restricted to the siphon withdrawal circuit or to a more general change in the whole animal. One way to examine this question is to analyze the development of sensitization in other response systems; thus we turned our attention to escape locomotion, a dramatic stereotypic response in which an animal rapidly locomotes away from a source of noxious stimulation. This response offers a variety of advantages for a developmental analysis: (1) it is expressed very early in development (as early as stage 8; unpublished observations); (2) it is simple to quantify in an unrestrained animal (Hening, Walters, Carew, & Kandel, 1979; Walters, Carew, & Kandel, 1979); (3) the response in the adult is known to be modulated by several different forms of both nonassociative and associative learning (Carew, Walters, & Kandel, 1981; Walters, Carew, & Kandel, 1981); and (4) the neural circuitry underlying escape locomotion in the adult has been examined in some detail (Hening et al., 1979; Jahan-Parwar & Fredman, 1978a, 1978b).

We examined the development of escape locomotion in juvenile stages 10, 11, and early and late 12, as well as in adults (Stopfer & Carew, 1988). Juvenile animals were observed through a stereomicroscope in appropriately scaled open-field test chambers (Fig. 2.8). There were three phases to the experiment: (1) pretesting, (2) training, and (3) testing. In the pretest phase, animals first received two weak pretest stimuli (mild tail shock), each followed by an observation period during which the distance traveled by the animal was recorded. For each developmental stage two groups of animals were run: a sensitization group, which received sensitization training (strong electric shocks to the tail); and a control group, which received another weak test stimulus. Following training, in the test phase, both groups received another two test stimuli, identical to pretest.

In stage 10, stage 11, and early stage 12 there were no significant differences between animals that received sensitization training and animals that received the control procedure; that is, there was no sensitization in these early juvenile stages. However, in late stage 12 animals there was significant sensitization as a result of strong tail shock (Fig. 2.9). Thus sensitization of escape locomotion appears to emerge between early and late stage 12 of juvenile development.

The emergence of sensitization of escape locomotion in late stage 12 is strikingly similar to the timetable for sensitization in the siphon withdrawal reflex.

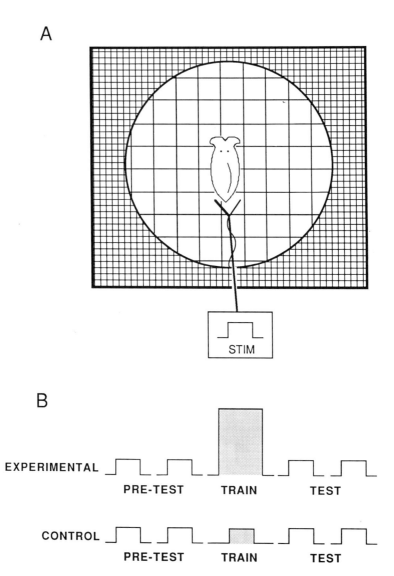

FIGURE 2.8. Experimental procedure for studying escape locomotion. (A) Test arena. Different-sized open-field test arenas were appropriately scaled for each developmental stage. Juvenile stages 10 to early 12 were observed through an adjustable stereomicroscope which could be kept centered over the animal. Escape locomotion was quantified by the number of boxes entered during an observation period. (B) Experimental procedure. Both experimental and control groups received two mild pretest stimuli and the distance traveled after each stimulus was recorded. A second experimenter then delivered a training stimulus to each animal. All animals were then tested with two mild stimuli (test) identical to the pretest. Each animal contributed a single score, the mean test response expressed as a percentage of the mean pretest response. (From Stopfer and Carew, 1988)

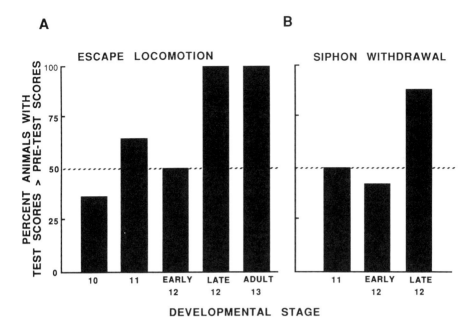

FIGURE 2.9. Sensitization of escape locomotion (A) emerges in the same juvenile stage as sensitization of siphon withdrawal (B). Data are expressed as the percentage of experimental animals within each stage exhibiting test scores greater than their prescores. The dashed line through the 50% level represents the percentage of animals that would be expected to show an increase in responding on the basis of chance alone. A clear developmental trend is exhibited, indicating that sensitization of both escape locomotion and siphon withdrawal emerges in late stage 12 of juvenile development.

Figure 2.9 compares the development of sensitization in escape locomotion with that of the siphon withdrawal reflex. The data are expressed as the percentage of animals in the experimental groups that exhibited sensitization (i.e., mean postshock score higher than their mean preshock scores). The dashed line through 50% indicates the proportion of preparations that would be expected to show an increase in response amplitude by chance alone. In both siphon withdrawal and escape locomotion there is no significant increase above the chance level until late stage 12 of juvenile development, when significant sensitization emerges in both response systems.

The fact that sensitization emerges within the same developmental stage in the escape locomotion system and the siphon withdrawal reflex is additionally interesting because the siphon withdrawal reflex and escape locomotion represent very different classes of response systems: siphon withdrawal is a graded response that involves a restricted effector organ system (the mantle organs: gill, siphon, and mantle shelf), whereas escape locomotion involves a widespread effector organ system (involving virtually the entire body, including the head and neck, the whole foot, the bilateral body walls, and the two parapodia). In addition, the two response systems have very different underlying neural circuits: the gill and siphon withdrawal reflex is mediated by a relatively simple circuit located in the abdominal ganglion (for review, see Hawkins et al., 1987), whereas escape locomotion is mediated by more complex circuitry involving the coordination of triggering, oscillatory, and effector circuits in the cerebral, pleural, and pedal ganglia (Hening et al., 1979; Jahan-Parwar & Fredman, 1978a, 1978b). Thus despite several differences in ontogeny, response topography, and underlying circuit complexity, both response systems begin to express sensitization within the same developmental stage.

DEVELOPMENT OF THE CELLULAR ANALOGUES OF HABITUATION, DISHABITUATION, AND SENSITIZATION

The developmental separation of different learning processes that we have observed in the siphon withdrawal reflex of *Aplysia* affords the opportunity to examine the unique contributions of different cellular and molecular mechanisms to each form of learning. A first step in this analysis is to establish that cellular analogues of these forms of learning can be identified and analyzed in the central nervous system of juvenile *Aplysia* at the same stages of development that these forms of learning are first behaviorally expressed. Although the neural circuit in the abdominal ganglion that controls siphon and gill withdrawal is relatively well understood in adult *Aplysia,* it has not yet been mapped in juvenile animals. However, the giant mucus motor neuron R2, also found in the abdominal ganglion, can provide an excellent system in which to explore cellular analogues of learning. This neuron is readily identifiable as a unique individual throughout juvenile development (Kriegstein, 1977b). In addition, R2 receives afferent input from the siphon (Kandel & Tauc, 1965; Rayport, 1981). Thus R2 can serve as a cellular vantage point to monitor plastic changes that emerge in the reflex pathways for gill and siphon withdrawal.

The development of cellular analogues of habituation and dishabituation in R2 was first examined by Rayport (1981) and by Rayport and Camardo (1984). They found that the analogue of habituation (synaptic decrement) was present at a very early stage in juvenile development, stage 9, and that the analogue of dishabituation (facilitation of decremented synaptic potentials) emerged in stage 10, about one week later. These findings are consistent with the behavioral observations of Rankin and Carew (1987a) that habituation in the siphon withdrawal reflex was present in stage 9 and dishabituation emerged in stage 10.

Since behavioral studies indicated that sensitization emerged during stage 12 of juvenile development, Nolen and Carew (1988) focused on this stage for their studies on the developmental emergence of the cellular analogue of sensitization, the facilitation of nondecremented excitatory postsynaptic potentials (EPSPs). The physiological preparation is shown in Figure 2.10. While recording intracellularly from R2, stimulation of the siphon skin was mimicked by brief

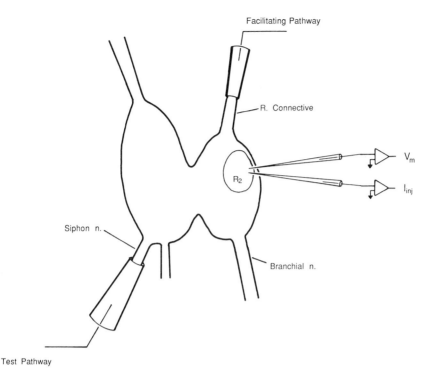

FIGURE 2.10.   Physiological preparation for the examination of the development of the cellular analogues of dishabituation and sensitization. Intracellular electrodes were used to record the membrane potential (V_m) of the identified mucus motor neuron R2 in the abdominal ganglion of stage 12 animals. In late stage 12 animals, a second electrode (I_{inj}) was used to hyperpolarize the cell. Afferent input from the siphon was activated by a brief shock to the siphon nerve, which evoked a complex EPSP in R2. Input from the tail pathway was activated by a train of brief shocks to the right connective. (From Nolen and Carew, 1988)

electrical pulses delivered to the siphon nerve, which evoked a complex EPSP in R2. To mimic tail shock, a train of electrical pulses was delivered to the pleural–abdominal connective (which carries the input from the tail to the abdominal ganglion). The analogue of sensitization was examined by analyzing the ability of connective stimulation to facilitate nondecremented complex synaptic potentials in R2. In behavioral studies stage 12 had been divided into two substages, early stage 12 and late stage 12; sensitization was absent in early stage 12 but present in late stage 12 (Rankin & Carew, 1988). To permit greater resolution of temporal emergence of the analogue of sensitization for the cellular analyses, stage 12 was divided into three substages: early, mid-, and late stage 12.

As would be predicted on the basis of the behavioral findings on the development of sensitization in both the siphon withdrawal reflex and escape locomotion, the analogue of sensitization was clearly present in late stage 12 animals.

Specifically, connective stimulation produced significant facilitation of nondecremented EPSPs. Moreover, in mid-stage 12 animals, connective stimulation also produced clear facilitation of nondecremented EPSPs. Thus the analogue of sensitization was present in both late and mid-stage 12 of juvenile development (Fig. 2.11). However, in contrast to the older substages, connective stimulation produced no significant facilitation of nondecremented EPSPs in early stage 12. Thus the analogue of sensitization was absent in this early stage. In fact, at this stage the connective stimulation actually produced significant depression of PSP amplitude (Fig. 2.11). These cellular results therefore show a clear developmental trend in the emergence of the cellular analogue of sensitization, which supports the behavioral observation that sensitization is absent in early stage 12 of juvenile development (Fig. 2.6; and Rankin & Carew, 1988).

Since the emergence of the analogue of sensitization occurs between early and

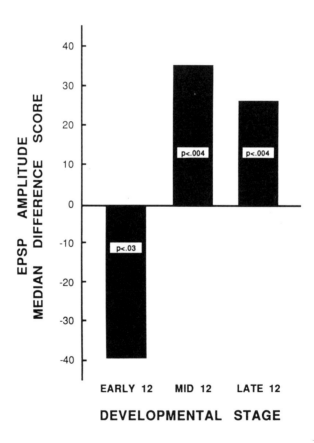

FIGURE 2.11.   Emergence of the cellular analogue of sensitization. The median difference score in EPSP amplitude (percent post minus pre) in R2 is shown for each developmental substage. While significant facilitation was present in middle and late stage 12, significant inhibition was present in early stage 12. (From Nolen and Carew, 1988)

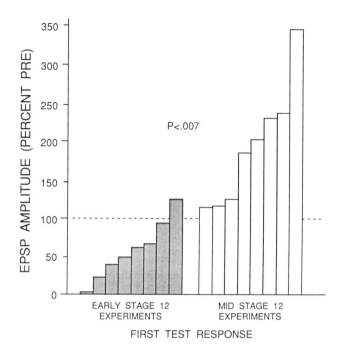

FIGURE 2.12.   Comparison of the effects of connective stimulation in early and mid-stage 12. The amount of facilitation of the first test response after connective stimulation is plotted for each preparation. All mid-stage 12 preparations (clear bars) exhibited facilitation, whereas all but one early stage 12 preparation showed depression (shaded bars). There was a highly significant difference between the two substages. (From Nolen and Carew, 1988)

middle stage 12, a detailed comparison of the effects of connective stimulation in these two developmental substages is instructive. Such a comparison is seen in Figure 2.12, in which the amplitude of the test EPSPs following connective stimulation is expressed as a percentage of its amplitude before connective stimulation. There was a clear and significant difference between the two substages: whereas all mid-stage 12 preparations exhibited *facilitation,* all but one early stage 12 preparation exhibited *depression;* and there was virtually no overlap between the groups.

   In summary, there are two striking parallels between the development of behavioral sensitization and the development of its cellular analogue. First, the cellular analogue of sensitization (produced by activation of the tail pathway) emerges in the same late juvenile stage of development as the appearance of behavioral sensitization (Rankin & Carew, 1988). Second, the cellular analysis of sensitization revealed an inhibitory process produced by connective stimulation similar to the behavioral depression produced by tail shock in animals prior to the emergence of behavioral sensitization (Figs. 2.6 and 2.7); specifically, prior to the emergence of the cellular analogue of sensitization, activation of the tail pathway produced significant depression of the afferent reflex input. Thus there is a close temporal correspondence between the development and maturation of behavioral sensitization and a cellular representation of that process in the CNS of juvenile *Aplysia*.

DISHABITUATION, SENSITIZATION, AND INHIBITION CAN BE BEHAVIORALLY DISSOCIATED IN ADULT *APLYSIA*

The developmental studies we have described thus far show that dishabituation and sensitization, as well as a novel inhibitory process, can be dissociated behaviorally in juvenile animals. Moreover, cellular analogues of each of these behavioral phenomena can also be dissociated during juvenile development. It is possible, however, that these processes, although separable during ontogeny, are not dissociable in the adult. Thus an important question was whether the same forms of behavioral plasticity could be identified and separated in adult animals. Marcus et al. (1987; 1988) addressed this possibility by examining the effects of a wide range of tail shock intensities, at several times after tail shock, on both habituated and nonhabituated siphon withdrawal reflex responses. They found that dishabituation and sensitization were clearly dissociable in adult animals in two independent ways: (1) on the basis of their differential time of onset, and (2) on the basis of their differential sensitivity to stimulus intensity.

Dishabituation and Sensitization Have Different Times of Onset

The dissociation of dishabituation and sensitization on the basis of their differential time of onset is shown in Figure 2.13A, which illustrates results obtained in a test session 90 sec after tail shock. The data are expressed as difference scores comparing postshock to preshock responses. Dishabituation was significantly expressed at a variety of stimulus intensities, whereas in this early test, sensitization was not exhibited at *any* stimulus intensity (in fact, examining nondecremented responses revealed that tail stimulation produces inhibition of reflex amplitude). Although sensitization was not expressed in the 90-sec tests, when nondecremented responses were examined in later tests, for example, 20 min and 30 min after tail shock, significant reflex facilitation was observed (data not shown). Therefore, dishabituation has an early onset, within 90 sec after tail shock, whereas sensitization has a very delayed onset, 20 to 30 min after tail shock.

An interesting aspect of the data seen in Figure 2.13A is that the strongest stimulus (4X, see below) produces no dishabituation, and in parallel, the same stimulus intensity produces significant inhibition. This suggests that the recruitment of an inhibitory process (by strong stimuli) competes with the expression of dishabituation. As mentioned earlier, a very similar result was recently obtained in juvenile *Aplysia* by Rankin and Carew (1987b; 1989), who found that increasing tail shock produced progressively *greater* reflex inhibition and also in parallel, progressively *less* dishabituation.

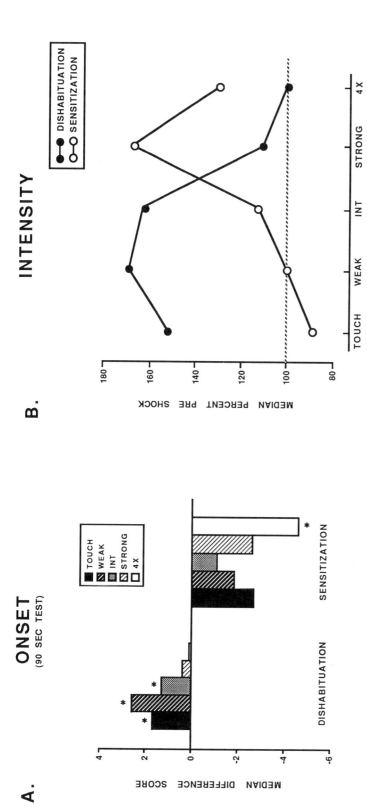

FIGURE 2.13. Behavioral dissociation of dishabituation and sensitization in adult *Aplysia*. (A) Significant dishabituation (asterisks) at a number of stimulus intensities is produced soon after the tail stimulus in the 90-sec test. In contrast, in this early test, no sensitization is produced at any intensity; in all cases, tail stimulation produced suppression of nondecremented responses, with the strongest stimulus (4X) producing significant inhibition. Data are expressed as median difference scores (post–pre). (B) Reflex magnitude as a function of tail shock intensity for dishabituation and sensitization is shown. The dashed line through 100% indicates baseline. Maximal dishabituation is produced by weak stimuli (which produces no sensitization), and maximal sensitization is produced by strong stimuli (which produces no dishabituation).

Dishabituation and Sensitization Are Differentially Sensitive to Stimulus Intensity

The dissociation of dishabituation and sensitization on the basis of stimulus intensity is seen in Figure 2.13B. A range of stimulus intensities to the tail was employed, from a mild tactile stimulus (touch) to increasing amplitudes of a single electric shock (weak, int, and strong), and, finally, to multiple tail shocks (4X). Maximal dishabituation was produced by weak tail stimuli, whereas maximal sensitization was produced by strong stimuli. Moreover, the stimulus intensity that was most effective in producing dishabituation (weak) produced *no* sensitization, and the stimulus intensity that was most effective in producing sensitization (strong) produced *no* significant dishabituation. These behavioral observations show that the processes of dishabituation, sensitization, and inhibiton, first behaviorally dissociated developmentally, could also be dissociated in adult animals.

CONCLUSIONS

The experiments that we have described in this chapter allow us to draw five principal conclusions. We will briefly discuss each of them in turn.

1. Habituation, Dishabituation, and Sensitization and Their Cellular Analogues Have Different Developmental Timetables in Aplysia

Figure 2.14 compares the developmental timetables for behavioral habituation, dishabituation, and sensitization and their cellular analogues. Habituation is present as early as we can study the siphon, in stage 9, and continues to develop in terms of the maximal ISI that produces habituation throughout the juvenile life of the animal. Dishabituation emerges approximately one week later in stage 10. Finally, sensitization emerges several weeks after dishabituation, during stage 12. A clear parallel between each of these forms of learning and its respective cellular analogue is apparent: habituation and its analogue, synaptic decrement, are present in stage 9 (Rayport & Camardo, 1984), the earliest stage tested; dishabituation and its analogue, facilitation of decremented EPSPs, emerge in stage 10 (Rayport & Camardo, 1984); and sensitization and its analogue, facilitation of nondecremented EPSPs, emerge considerably later, during stage 12 (Nolen & Carew, 1988; Rankin & Carew, 1987b; 1988). The developmental parallel between the emergence of each form of learning and its respective cellular analogue is striking; it suggests that gaining an understanding of the cellular mechanisms underlying the expression of the synaptic plasticity we have observed, prior to the emergence of additional processes that develop later in time, may contribute importantly to an understanding of the mechanisms underlying the expression of the learning processes themselves.

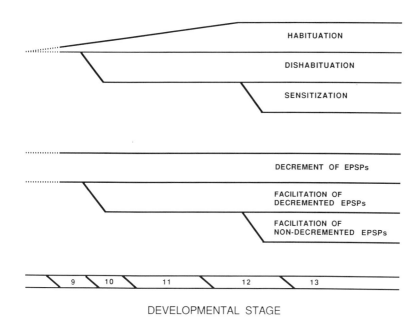

DEVELOPMENTAL STAGE

FIGURE 2.14.   Comparison of the developmental timetables of behavioral habituation, disha-bituation, and sensitization and their cellular analogues. Habituation and its cellular analogue (ho-mosynaptic decrement of EPSPs) emerge by stage 9; dishabituation and its analogue (facilitation of decremented EPSPs) emerge in stage 10. Sensitization and its cellular analogue (facilitation of nondecremented EPSPs) emerge much later (approximately 60 days) in mid- to late stage 12. (From Nolen and Carew, 1988)

2. The Simultaneous Emergence of Sensitization in Different Response Systems Suggests the Development of a General Process

The observation that sensitization or its cellular analogue emerges at the same time in development in at least two different systems (siphon withdrawal and escape locomotion) suggests the intriguing possibility that a set of integrating mechanisms responsible for an animal-wide activation of this form of learning may be expressed during stage 12 of juvenile development. Consistent with this general idea is the recent observation that in this same stage of juvenile devel-opment there is a dramatic and highly nonlinear proliferation of neurons throughout the entire CNS (Cash & Carew, 1989), raising the possibility that some aspect of the developmental trigger for neuronal proliferation might also contribute to the general expression of sensitization. Such integrating mecha-nisms for the coordinated expression of sensitization might include the induc-tion of particular hormones, neurotransmitters, or facilitatory interneuronal sys-tems, or the expression of one or more second messenger systems, which are important for neuromodulation in the different response systems. Finally, if such integrating facilitatory mechanisms exist, they are likely to be important not only for the coordinated expression of sensitization in different response systems during ontogeny, but also for the integration of sensitization in multiple response systems in the adult animal as well.

3. Analysis of Nondecremented Responses Prior to the Emergence of Sensitization Reveals a Novel Inhibitory Process

Our behavioral and cellular studies examining the development of sensitization have shown that in young animals, tail shock actually produces an inhibition of response amplitude. In the behavioral analysis of the siphon withdrawal reflex, Rankin and Carew (1987a, 1987b, 1988, 1989) found that before the emergence of sensitization in late stage 12, tail shock actually produced a modest but significant depression of nondecremented reflex responses. Similarly, Nolen and Carew (1988) identified a cellular analogue of this depressive effect of tail shock in nondecremented EPSPs in R2 prior to the development of sensitization. A similar observation of inhibition in R2 was made by Rayport and Camardo (1984) in stage 9 juvenile animals in their analysis of the emergence of the cellular analogue of dishabituation. They found that when facilitation of decremented EPSPs in R2 was absent in this early developmental stage, connective stimulation produced a short-lived depression of peak EPSP amplitude. Thus in both stage 9 and early stage 12, when the facilitatory processes underlying dishabituation and sensitization respectively have not yet emerged, an inhibitory effect of connective stimulation is revealed.

To further examine this inhibitory process, Rankin and Carew (1987b, 1989) recently studied the effects of different intensities of tail shock (very weak and very strong) on the amplitude of siphon withdrawal in stage 11 and early stage 12 animals. Not surprisingly, they found that greater inhibition was produced by the strong tail shock than by the weak shock. However, counterintuitively, they found that significantly *less* dishabituation was produced by strong tail shock than by weak tail shock, a finding also confirmed in adult animals (Marcus et al., 1987, 1988). This observation is consistent with the hypothesis that the inhibition produced by the strong tail shock actually competes with the expression of a facilitatory process (dishabituation) that is present in early developmental stages. Taken collectively, these data suggest that two antagonistic processes, one facilitatory (dishabituation) and the other inhibitory, emerge early in development, and that at a later stage another facilitatory process (sensitization) emerges.

4. Dishabituation, Sensitization, and Inhibition Can Be Separated in Adult Aplysia

The behavioral separation of dishabituation and sensitization, as well as the identification of an inhibitory process in developing juvenile *Aplysia,* raised the interesting question of whether these processes can be identified behaviorally and dissociated in adult animals as well. Recent experiments by Marcus et al.

(1987, 1988) show that they can. By examining a variety of intensities of tail shock, at several test intervals after shock, they found (1) that dishabituation has an early onset (within 90 sec), whereas sensitization has a very delayed onset (20–30 min) and (2) that dishabituation is produced by weak stimuli, whereas sensitization is produced by strong stimuli. Moreover, tail shock intensities that produced significant facilitation of habituated responses produced depression of nonhabituated responses.

A similar tail shock induced inhibitory process has recently been described by Mackey and colleagues (1987) and by Krontiris-Litowitz, Erikson, and Walters (1987). Moreover, Mackey et al. (1987) identified an interneuron in *Aplysia* that produces presynaptic inhibition of siphon sensory neurons, which is thought to contribute to behavioral inhibition in the siphon withdrawal reflex. Thus there is clear behavioral and cellular evidence that the inhibitory process we have found in juvenile animals persists in adult *Aplysia* as well.

5. A Dual-Process View of Nonassociative Learning Requires Reevaluation

As described earlier in this chapter, until recently, a commonly held view was that habituation, dishabituation, and sensitization could be accounted for by two opposing processes: a decrementing process that produces habituation and a *single* facilitatory process that produces both dishabituation and sensitization (Carew et al., 1971; Carew & Kandel, 1974; Groves & Thompson, 1970). Our experiments show that this view requires revision. Specifically, a key prediction of the dual-process view is that dishabituation and sensitization should invariably occur together. However, we showed that dishabituation and sensitization (as well as an additional process, inhibition) can be dissociated behaviorally in the siphon withdrawal reflex of *Aplysia* in three independent ways: (1) on the basis of their differential time of onset; (2) on the basis of their differential sensitivity to stimulus intensity; and (3) on the basis of their differential developmental timetables. Moreover, previous theoretical and behavioral work by Whitlow (1975) and Wagner (1976) suggested that dishabituation might be different from sensitization, and more recent cellular evidence by Hochner and colleagues (1986a, 1986b) shows that two cellular processes in *Aplysia* sensory neurons (transmitter mobilization and spike broadening) may contribute differentially to behavioral dishabituation and sensitization. Based on these collective results, we suggest that a dual-process view involving a single decrementing and a single facilitatory process requires revision, and a multiprocess view, perhaps involving inhibitory as well as facilitatory interactions, is better suited to explain the interactive mechanisms underlying nonassociative learning.

Acknowledgments

We are very grateful to the Howard Hughes Medical Institute for their generous support in supplying juvenile *Aplysia.* This research has been supported by an NSF predoctoral fellowship (to E.A.M.), by NIH NRSA grant 5-F32-NS-07480 (to T.G.N.), and by NSF grant BNS 8614961, NIMH grant MH 41083, and ONR grant N0014-87-K-0381 (to T.J.C.).

REFERENCES

Byrne, J. H. (1987). Cellular analysis of associative learning. *Physiological Review, 67*(2), 329–439.

Carew, T. J. (1987). Cellular and molecular advances in the study of learning in *Aplysia*. In J. P. Changeaux & M. Konishi (Eds.), *The neural and molecular basis of learning* (pp. 177–204). New York: Wiley.

Carew, T. J., Castellucci, V. F., & Kandel, E. R. (1971). An analysis of dishabituation and sensitization of the gill-withdrawal reflex in *Aplysia*. *International Journal of Neuroscience, 2,* 79–98.

Carew, T. J., & Kandel, E. R. (1974). A synaptic analysis of the interrelationship between different behavioral modifications in *Aplysia*. In E. R. Kandel & M. V. L. Bennett (Eds.), *Synaptic transmission and neuronal interaction* (pp. 187–215). New York: Raven.

Carew, T. J., & Sahley, C. L. (1986). Invertebrate learning and memory: From behavior to molecules. *Annual Review of Neuroscience, 9,* 435–487.

Carew, T. J., Walters, E. T., & Kandel, E. R. (1981). Associative learning in *Aplysia:* Cellular correlates supporting a conditioned fear hypothesis. *Science, 211,* 501–504.

Cash, D., & Carew, T. J. (1989). A quantitative analysis of the development of the CNS in juvenile *Aplysia*. *Journal of Neurobiology, 20,* 25–47.

Groves, P. M., & Thompson, R. F. (1970). Habituation: A dual process theory. *Psychological Review, 77,* 419–450.

Hawkins, R. D., Clark, G. A., & Kandel, E. R. (1987). Cell biological studies of learning in simple vertebrate and invertebrate systems. In F. Plum (Ed.), *Handbook of physiology: Sec. 1. The nervous system: Vol. 5. Higher functions of the brain* (pp. 25–83). Bethesda, Md.: American Physiological Society.

Hening, W. A., Walters, E. T., Carew, T. J., & Kandel, E. R. (1979). Motorneuronal control of locomotion in *Aplysia*. *Brain Research, 179,* 231–253.

Hochner, B., Klein, M., Schacher, S., & Kandel, E. R. (1986a). Action-potential duration and the modulation of transmitter release from the sensory neurons of *Aplysia* in presynaptic facilitation and behavioral sensitization. *Proceedings of the National Academy of Sciences USA, 83,* 8410–8414.

Hochner, B., Klein, M., Schacher, S., & Kandle, E. R. (1986b). Additional component in the cellular mechanism of presynaptic facilitation contributes to behavioral dishabituation in *Aplysia*. *Proceedings of the National Academy of Sciences USA, 83,* 8794–8798.

Jahan-Parwar, B., & Fredman, S. M. (1978a). Control of pedal and parapodial movements in *Aplysia*, I. Proprioceptive and tactile reflexes. *Journal of Neurophysiology, 41,* 600–608.

Jahan-Parwar, B., & Fredman, S. M. (1978b). Control of pedal and parapodial movements in *Aplysia*. II. Cerebral ganglion neurons. *Journal of Neurophysiology, 41,* 609–620.

Kandel, E. R., & Tauc, L. (1965). Mechanism of heterosynaptic facilitation in the giant cell of the abdominal ganglion of *Aplysia depilans*. *Journal of Physiology, 181,* 28–47.

Kriegstein, A. R. (1977a). Stages in the post-hatching development of *Aplysia californica*. *Journal of Experimental Zoology, 199,* 275–288.

Kriegstein, A. R. (1977b). Development of the nervous system of *Aplysia californica*. *Proceedings of the National Academy of Sciences USA, 74,* 375–378.

Krontiris-Litowitz, J. K., Erikson, M. T., & Walters, E. T. (1987). Central suppression of defensive reflexes in *Aplysia* by noxious stimulation and by factors released from the body wall. *Society for Neuroscience Abstracts, 13,* 815.

Mackey, S. L., Glanzman, D. L., Small, S. A., Dyke, A. M., Kandel, E. R., & Hawkins, R. D. (1987). Tail shock produces inhibition as well as sensitization of the siphon-withdrawal reflex of *Aplysia:* Possible behavioral role for presynaptic inhibition mediated by the peptide Phe-Met-Arg-Phe-NH$_2$. *Proceedings of the National Academy of Sciences USA, 84,* 8730–8734.

Marcus, E. A., Nolen, T. G., Rankin, C. H., & Carew, T. J. (1987). Behavioral dissociation of dishabituation, sensitization and inhibition in the siphon withdrawal reflex of adult *Aplysia. Society for Neuroscience Abstracts, 13,* 816.

Marcus, E. A., Nolen, T. G., Rankin, C. H., & Carew, T. J. (1988). Behavioral dissociation of dishabituation, sensitization, and inhibition of *Aplysia. Science, 421,* 210–213.

Mpitsos, G. J., & Lukowiak, K. (1985). Learning in gastropod molluscs. In A. O. D. Willows (Ed.), *The mollusca* (Vol. 8, pp. 96–267). Orlando, Fla.: Academic Press.

Nolen, T. G., & Carew, T. J. (1988). The cellular analog of sensitization in *Aplysia* emerges at the same time in development as behavioral sensitization. *Journal of Neuroscience. 8,* 212–222.

Nolen, T. G. Marcus, E. A., & Carew, T. J. (1987). Development of learning and memory in *Aplysia.* III. Central neuronal correlates. *Journal of Neuroscience, 7,* 144–153.

Rankin, C. H., & Carew, T. J. (1987a). Development of learning and memory in *Aplysia.* II. Habituation and dishabituation. *Journal of Neuroscience, 7,* 133–143.

Rankin, C. H., & Carew, T. J. (1987b). Analysis of the development emergence of sensitization in *Aplysia* reveals an inhibitory effect of a facilitatory stimulus. *Society for Neuroscience Abstracts, 13,* 816.

Rankin, C. H., & Carew, T. J. (1988). Dishabituation and sensitization emerge as separate processes during development in *Aplysia. Journal of Neuroscience. 8,* 197–211.

Rankin, C. H., & Carew, T. J. (1989). Developmental analysis in *Aplysia* reveals inhibitory as well as facilitatory effects of tail shock. *Behavioral Neuroscience, 103,* 334–344.

Rankin, C. H., Stopfer, M., Marcus, E. A., & Carew, T. J. (1987). Development of learning and memory in *Aplysia.* I. Functional assembly of gill and siphon withdrawal. *Journal of Neuroscience, 7,* 120–132.

Rayport, S. G. (1981). *Development of the functional and plastic capabilities of neurons mediating a defensive behavior in* Aplysia. Unpublished doctoral dissertation, Columbia University, New York.

Rayport, S. G., & Camardo, J. S. (1984). Differential emergence of cellular mechanisms mediating habituation and sensitization in the developing *Aplysia* nervous system. *Journal of Neuroscience, 4,* 2528–2532.

Stopfer, M., & Carew, T. J. (1988). Development of sensitization in the escape locomotion system in *Aplysia. Journal of Neuroscience, 8,* 223–230.

Wagner, A. R. (1976). Priming in STM: An information-processing mechanism for self-generated or retrieval-generated depression of performance. In T. J. Tighe & R. N. Leaton (Eds.), *Habituation: Perspectives from child development, animal behavior, and neurophysiology* (pp. 95–128). Hillsdale, N.J.: Erlbaum.

Walters, E. T., Carew, T. J., & Kandel, E. R. (1979). Classical conditioning in *Aplysia californica. Proceedings of the National Academy of Sciences USA, 76,* 6675–6679.

Walters, E. T., Carew, T. J., & Kandel, E. R. (1981). Associative learning in *Aplysia:* Evidence for conditioned fear in an invertebrate. *Science, 211,* 504–506.

Whitlow, J. W. (1975). Short-term memory in habituation and dishabituation. *Journal of Experimental Psychology, Animal Behavioral Processes, 1,* 189–206.

3

Synaptic Plasticity, Neural Architecture, and Forms of Memory

RICHARD G. M. MORRIS

This chapter deals with the relationship between synaptic plasticity and learning, with particular reference to the work of Kandel and his colleagues on *Aplysia*. After summarizing several general principles that may be derived from this work, I argue that the claim that the neural mechanisms of conditioning involve altering the efficacy of existing synapses does not require that all forms of conditioning elaborate existing reflexes. I argue further that a neural mechanism which detects the conjunction of two events will allow the nervous system to represent this temporal relationship only if the conjunction mechanism is embedded into appropriate circuitry. These arguments are relevant to efforts to understand the relationship between psychological and neurobiological accounts of conditioning, and they offer a new way of thinking about the significance of parallel distributed memory systems.

The idea that synaptic plasticity plays a role in the neural mechanisms of learning and memory has a long history. Tanzi (1893, cited by Ramón y Cajal, 1911, p. 886) was the first to propose that learning involved alterations in the efficacy of existing connections from one neuron to another. Ramón y Cajal (1911), however, argued that although such changes would be sufficient to account for the perfection of existing skills, they would be insufficient to account for the acquisition of new skills: "En admettant tout d'abord que les voies organiques prexistantes sont renforcées par l'exercice; en supposant ensuite que de nouvelles voies s'etablissent, gracé a une ramification et une croissance de plus en plus grande des arborisations dendritiques et cylindre-axiles" (p. 897).

This passage might allow two interpretations, but the context makes it clear that Ramón y Cajal believed that learning involved the formation of new connections between hitherto unconnected neurons. In 1949 Hebb elaborated the older of these ideas in his theory of cell assemblies and proposed his now well-known rule concerning the conditions under which alterations of synaptic efficacy might occur: "When an axon of cell A is near enough to excite a cell B and repeatedly or persistently takes part in firing it, some growth process or metabolic change takes place in one or both cells such that A's efficiency, as one of the cells firing B, is increased" (p. 62). Hebb's (1949) monograph is usually taken as the starting point for the modern assumption, widely held by many neuroscientists, that synaptic plasticity has a role in learning as a mechanism for storing information. However, the first definitive evidence that alterations of synaptic efficacy play a causal role in learning did not come until 20 years later, with the discovery, by Pinsker, Kupfermann, Castellucci, and Kandel (1970) and Castellucci and Kandel (1974) that behavioral habituation of the gill and siphon withdrawal reflex of *Aplysia* was mediated by a reduction in transmitter release at a defined synaptic locus. Subsequently, Bailey and Chen (1983) showed that habituation was accompanied by alterations in the morphology of electrophysiologically identified synapses. Greenough and Bailey (1988) offer an excellent review of the current state of the art concerning the relationship between learning and morphological alterations of synapses in both vertebrates and invertebrates.

Given that it is now feasible to study isolated synapses in some nervous systems through the use of a variety of ingenious techniques, it is tempting to believe that the major remaining problems in understanding the relationship between plasticity and learning are essentially cell biological. Implicit in the arguments presented in this chapter is a note of caution about whether these are the only major problems left. To be sure, understanding the physical basis of memory—the sequence of cellular and molecular events that give rise to the various forms of synaptic and neural plasticity—is both a formidable goal and a major one for many investigators (Horn, 1985; Kandel & Schwartz, 1982; Lynch & Baudry, 1984; Rose, 1984; Routtenberg, 1987). However, I shall argue that a full understanding of the relationship between synaptic plasticity and learning requires an appreciation of different *forms of learning* and of the role of different kinds of *neural architecture* within which a given type of *synaptic plasticity* is embedded.

TWO ARGUMENTS OF THIS CHAPTER

Specifically, I shall argue that while neurobiological data favor the view that the neural mechanisms of conditioning involve altering the efficacy of existing synapses, accepting this need not commit us to view all conditioning as a process through which existing reflexes are modulated. Here I must emphasize the phrase "need not commit us," because certain well-described forms of conditioning do involve no more than the alteration of existing reflexes. However, not all forms of conditioning are of this kind. Importantly, it is possible to imagine neurobiologically realistic schemes in which two hitherto unrelated events can be associated through a neural mechanism that involves changing the efficacy of existing neural connections but that can in no way be construed as a modulation of existing reflexes. This possibility may seem paradoxical, but it is feasible provided the stimuli to be associated are represented in the nervous system in a distributed code.

The second argument of this chapter is that the type of learning mediated by a particular form of synaptic plasticity is a function of the neural architecture within which it is embedded. Such an argument may at first seem trivial, since few if any neuroscientists would deny that knowledge of neuroanatomy is essential for understanding the functioning of the nervous system. However, my emphasis is not on the indubitable and uncontroversial fact that knowledge of neural architecture is useful (e.g., for the technical purpose of doing neurophysiological experiments properly), but on the idea that different kinds of neural architecture allow different logical functions to be computed by particular types of plasticity. That is, a particular type of plasticity will enable one logical function to be computed in one circuit and another in a different circuit. Clearly, a corollary of this second argument is that there need be no simple relationship—no isomorphism—between a particular type of synaptic plasticity and a particular form of learning. Again, it may often turn out that nature's secrets are simple and that a one-to-one relationship between learning and plasticity generally holds, but the principle I want to establish is that a simple relationship is not logically demanded. Examples will be offered both from recent work on *Aplysia* and from one type of distributed memory system.

THE NECESSITY FOR THREE LEVELS OF INQUIRY IN THE NEUROSCIENCES

In this chapter I follow Marr (1982) in recognizing the necessity for three different levels of explanation in the neurosciences. Marr refers to these as the computational, the algorithmic, and the neural implementational levels (Table 3.1). The computational level (which is hereafter referred to as level 1) is used for describing the task to be performed. In the case of learning, this might be to ignore irrelevant stimuli (habituation) or to associate two events (conditioning). The algorithmic level (level 2) describes the processes (but not the mechanisms)

TABLE 3.1   Levels of Inquiry in the Neurosciences

Computational Theory	Representation and Algorithm	Hardware Implementation
What is the goal of the computation, why is it appropriate, and what is the logic of the strategy by which it can be carried out?	How can this computational theory be implemented? In particular, what is the representation for the input and output, and what is the algorithm for the transformation?	How can the representation and algorithm be realized physically?

Source: From Marr (1982).

with which these tasks are accomplished. Thus we might have a procedural algorithm such as "reduce response amplitude to all stimuli not followed by biologically significant events" (the conventional view of habituation) or, to take a different theory of habituation, "learn what stimuli are to be expected in a given context and do not process predictable stimuli in short-term memory" (Wagner, 1978). The algorithmic level is the level at which most psychological theories are couched. Finally, the neural implementation (level 3) is the tangible description of the neurons, the essential circuitry, the mechanisms of plasticity, etc., which are hypothesized to underlie a given form of learning. It is the level concerning itself with the physical machinery of the brain.

Each of these different levels of inquiry is important, each is characterized by a particular type of discourse, and each has its own terminology. In this chapter, for reasons that I hope to make clear, I shall maintain a particularly sharp distinction between processes (level 2) and mechanisms (level 3).

SOME GENERAL PRINCIPLES ABOUT LEARNING THAT HAVE EMERGED FROM RESEARCH ON *APLYSIA*

The idea that many—perhaps all—forms of conditioning are the modulation of existing reflexes has its origins in research on the neurophysiological basis of simple forms of learning in *Aplysia*. The "basic circuitry" for habituation, dishabituation, sensitization, and a particular form of classical conditioning is discussed by Carew and colleagues (Chapter 2, this volume) and is shown in Figure 3.1. An appreciation of this basic circuit is sufficient for understanding certain general principles that are widely held to have emerged from the remarkable studies of learning in *Apylsia* since the early 1960s. However, this is by no means the complete circuit responsible for these different forms of learning; Hawkins, Castellucci, and Kandel (1981) described several other interconnections now known to be important. Moreover, this is not the complete circuit for explaining the learning of different aspects of responsiveness (duration, amplitude, etc.) in even one of these forms of learning, namely sensitization (see Frost, Clark, & Kandel, 1988). In a later section, I shall refer to these more complex aspects of circuitry but the discussion here is restricted to the "basic circuit."

Reductions in transmitter release at the terminals from the sensory neurons onto both interneurons and motorneurons are held to be the basis for habituation. Sensitization may be explained in terms of the activity in facilitator neurons synapsing onto these same presynaptic terminals, causing a cascade of intracellular events resulting in increased transmitter release. Classical conditioning involves an activity-dependent modulation of this presynaptic facilitation, a modulation induced by the temporal contiguity of neural activity in the sensory neuron with neural activity in the facilitator neuron (Kandel & Schwartz, 1982).

In effect, there is a relatively simple isomorphism between the type of plastic-

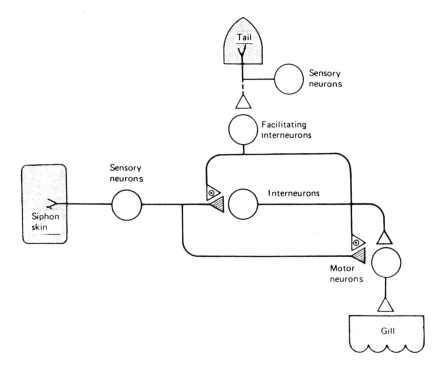

FIGURE 3.1.   Basic circuit diagram used by Kandel to explain the essential mechanisms of habituation, dishabituation, sensitization, and classical conditioning in *Aplysia*. This diagram is not the complete circuit of even part of the abdominal ganglion. (From Kandel and Schwartz, 1985, Fig. 62–3)

ity and the form of learning it mediates. There are three different types of synaptic plasticity mediating three different forms of learning with, as Kandel and Schwartz (1982) emphasized, one of these types (activity-dependent modulation of presynaptic facilitation) being closely related to and perhaps evolved from another (presynaptic facilitation). To the extent that ontogeny recapitulates phylogeny (Haekel, 1864, cited in Boakes, 1984), the intriguing proposal that the neural mechanism of classical conditioning may have evolved from the mechanism of sensitization is supported by Carew and his colleagues' (Chapter 2, this volume) studies of their time course of emergence during development—an ordered time course which they refer to as functional assembly. As each successive mechanism of plasticity emerges, so does a corresponding form of learning. Moreover, in developing their concept of a cellular alphabet of conditioning, Hawkins and Kandel (1984) described how these cellular mechanisms of plasticity can, when considered together and in the context of this basic circuitry, explain various aspects of acquisition, extinction, and discrimination in conditioning. Reference to the additional aspects of known circuitry referred to previously (Hawkins et al., 1981) is, however, essential to explain various other conditioning phenomena such as second-order conditioning and blocking. Recently Gluck and Thompson (1987) and Hawkins (1989) have extended Hawkins and Kandel's (1984) analysis with a quantitative model that postulates an S-shaped learning function to explain blocking.

What general principles have emerged from this work? First, it implies that information storage is intrinsic to sensorimotor pathways mediating a particular learned behavior. A second principle is the idea that information storage is an alteration in the efficacy of existing neural pathways. Kandel repeatedly stressed this second point in numerous papers and the evidence strongly supports his view, subject to one qualification. Bailey and Chen (1986) found that long-term memory for sensitization can involve new connections being formed de novo—an increase in the number of varicosities per sensory neuron. That this sprouting occurs can perhaps be best understood in relation to the quantal release equation ($m = n \times p$). Greater overall synaptic throughput may, statistically, be more easily achieved by having more presynaptic terminals available to release transmitter (an increase in n) than by a modest increase in the probability of release (an increase in p). If this presumption is correct, the sprouting of new terminals is better seen as a special case of increasing the efficacy of existing connections than as the formation of new connections between hitherto unconnected neurons. Subject to this qualification, the evidence from *Aplysia* (as well as from several other preparations, e.g., *Hermissenda* [Alkon & Farley, 1984] and nictitating membrane conditioning in rabbits [Thompson, 1986]) supports the principle that the underlying mechanism of learning involves altering the efficacy of preexisting neural pathways.

A third general principle of the work on *Aplysia* is the possibility that the detection of contiguity in classical conditioning is a cell-biological property of neurons, not a system property. Thus activity-dependent modulation of presynaptic facilitation is a mechanism for detecting the contiguity of CS and US events. Specifically, prior depolarization of the sensory neuron presynaptic terminals (i.e., CS activity) coupled with activation of the 5-HT receptor approximately 500 msec later is detected as an allosteric modification of a membrane-bound adenylate cyclase (Abrams & Kandel, 1988). This is believed to happen because of the possibility of dual activation of the cyclase by calcium-calmodulin (representing the CS) and a G-protein (representing the US). The consequence of the allosteric modification of the adenylate cyclase is that its subsequent activation by USs will result in a greater production of cAMP and, in turn, enhanced phosphorylation of presynaptic K^+ channels. Later CSs will then cause even greater transmitter release than occurs after presynaptic facilitation on its own. The detection of contiguity of CS and US is therefore not a property of circuitry except in the trivial sense that the two neurons carrying CS and US information must have a synapse between them. Rather it is a cell-biological property arising out of the capacity for dual activation of adenylate cyclase. This third principle is a brilliant discovery. It is perhaps not entirely without problems, notably in dealing with long-delay learning in classical conditioning (Garcia & Koelling, 1966) and effects of interstimulus interval (not CS–US interval) on conditioning (Yeo, 1974). However, long-delay learning is explicitly held to be outside the scope of the principle and I shall not dwell on the point further (see Abrams & Kandel, 1988).

Several other principles have emerged from the work on *Aplysia* but the three just summarized provide a sufficient basis for introducing the detailed arguments of this paper.

NOT ALL FORMS OF CONDITIONING INVOLVE THE MODULATION OF PREEXISTING REFLEXES

As stated earlier, the first argument of this chapter is that we need not view all forms of conditioning as a process through which preexisting reflexes are modulated even if we accept the premise that the neural mechanisms of conditioning involve altering the efficacy of preexisting neural connections.

It has often been noted that the classical conditioning displayed by the abdominal ganglion circuitry of *Aplysia* is what is generally known as *alpha-conditioning*. The CS of tactile stimulation to the siphon is not a neutral CS at the start of conditioning. It already elicits the CR of siphon withdrawal. The effect of pairing this CS with a tail shock US is to increase the strength of this preexisting CR.

Opinion is divided about whether alpha-conditioning is qualitatively different from beta-conditioning (in which the learned CR is different from any responses the CS elicits prior to conditioning). Kandel and his colleagues are well aware of this division of opinion—tired of it even—because they have repeatedly asserted that any differences between these types of conditioning are unimportant (e.g., Hawkins & Kandel, 1984, p. 379n1). The position I shall adopt is that at the level of neural mechanism the issue is trivial, whereas at the level of psychological process it is of some importance. Furthermore, I believe that despite many years of argument about alpha-conditioning, extending back to Hull (1934), the position I am presenting is a novel one.

The first step is to understand why Kandel looks on the issue of alpha-conditioning as unimportant. One reason is his belief, given the current state of our knowledge, that any insights into any forms of learning are useful. Even if alpha-conditioning should later prove not to be a particularly interesting form of learning, profitable research begins with a tractable problem (Medawar, 1966). The study of alpha-conditioning is just such a problem and it is therefore right to study it. I concur with this argument and my concern about alpha-conditioning lies elsewhere.

The second and main reason Kandel regards the alpha-conditioning issue as unimportant is because he sees no qualitative difference between alpha- and beta-conditioning. To understand why he takes this view, it is helpful to contrast a long-abandoned psychological theory of conditioning, the S–R version of "stimulus substitution" (Hull, 1934), with Kandel's (1965, 1976) differential facilitation hypothesis. In a typical classical conditioning task (level 1 description), the procedure is to pair an initially neutral CS with a US which elicits a UR. This results in the development of a CR, which in many cases resembles the UR. According to S–R stimulus substitution theory (level 2 algorithm), the new CR can be evoked by the CS because a "connection" is formed (dashed line in Fig. 3.2) from CS to UR. This process account must, however, worry anyone attempting to understand the neural mechanisms of learning (a level 3 implementation), because the new connection from CS to UR seems to require a new neural pathway. As Kandel (1976) points out, "Presumably this involves the development of a new neural pathway [dotted line in Fig. 3.2] through which the CS (which previously did not have access to the UR) now produces responses similar to the UR" p. 639, Fig. 13-20). Although not stated explicitly, it is clear that Kandel is rightly skeptical about the possibility of such new connections being formed. He therefore rejects stimulus substitution as neurally implausible.

Kandel's differential facilitation hypothesis is radically different. Following Marr's (1982) terminology, I shall refer to this hypothesis as the "differential facilitation algorithm" in order to maintain the sharp distinction between process accounts (level 2) and accounts in terms of mechanism (level 3). Strictly speaking, differential facilitation is a process account (a level 2 account), which could be implemented in neural hardware in any of a variety of ways. According to the hypothesis, a CS covertly elicits a wide variety of CRs and the effects of pairings of the CS with the US is to facilitate one (or more) of these CRs at the expense of the others (Fig. 3.3). The implication of this hypothesis is absolutely clear in Kandel's (1976) description: "Prior to pairing with a US, a CS may be capable of eliciting, if only in subthreshold form, all the responses to which it can subsequently become conditioned" (p. 638). This extraordinary feature of the differential facilitation hypothesis raises various problems that I shall discuss shortly. Its great virtue, of course, is that it can more easily be translated into a plausible account at the level of neural mechanism. Connections from CS to CR become pathways, and differential facilitation becomes activity-dependent modulation of presynaptic facilitation. Interestingly, the differential facilitation hypothesis was not developed after the fact—it predated the discoveries about

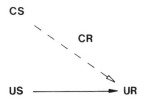

FIGURE 3.2. Pairing of a CS with a US, which elicits a UR, is held, according to Hull's S–R version of stimulus substitution, to result in the formation of a new connection between the CS and UR.

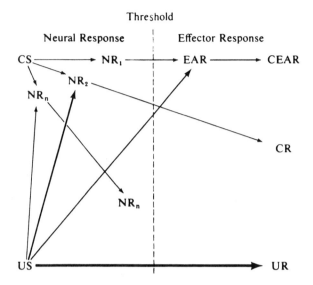

FIGURE 3.3.   Kandel's (1965) differential-facilitation hypothesis of conditioning. According to the model, the CS gives rise to a family of responses many of which will initially be below threshold for behavioral expression. Pairing of the CS and US results in a differential facilitation of certain CRs depending on the particular US with which a given CS is paired. As the strength of these covert CRs increases, one CR may rise above threshold and so be expressed in the form of overt behavior. (From Carew et al., 1984, Fig. 8.4)

the mechanisms of conditioning in *Aplysia* by several years (Kandel, personal communication, 1987).

Kandel's idea that all conditioning is the elaboration of existing reflexes was first presented in an unpublished paper dating from 1965, which he has kindly made available to me. This paper outlines the relation between alpha-conditioning and other forms of learning. Table 3.2, adapted from that paper, summarizes the differences between four different forms of learning: alpha-conditioning, beta-conditioning, pseudoconditioning, and sensitization. Hull's (1934) distinction between alpha- and beta-conditioning is shown on the left. For Hull, "true" conditioning is pairing-specific (and is therefore in the top row) and involves the emergence of a new response (lefthand column). Hull saw alpha-conditioning as akin to sensitization because the CR is an amplification of a preexisting response (righthand column), but he failed to emphasize that they differed with respect to pairing specificity. Grether (1938) introduced the distinction between conditioning and pseudoconditioning. In both of these forms of learning, the conditioned response is a new one (lefthand column). For Grether, the important difference between conditioning and pseudoconditioning lay in only the former being pairing-specific. In pseudoconditioning, US presentations in the absence of a CS subsequently result in the CS evoking a CR that resembles the UR, even though

TABLE 3.2 Differences Between Forms of Learning

	Hull (1934)	
Learning	New Response	Preexisting Response
Specific	Beta-conditioning	
Nonspecific		Alpha-conditioning

	Grether (1938)	
Learning	New Response	Preexisting Response
Specific	Beta-conditioning	
Nonspecific	Pseudo-conditioning	

	Kandel (1965)	
Learning	New Response	Preexisting Response
Specific	Beta-conditioning	Alpha-conditioning
Nonspecific	Pseudo-conditioning	Sensitization

there has been no pairing of the CS and US. However, Grether failed to emphasize any distinction between sensitization and pseudoconditioning and in many textbooks since that date, the two phenomena have frequently been confused. Kandel's (1965) contribution was to see these two distinctions, for the first time, as components of a 2 × 2 table in which *specificity of pairing* was one dimension and *newness of the conditioned response* was the other. In such a 2 × 2 table, a new box emerges (top right), specific alpha-conditioning, the type of conditioning displayed by *Aplysia*. It is true conditioning because it is pairing-specific, but the CR that emerges is the same as that originally elicited by the CS (i.e., a preexisting response). For Kandel, the two rows of this 2 × 2 table are qualitatively different: they reflect the cell-biological mechanism of activity-dependent modulation. But the two columns differ only quantitatively. New responses are merely CRs that were below threshold before conditioning.

My purpose in comparing the S–R version of stimulus substitution with differential facilitation is threefold. First, it makes clear that Kandel's theorizing occupies two very different domains, level 2 *and* level 3: (1) he has an essentially psychological hypothesis about the kind of algorithm being computed in a conditioning task and (2) he has a wide range of ideas (and evidence!) about the neural mechanisms involved (the general principles summarized above). Second, the comparison suggests a plausible reason why Kandel developed the differential facilitation hypothesis. I surmise that he wanted to avoid what he cor-

implausibility. In effect, he was accepting that aspect of the Ramón y Cajal heritage which supposed that synapses were important for information storage while rejecting the "strong interpretation" of Ramón y Cajal's position—the necessity for new connections between hitherto unconnected neurons. Kandel frequently writes that he sees learning as "fundamentally different" from other plastic neural processes in which new connections are formed (such as reactive synaptogenesis; see Lynch & Baudry, 1984, who take the opposite view). Indeed, in Chapter 62 of *Principles of Neural Science,* work on learning in *Aplysia* is juxtaposed with work on the unmasking of silent synapses in cat spinal cord (Wall, 1975) and primate somatosensory cortex (Merzenich et al., 1983). Thus the common feature of activity-dependent modulation and the sectioning of afferent nerves is that they both have functional consequences which reflect the intricacy of prewiring in the nervous system. Kandel's perspective echoes that of Sherrington (1951): the nervous system is an "enchanted loom," and we should respect its intricate prewiring.

The third point served by the comparison of stimulus substitution and differential facilitation is that it makes clear why Kandel regards the alpha-conditioning issue as trivial. According to the differential facilitation hypothesis, there never are any new responses. Everything is prewired.[1] In his view, the behavioral scientist is misled by the emergence of *apparently* new responses during certain conditioning procedures (see Carew, Abráms, Hawkins, & Kandel, 1984, pp. 175–177) because the underlying process of conditioning is a gradual increase in the efficacy of CRs to which the CS has *always* been wired up. Eventually these CRs cross a behavioral threshold and emerge as apparently novel responses.

It is on this third point that I have to part company with Kandel, because this feature of the differential facilitation hypothesis—reflex prewiring—is psychologically implausible. It cannot be correct to say that *all* the responses a CS can *ever* elicit already exist as reflexes to that CS, albeit in subthreshold form. My reasons for rejecting such a possibility are (1) its intuitive implausibility and (2) the fact that conditioning is a process through which animals learn about the predictability of the environment.

Consider the issue of plausibility first. Is it plausible to suppose that all the responses that can ever be conditioned to a CS are already reflexly wired up to it? That Pavlov's dog salivated to the metronome because the metronome stimulus was covertly wired up to salivation? Kandel's work on the underlying neural mechanisms of learning seems to require this conclusion. However, several phenomena in the behavioral literature render "reflex prewiring" particularly implausible. One is the emergence of US-relevant responses during autoshaping (Jenkins & Moore, 1973). Approach and contact may well be prewired investigatory responses to a focal light stimulus, such as a key light in an operant chamber, but it is hard to accept that the "drinking" keypecks which birds elicit when autoshaped for water are also reflexively prewired. Another is the phenomenon of counterconditioning in which, for example, weak electric shock is used as a CS for food. Initially the shock elicits unconditional responses of flinching, freezing, and defecation. However, as conditioning proceeds, these responses subside (although they need not be totally obscured; see Dickinson & Dearing, 1979) and come to be replaced by behavior reflecting the anticipation of food: general activity and, in the case of the study by Erofeeva cited by Pavlov (1927), salivation. It is hard to believe that salivation is reflexively prewired to electric shock.

The second reason for being suspicious of the generality of differential facilitation is that nothing in the algorithm captures the sense that conditioning is a process through which an animal comes to learn about the predictability of the environment. Any sense that salivation happens because the CS *predicts* the meat (Zener, 1937) is, strictly speaking, absent from the hypothesis. Here, however, I confess to being confused by Kandel's writings. Several passages in Kandel and Schwartz (1985) make it abundantly clear that Kandel fully appreciates the revolution in our thinking about the processes of conditioning that began in the 1960s (Dickinson, 1980; Mackintosh, 1983; Rescorla, 1988; Rescorla & Wagner, 1987). Thus Kandel writes:

> Classical conditioning is fascinating because, as we saw earlier, it represents the learning of a fundamental causal relationship. When an animal has been conditioned, it has learned that the conditioned stimulus predicts the unconditioned stimulus. Thus, through classical conditioning, an organism is able to discriminate cause and effect relationships in the environment. (Kandel & Schwartz, 1985, pp. 823–824)

The problem is that the differential facilitation algorithm cannot realize the process of predicting the environment. It is an algorithm for differentially increasing the strength of existing CRs when the CS and a particular US occur in temporal contiguity. *In no sense does the learned CR predict the US.* A particularly striking way of seeing this problem is with reference to the phenomenon of sensory preconditioning in which two initially neutral CSs are paired and one of them is later paired with a US (Rescorla, 1980). In a standard conditioning procedure, a CS is arranged to predict the US. In sensory preconditioning, this procedure is broken down into two stages: CS_1 is arranged to predict CS_2, and CS_2 subsequently is arranged to predict the US. In a final test phase, CS_1 is presented, and the question at issue is whether the animal behaves in a manner reflecting the anticipation of the US. The problem for differential facilitation here is that the pairing of CS_1 and CS_2 (stage 1) occurs before the CS_2 is paired with *either* an aversive *or* an appetitive stimulus (stage 2). As there is no way of the animal knowing, in the first stage of the experiment, what kind of event CS_2 will be paired with in stage 2, there is no obvious way, short of serendipity, of selectively facilitating defensive or consummatory reflexes in stage 1. Although sensory preconditioning might be put aside as an example of a particularly complex form of conditioning and therefore outside the scope of differential facilitation, it is, in my view, the sort of phenomenon that brings us closer to an understanding of the kind of process conditioning really is. In a recent book largely devoted to work on invertebrate simple systems, Rescorla (1984) drew particular attention to sensory preconditioning: "My view is that neurobiologists studying learning could profit considerably by including this paradigm in their armoury of procedures" (p. 43).

Thus far in this section I have endeavored to suggest (1) an explanation of why Kandel was led to propose his differential facilitation theory of conditioning, and (2) why it is psychologically implausible. However, the argument is incomplete in two very different ways. First, Hawkins and Kandel (1984) are well aware that the "basic circuit" of the abdominal ganglion is incapable of explaining several higher forms of conditioning and they point out that it is essential to refer to additional aspects of known circuitry to explain these. I turn to these arguments in a later section where I consider the relationship between synaptic plasticity and neural architecture. Second, because I have no quarrel with the idea that learning involves no more than changing the efficacy of pre-existing neuronal connections, the final part of this section has to be the more constructive task of outlining one way in which this principle can be made compatible with a more plausible process account of conditioning. One such way is the distributed associative matrix (Willshaw, Buneman, & Longuet-Higgins, 1969), the earliest and most frequently "rediscovered" system for storing information in a distributed manner. Although some of the newer networks of contemporary work on parallel distributed processing involve more sophisticated algorithms (Rumelhart & McClelland, 1986), the principle I wish to establish in this section can be made with reference to the associative matrix alone.

Consider a matrix of wires intersecting at nodes (analagous to synapses) that can be either OFF or ON (Fig. 3.4). If a node is ON, activity in a horizontal wire can induce activity in a vertical wire. If a node is OFF, activity in a horizontal wire has no effect on activity in a vertical wire. In the initial state of the matrix, all nodes are OFF (Fig. 3.4a). Thus no pattern of activity on the horizontal wire will cause any activity whatsoever in the vertical wires. This matrix can be made to store information according to the "Hebbian" rule that a node is turned permanently from OFF to ON when there is simultaneous (i.e., conjunctive) activity in both a horizontal and a vertical wire. Information is stored as a change of state of the corresponding node when such conjunctions are detected. Stimuli are presented to this matrix as spatial patterns of activity on either the horizontal or the vertical wires. Thus 000111 might be one stimulus of a pair and 110100 the other. Notice that these stimuli differ in their spatial pattern, but they overlap in one of their elements (in this instance, the fourth digit). The association between these two stimuli is stored as a distributed pattern of changed nodes (Fig. 3.4b). After one pair of stimuli has been stored, the matrix assumes a particular pattern, and as further pairs of stimuli are presented in succession, the matrix alters progressively (Fig. 3.4c and 3.4d). Numerous nodes are involved in each association, and there is substantial overlap between different pairs of associations. Thus a given node may be involved in the storage of several associations. However, if an attempt is made to store too much information, the matrix will become saturated and cause errors in recall.

Storage of associations is of use only if the information can be retrieved. This

The Matrix

Storage of three pairs of associations

Recall

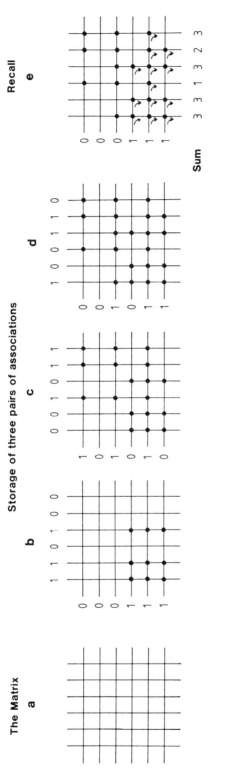

Integer division by number of active elements of recall cue (ie. 3) yields...

FIGURE 3.4. Associative matrix memory system in which storage depends on conjunctive activation of orthogonal wires intersecting at modifiable nodes (after Willshaw et al., 1969). Information to be associated is presented simultaneously to the matrix during storage, and those nodes at which there is simultaneous activation become irreversibly switched from OFF to ON (heavy dots). Several pairs of associations can be stored within the matrix without saturation. Retrieval results in activation of one member of an associative pair upon presentation of the other. A thresholding operation analogous to integer division is required for correct recall. Such a system might be realized in a real nervous system in which NMDA receptors detect the conjunction of afferent activity and postsynaptic depolarization, the resulting intracellular calcium signal triggers an alteration of synaptic efficacy, and feedforward inhibition serves the function of thresholding during recall (see McNaughton and Morris, 1987).

is achieved by presenting one member of any associative pair and attempting to activate ("remember") the other. In Figure 3.4e, the retrieval cue 000111 is presented to the horizontal wires. The retrieval rule is to allow activity in a horizontal wire to induce activity in a vertical wire only at switches that are ON. Adding things up, 000111 will therefore induce the output pattern 331321. At first sight, this pattern in no way resembles the stimulus with which 000111 was initially presented. However, integer division by the number of active elements in the recall cue (i.e., 3) gives the number 110100—the stimulus with which 000111 was originally associated.

Numerous fascinating properties of matrix memories have been explored formally over many years (Kohonen, 1977; Palm, 1982; Rumelhart & McClelland, 1986; Willshaw et al., 1969). I shall not dwell on these, except to say that their storage capacity is a function of (1) how stimuli are represented across the input array, and (2) the "local synaptic rules" governing changes at the nodes comprising the matrix (Palm, 1982). The Hebbian rule is one effective synaptic rule, but there are others (Levy, Andersen, & Lehmkule, 1985). In the present context, three principles of matrix memory systems must be stressed:

1. The matrix concept is not an obscure invention of computer science of no biological relevance. It is biologically feasible and McNaughton and Morris (1987) and Morris (1988) have tentatively explored the possibility that the mammalian hippocampus (or at least parts of it) is a type of associative matrix memory.
2. If implemented in neural hardware, the mechanism of storage would involve no more than changing the efficacy of preexisting synapses. Thus the matrix concept shares with the neural mechanisms of learning displayed by *Aplysia* the fact that no new neural connections have to be formed.
3. Any stimulus that can be represented as a pattern of activity over the horizontal wires can be paired with any stimulus represented as activity on the vertical wires. Of course, a potentiality for association must exist; it must be possible to represent stimuli in the form of a pattern of activity across the wires of the matrix in order for the stimuli to enter into associations (this potentiality might be thought of as a "biological constraint" on learning in exactly the same sense as Carew et al. (1984) proposed; see note 1). However, subject to this qualification, any stimulus can be arbitrarily paired with any other and, in recall, the "memory" of one stimulus will be activated by presentation of the other. Such a storage principle captures the essential notion of "representation," which, as described above, is so central to modern accounts of conditioning.

FORMS OF LEARNING ARE A FUNCTION OF NEURAL ARCHITECTURE

The second argument of this chapter is that the form of learning mediated by a particular type of synaptic plasticity is a function of the neural architecture within which it is embedded.

A mechanism for detecting the conjunction of two events is clearly an essential feature of any implementational theory of classical conditioning (level 3). However, a synaptic mechanism that detects contiguity will allow the nervous system to represent this temporal relationship only if the conjunction mechanism is embedded into appropriate circuitry.

Consider the "basic circuit" for *Aplysia* seen in Figure 3.1. The facilitator neuron synapses onto both the sensory neuron–interneuron pathway and the sensory neuron–motor neuron pathway. Activity in the facilitator neuron can therefore modulate the effectiveness of these synapses (in both sensitization and classical conditioning). However, the CS cannot evoke any neural representation of the US because the circuitry apparently does not permit it. The basic circuit will detect the contiguity of CS and US events during conditioning through activity-dependent modulation of presynaptic facilitation, but it cannot represent this relationship, where "representation" is taken to mean the CS being capable of evoking activity in the US pathway.

Hawkins and Kandel (1984) are well aware of the problem. In the second half of their paper, they draw attention to various additional aspects of known circuitry in *Aplysia* and, in particular, to neural pathways from the sensory neurons to the facilitator neurons (Fig. 3.5). These synapses are modifiable according to a quasi-Hebbian principle by virtue of feedback modulation from the facilitator neuron collaterals onto the presynaptic terminals of the sensory neuron input (Fig. 3.5B). Accordingly, in the real circuit of the abdominal ganglion, if sensory neuron activity impinges on the facilitator just before US activity, the synaptic connection between the sensory neuron and the facilitator neuron will be subject to activity-dependent modulation. As a result, subsequent activation of the sensory neuron can drive the motor neuron via the US pathway. Hawkins and Kandel (1984) make reference to these additional aspects of circuitry to explain higher order conditioning. However, this additional pathway—the pathway from sensory neuron to facilitator neuron—has wider ramifications. Specifically, the real circuit differs from the "basic circuit" in that it both detects and can, in principle, represent contiguity. The reason is as follows. Activity in the US pathway, as a consequence of facilitator neuron activation, can be regarded as an elementary kind of representation of the US. The CS now has the capacity to evoke this representation. The real circuit may therefore, as Hawkins and Kandel (1984) point out, be regarded as one way to implement a completely different theory of stimulus substitution, namely Pavlov's (1927) and Konorski's (1948) S–S version of stimulus substitution. However, in describing a circuit in *Aplysia* compatible with a different version of stimulus substitution theory, a version that does not require the formation of new neural pathways between hitherto unconnected neural elements, Hawkins and Kandel have broken the ostensibly intimate connection between sensitization and classical conditioning.

Consider what would happen in the real circuit if US presentations occurred alone. Strong stimulation of the tail region would activate tail sensory neurons, drive the facilitator neurons, and, by the feedback pathway on the presynaptic terminals of the sensory neuron–facilitator neuron pathway, increase the strength of these terminals by the process of presynaptic facilitation. That is, US

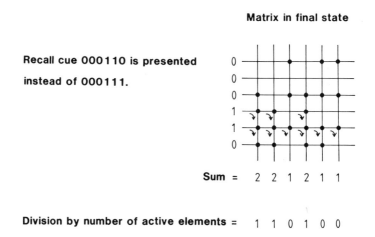

Recall cue 000110 is presented
instead of 000111.

Sum =   2 2 1 2 1 1

Division by number of active elements =   1 1 0 1 0 0

FIGURE 3.5.   A particularly important property of distributed memories is their capacity to recall stimuli accurately from fragmentary input. This property is a function of the neural architecture and independent of the particular cell-biological mechanism through which nodes are modified.

rectly judged to be the fatal weakness of Hull's (1934) account—its neural presentations alone could, at least in principle, increase the tendency of the CS to evoke responses similar to the UR without any necessity for pairing of the CS and US. This, as we saw earlier, is the process of "pseudoconditioning." That is, presynaptic facilitation may be the underlying mechanism of pseudoconditioning as well as the underlying mechanism of the process with which it is usually discussed, sensitization. Whether the behavioral outcome is sensitization or pseudoconditioning will depend on the circuitry within which presynaptic facilitation is embedded. Further, given that there is no a priori reason to regard the basic circuit as any more fundamental than the real circuit, it would surely be as appropriate for Hawkins and Kandel (1984) to describe classical conditioning as an elaboration of pseudoconditioning as to describe it as an elaboration of sensitization. The nature of the response that could be conditioned to a CS by activity-dependent modulation of presynaptic facilitation would then be determined by the efferent connections of the facilitator neuron, not the efferent connections of the CS pathway.

The breaking of the connection between classical conditioning and sensitization in favor of an equally plausible one between classical conditioning and pseudoconditioning might be thought to be of little consequence. Indeed, Kandel argued in his unpublished paper of 1965 that the difference between the columns of Table 3.2 may only be quantitative. In my opinion, such a position is untenable, first, because the link between classical conditioning and sensitization is axiomatic within differential facilitation—the whole point of the algorithm being that conditioning is to be viewed as a process through which existing reflexes to a CS are modulated by CS–US conjunctions. And it is untenable because describing a critical change in the neural architecture within which activity-dependent modulation is embedded as "quantitative" gives unreasonable priority to the importance of cell-biological principles over those at the system level.

The idea that the relationship between plasticity and learning depends critically on the neural architecture within which it is embedded can also be seen in relation to matrix memories. I shall consider this principle with reference to one positive feature and one weakness of matrix memories.

The positive feature is the capacity of matrix memories to achieve accurate recall despite being given only an incomplete or inaccurate input. A corollary of this feature is that matrix memories may continue to function quite well when partially damaged, a feature which Kohonen (Chapter 16, this volume) refers to as "graceful degradation" and which has been explored by Wood (1978). In the description given earlier, I outlined how the association of 000111 with 110100 in the learning phase would allow the stimulus 000111 to reactivate a memory representation of 110100 during retrieval even if several other associations are overlaid in the same matrix. Consider now what happens if, after learning, the retrieval cue 000110 was presented instead of 000111. The two stimuli are similar, differing only in the last digit. Adding things up, as in Figure 3.6, 000110 causes a pattern of activity in the vertical wires amounting to 221211. Remember, however, that this number must be divided by the total number of active elements in the retrieval cue to achieve accurate recall. Previously this number was 3 (the total number of 1's in 000111). Now the total number is 2 because the incomplete cue is being presented (000110). Integer division of 220211 by 2 yields 110100, the stimulus with which 000111 was originally associated. Thus an important "emergent" property of matrix circuitry is its capacity to continue to function effectively in recall despite incomplete or fragmentary input. This property of matrix memories has received extensive analysis elsewhere (e.g., Willshaw, 1981).

The weakness of matrix memories, which is also a property of the architecture rather than the particular cell-biological mechanism with which the constituent Hebb synapses are implemented in the nervous system, is that they fail to offer a satisfactory account of predictability or contingency. This may be seen most easily in relation to the phenomenon of blocking first described by Kamin (1968). The basic paradigm involves two groups of animals and a three-phase experiment (Fig. 3.7). In phase 1, one group learns that a stimulus (A) is paired with a US; the other group is given no training. In phase 2, a second stimulus (B) is added and the compound A + B is paired with the same US that was used in phase 1. Identical training procedures are used for both groups in phase 2. In a final test phase, B is presented alone and the question at issue is whether B evokes a memory of the US. Kamin's (1968) discovery was that learning of the B–US association was "blocked" in group 1. Blocking is not an inevitable consequence of compound training because satisfactory learning of the B–US association occurred in group 2. Kamin's original account of this phenomenon emphasized the sense in which the US was already predicted in group 1 at the

A

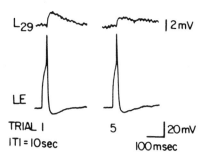

L29

LE

TRIAL 1   5
ITI = 10 sec

|2 mV

|20 mV
100 msec

B

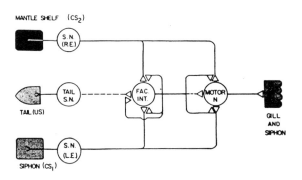

MANTLE SHELF (CS₂)

S.N.
(R.E.)

TAIL
S.N.

FAC.
INT.

MOTOR
N

GILL
AND
SIPHON

TAIL (US)

S.N.
(L.E.)

SIPHON (CS₁)

C

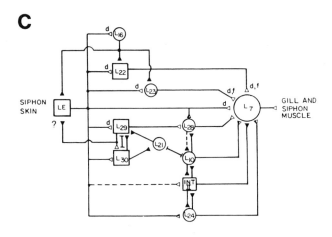

SIPHON
SKIN

LE

L-16

L-22

L-23

L-29

L-21

L-30

L-26

L-19

INT

L-24

L 7

GILL AND
SIPHON
MUSCLE

	Phase 1	Phase 2	Test Phase
Group 1	A⇨US	A+B⇨US	B?
Group 2		A+B⇨US	B?

FIGURE 3.7.   Basic stimulus arrangements for an experiment on blocking (after Kamin, 1968).

start of phase 2 and that, in some way, this prevented any new learning from happening. Clearly the US is not predicted at the start of phase 2 for group 2 and thus learning proceeds normally. Rescorla and Wagner (1972) formalized this intuition in a simple equation according to which conditioning occurs whenever there is a discrepancy between the total associative strength of all stimuli present on a trial and the total associative strength that a given US can support. Other acocunts of blocking have also been offered (Mackintosh, 1975; Pearce & Hall, 1980).

The distributed matrix cannot compute the essential difference algorithm of Rescorla and Wagner (1972) in order to account for blocking. This is because the Hebbian rule operates *locally* at nodes throughout the matrix in the absence of global information about the extent to which one stimulus adequately predicts the other with which it is paired. Figure 3.8 shows how pairings of a stimulus A (e.g., 10011) and the US (e.g., 11010) might produce a particular matrix of altered nodes (in a 5 × 5 matrix), how the compound of A + B would result in the matrix changing at those nodes where the B stimulus interacts with the US and which had not already been modified, and how subsequent presentations of B would therefore result in a memory representation of the US being evoked. Thus, as described, the matrix concept fails to account for blocking. The central problem is that there appears to be no way to prevent the additional B–US nodes from being altered because of the prior association of A with the US.

←_____

FIGURE 3.6.   Synaptic connections of L_{29}, one of the facilitator neurons. (A) A spike elicited by intracellular stimulation in an LE neuron produces an EPSP in L_{29}. (From Hawkins et al., 1981, Fig. 7A) (B) More complete circuit for gill- and siphon-withdrawal reflex and its modification by tail stimulation and differential conditioning. Note feedback innervation from the facilitator interneuron onto terminals from the LE neurons onto the facilitator neuron itself. (From Hawkins and Kandel, 1984, Fig. 5A) (C) More complete summary diagram of the synaptic connections of interneurons involved in the gill-withdrawal reflex. (From Hawkins et al., 1981, Fig. 9, where details of the interconnections are given) The recent paper by Frost et al. (1988) confirms that the siphon-withdrawal reflex is also mediated by highly complex circuitry and discusses the idea that different components of responsiveness are represented at different points of this circuitry.

There may be a number of ways to get around the problem and these fall naturally into two classes: (1) solutions that add extra circuitry, which "gates" input to the matrix by solving what is known as the "exclusive-or" problem (see Rumelhart & McClelland, 1986, Chapter 2); and (2) solutions that alter the local synaptic rule operating at individual nodes (e.g., Bear, Cooper, & Ebner, 1987). I shall not pursue these detailed matters here.

Some readers may find it confusing to have a discussion of conditioning in an animal whose circuitry has been worked out through painstaking anatomical and electrophysiological experimentation together with discussion of an idealized system whose implementation within the nervous system has never been established. However, my aim is to establish a principle that applies equally to both systems: the form of learning mediated by a particular type of synaptic plasticity is a function of the neural architecture within which it is embedded. In this final section, I have attempted to show how the basic circuit of *Aplysia,* widely used by Kandel and his colleagues for the pedagogical purpose of explaining their ideas about synaptic plasticity, is a circuit that cannot represent the relationship between the CS and US in classical conditioning. The real circuitry of *Aplysia* can represent contiguity (and predictability), but it does so awkwardly and at the cost of abandoning the relation between classical conditioning and sensitization that has been central to Kandel's approach for many years. In comparison, the matrix concept provides a much more straightforward way to explain how any stimulus can evoke a memory representation of any other stimulus, provided both stimuli can be presented to the matrix in a distributed code. However, the matrix concept fails to provide a satisfactory account of predict-

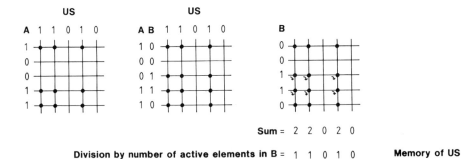

FIGURE 3.8.   The associative matrix operating according to a Hebbian conjunction rule is unable to explain blocking because the alteration of nodes from an OFF to an ON state is determined locally and unaffected by the global computation of the extent to which the US is already predicted by stimulus A.

ability because the local synaptic rule determining information storage is not error-correcting.

CONCLUSIONS

This chapter has reconsidered an old issue, the relation of alpha-conditioning to classical conditioning, with the aim of revealing insights into (1) the relationship between psychological and neurobiological accounts of conditioning and (2) the problem of representation by the nervous system. I argued that the algorithmic computations performed during learning are realized by particular mechanisms of synaptic plasticity embedded into particular types of neural architecture such that the nervous system's capacity to represent the association between events is an emergent property of circuitry. Thus there need be no simple mapping between cell biology and learning. A cellular alphabet of plasticity exists; a cellular alphabet of learning does not (Table 3.3).

Finally, as parts of this chapter might be wrongly construed as critical of the work on *Aplysia,* it may be worth clarifying the essential point of disagreement. It is not with respect to the experimental work itself, which has justly earned the respect of neuroscientists all over the world. Equally, I have no criticisms of Kandel's account of the mechanisms of those forms of conditioning that are displayed by the abdominal ganglion of *Aplysia.* Rather, in trying to think about how to apply the principles often drawn from this work, particularly in relation to the vertebrate nervous system, I find that it may be possible to accept the idea that learning involves the modulation of existing neural pathways without accepting the idea of reflex prewiring. The matrix idea is but one of a range of distributed information processing systems with the capacity to learn and, like others, it is a system for which it makes no sense to speak of a particular CR covertly prewired to a particular CS.

TABLE 3.3   Summary of Arguments

Changes in synaptic efficacy during learning can store information.
Presynaptic facilitation
Long-term potentiation
Cell-biological mechanisms may be responsible for detecting associations between temporally coincident events.
Activity-dependent modulation
NMDA receptors
Computations performed during learning depend on the anatomical circuitry within which cell-biological mechanisms are embedded.
Activity-dependent modulation detects but need not always represent contiguity.
Matrix memories represent contiguity but may not represent predictability.

Acknowledgments

I should like to thank E. R. Kandel, N. J. Mackintosh, J. N. P. Rawlins, I. C. Reid, and D. J. Willshaw for their detailed comments on an earlier draft of this chapter. I should particularly like to thank Eric Kandel for sending me the unpublished manuscript of 1965 referred to in the text and for his permission to reproduce certain previously published figures. This work was supported by an MRC Programme Grant to R. G. M. Morris and D. J. Willshaw.

Note

1. A careful reading of Carew et al. (1984) points to a qualification of this claim: "We should emphasize that this does not imply that every potential stimulus is pre-wired to every potential motor response in the nervous system" (pp. 175–177). At first I wondered if this implied that they had in mind some other mechanism of learning than alpha-conditioning. However, the succeeding sentence makes it clear they do not, and that the qualification refers only to the fact that stimuli and responses with no neural connection between them cannot be learned.

REFERENCES

Abrams, T. W., & Kandel, E. R. (1988). Is contiguity detection in classical conditioning a systems or a cellular property? Learning in *Aplysia* suggests a possible molecular site. *Trends in Neurosciences, 11,* 128–135.

Alkon, D. L., & Farley, J. (1984). *Primary neural substrates of learning and behavioral change.* Cambridge: Cambridge University Press.

Bailey, C. H., & Chen, M. C. (1983). Morphological basis of long-term habituation and sensitization in *Aplysia. Science, 220,* 91–93.

Bailey, C. H., & Chen, M. C. (1986). Long-term sensitization in *Aplysia* increases the total number of varicosities of single identified sensory neurons. *Society for Neuroscience Abstracts, 12,* 860.

Bear, M. F., Cooper, L. N., & Ebner, F. F. (1987). A physiological basis for a theory of synapse modification. *Science, 237,* 42–48.

Boakes, R. A. (1984). *From Darwin to behaviourism: Psychology and the minds of animals,* Cambridge: Cambridge University Press.

Carew, T. J., Abrams, T. W., Hawkins, R. D., & Kandel, E. R. (1984). The use of simple invertebrate systems to explore psychological issues related to associative learning. In D. L. Alkon & J. Farley (Eds.), *Primary neural substrates and behavioural change* (pp. 169–183). Cambridge: Cambridge University Press.

Castellucci, V. F., & Kandel, E. R. (1974). A quantal analysis of the synaptic depression underlying habituation of the gill-withdrawal reflex in *Aplysia. Proceedings of the National Academy of Sciences, 71,* 5004–5008.

Castellucci, V. F., & Kandel, E. R. (1976). Presynaptic facilitation as a mechanism for behavioural sensitization in *Aplysia. Science, 194,* 1176–1178.

Dickinson, A. (1980). *Contemporary animal learning theory.* Cambridge: Cambridge University Press.

Dickinson, A., & Dearing, M. (1979). Appetitive-aversive interactions and inhibitory processes. In A. Dickinson & R. A. Boakes (Eds.), *Mechanisms of learning and motivation: A memorial volume to Jerzy Konorski* (pp. 203–231). Hillsdale, N.J.: Erlbaum.

Frost, W. N., Clark, G. A., & Kandel, E. R. (1988). Parallel processing of short-term memory for sensitization in *Aplysia. Journal of Neurobiology, 19,* 297–334.

Garcia, J., & Koelling, R. A. (1966). Relation of cue to consequence in avoidance learning. *Psychonomic Science, 4,* 123–124.

Gluck, M. A., & Thompson, R. F. (1987). Modeling the neural substrates of associative learning and memory: A computational approach. *Psychological Review, 94,* 176–191.

Greenough, W. T., & Bailey, C. H. (1988). The anatomy of a memory: Convergence of results across a diversity of tests. *Trends in Neurosciences, 11,* 142–146.

Grether, W. F. (1938). Pseudoconditioning without paired stimulation encountered in attempted backward conditioning. *Journal of Comparative Psychology, 25,* 91–96.

Hawkins, R. D. (1989). A biologically realistic neural network model for higher order features of classical conditioning. In R. G. M. Morris (Ed.), *Parallel distributed processing: Implications for psychology and neurobiology* (pp. 214–247). Oxford: Oxford University Press.

Hawkins, R. D., Castellucci, V. F., & Kandel, E. R. (1981). Interneurons involved in mediation and modulation of gill-withdrawal reflex in *Aplysia.* I. Identification and characterization. *Journal of Neurophysiology, 45,* 304–314.

Hawkins, R. D., & Kandel, E. R. (1984). Is there a cell-biological alphabet for simple forms of learning? *Psychological Review, 91,* 375–391.

Hebb, D. O. (1949). *The organization of behaviour.* New York: Wiley.

Horn, G. (1985). *Memory, imprinting and the brain.* Oxford: Clarendon Press.

Hull, C. L. (1934). Learning II. The factor of the conditioned reflex. In D. Murchison (Ed.), *A handbook of general experimental psychology* (pp. 392–455). Worcester, Mass.: Clark University Press.

Jenkins, H. M., & Moore, B. R. (1973). The form of the auto-shaped response with food or water reinforcers. *Journal of Experimental Analysis of Behavior, 20,* 163–181.

Kamin, L. J. (1968). Attention-like processes in classical conditioning. In M. R. Jones (Ed.), *Miami symposium on prediction of behavior; aversive stimulation* (pp. 9–33). Coral Gables, Fla.: University of Miami Press.

Kandel, E. R. (1965). *The relation of alpha conditioning to classical conditioning.* Unpublished manuscript.

Kandel, E. R. (1976). *Cellular basis of behavior: An introduction to behavioral neurobiology.* San Francisco: Freeman.

Kandel, E. R., & Schwartz, J. H. (1982). Molecular biology of learning: Modulation of transmitter release. *Science, 218,* 433–443.

Kandel, E. R., & Schwartz, J. H. (1985). *Principles of neural science* (2nd ed.). New York: Elsevier.

Kohonen, T. (1977). *Associative-memory.* Heidelberg: Springer-Verlag.

Konorski, J. (1948). *Conditioned reflexes and neuron organisation.* Cambridge: Cambridge University Press.

Levy, W. B., Andersen, J. A., & Lehmkule, S. (1985). *Synaptic modification, neuron selectivity and nervous system organization.* Hillsdale, N.J.: Erlbaum.

Lynch, G., & Baudry, M. (1984). The biochemistry of memory: A new and specific hypothesis. *Science, 224,* 1057–1063.

Mackintosh, N. J. (1975). A theory of attention: Variations in the associability of stimuli with reinforcement. *Psychological Review, 82,* 276–298.

Mackintosh, N. J. (1983). *Conditioning and associative learning.* Oxford: Clarendon Press.

Marr, D. (1982). *Vision.* San Francisco: Freeman.

McNaughton, B. L., & Morris, R. G. M. (1987). Hippocampal synaptic enhancement and information storage within a distributed memory system. *Trends in Neuroscience, 10,* 408–415.

Medawar, P. M. B. (1966). *The art of the soluble.* London: Methuen.

Merzenich, M. M., Kaas, J. H., Wall, J. T., Sur, M., Nelson, R. J., & Felleman, D. J. (1983). Progression of change following median nerve section in the cortical representation of the hand in areas 3b and 1 in adult owl and squirrel monkey. *Neuroscience, 10,* 639–665.

Morris, R. G. M. (1988). Elements of a hypothesis concerning participation of hippocampal NMDA receptors in learning. In D. Lodge (Ed.), *Excitatory amino acids in health and disease* (pp. 297–320). Chichester: Wiley.

Palm, G. (1982). *Neural assemblies: An alternative approach to artificial intelligence.* Heidelberg: Springer-Verlag.

Pavlov, I. P. (1927). *Conditioned reflexes.* Oxford: Oxford University Press.

Pearce, J. M., & Hall, G. (1980). A model for Pavlovian learning: Variations in the effectiveness of conditioned but not of unconditioned stimuli. *Psychological Review, 87,* 532–552.

Pinsker, H., Kupfermann, I., Castellucci, V. F., & Kandel, E. R. (1970). Habituation and dishabituation of the gill-withdrawal reflex in *Aplysia. Science, 167,* 1740–1742.

Ramón y Cajal, S. (1911). *Histologie du systeme nerveux de l'homme et des vertebrates* (Vol. 2). Paris: Maloine.

Rescorla, R. A. (1980). Simultaneous and successive associations in sensory preconditioning. *Journal of Experimental Psychology: Animal Behavior Processes, 4,* 267–275.

Rescorla, R. A. (1984). Comments on three Pavlovian paradigms. In D. L. Alkon and J. Farley (Eds.), *Primary neural substrates of learning and behavioural change.* Cambridge: Cambridge University Press.

Rescorla, R. A. (1988). Behavioural studies of Pavlovian conditioning. *Annual Review of Neuroscience, 11,* 329–352.

Rescorla, R. A., & Wagner, A. R. (1972). A theory of Pavlovian conditioning: Variations in the effectiveness of reinforcement and nonreinforcement. In A. H. Black & W. F. Prokasy (Eds.), *Classical conditioning* (Vol. 2, pp. 64–99). New York: Appleton-Century-Crofts.

Rose, S. P. R. (1984). Strategies in studying the cell biology of learning and memory. In L. R. Square & N. Butters (Eds.), *Neuropsychology of memory* (pp. 547–554). New York: Guilford.

Routtenberg, A. (1987). Synaptic plasticity and protein kinase C. In W. H. Gispen & A. Routtenberg (Eds.), *Progress in brain research* (Vol. 69, pp. 221–234). Amsterdam: Elsevier.

Rumelhart, D. E., & McClelland, J. (1986). *Parallel distributed processing* (Vols. 1, 2). Cambridge, Mass.: MIT Press.

Sherrington, C. S. (1951). *Man on his nature.* (The Gifford Lectures). (2nd ed.). Cambridge: Cambridge University Press.

Thompson, R. F. (1986). The neurobiology of learning and memory. *Science, 233,* 941–947.

Wagner, A. R. (1978). Expectancies and the priming of STM. In S. H. Hulse, H. Fowler, & W. K. Honig (Eds.), *Cognitive processes in animal behavior* (pp. 177–209). Hillsdale, N.J.: Erlbaum.

Wall, P. D. (1975). Signs of plasticity and reconnection in spinal cord damage. In *Outcome of severe damage to the central nervous system.* London: Ciba Foundation Symposium, 34.

Willshaw, D. J. (1981). Holography, associative-memory and inductive generalisation. In G. A. Hinton & J. A. Anderson (Eds.), *Parallel models of associative memory* (pp. 83–104). London: Academic Press.

Willshaw, D. J., Buneman, O., & Longuet-Higgins, H. C. (1969). Non-holographic associative memory. *Nature, 222,* 960–962.

Wood, C. (1978). Variations on a theme by Lashley: Lesion experiments on the neural model of Andersen, Silverstein, Ritz and Jones. *Psychological Review, 85,* 582–591.

Yeo, A. G. (1974). The acquisition of conditioned suppression as a function of interstimulus interval duration. *Quarterly Journal of Experimental Psychology, 26,* 405–416.

Zener, K. (1937). The significance of behaviour accompanying conditioned salivary secretion for theories of the conditioned response. *American Journal of Psychology, 50,* 384–403.

4

Forms of Memory
in Pavlovian Conditioning

PETER C. HOLLAND

Psychologists have made few compelling generalizations about memory as a whole, but a variety of satisfying statements about performances on particular memory tasks. The conventional psychological approach to this state of affairs was to view memory as a single system and each task as a way of illuminating a small set of its attributes. More recently psychologists have taken the view that there are several memory systems, which may serve different purposes and follow different rules of operation. Furthermore, it has been tempting to suggest that those systems have separate neural mechanisms and evolutionary histories.

A plethora of "divisions of memory" has been proposed, many based on exciting new evidence from neuropsychology and animal conditioning. These forms of memory are distinguished along many attributes, such as content (e.g., semantic vs. episodic), type of processing (e.g., working vs. reference), capacity (limited or unlimited), and endurance (transient vs. permanent). Considerable experimentation shows that memory tasks thought to engage these different systems are differentially sensitive to certain variables and manipulations.

I do not intend to examine any of the currently popular memory-form distinctions explicitly, but rather to describe a functional view of memory in animal conditioning, which links the study of memory to that of perception, motor skills, and other psychological and neurobiological processes. Within this view, much memory is an elaboration of sensory and motor processes, the consequence of plasticity and convergence at many steps in the pathways of perception and action. Thus at some level it begs a multisystems view; it would not be surprising if tasks that engaged different perceptual and/or motor systems, or engaged the same systems in different ways or at different loci, would be differentially responsive to certain variables or exhibit different functional characteristics. At another level, however, such a view demands a more integrating, unitary perspective. It is unlikely that *any* "memory system" would be completely independent: memory itself is likely to be both the consequence and the heart of integration of neural systems.

PAVLOVIAN CONDITIONING AS A MEMORY TASK

Many claims about memory are limited in applicability to certain tasks. Unfortunately, understanding of what many tasks in vogue are tapping, or what influences them, is vague. Theories of memory based on research with poorly understood tasks are on shaky ground at best. But limiting one's study to a single task, no matter how completely understood it may be, is unlikely to reveal much of the range of memory's functions. For me, the Pavlovian conditioning preparations described in this chapter are a reasonable compromise between understanding and diversity.

Considerable progress has been made since the late sixties in describing the nature of Pavlovian conditioning, at both psychological and neurobiological levels. Its determinants and effects are at least as well understood as any other psychological phenomenon. Furthermore, it is a rich phenomenon, with the diversity needed to permit a broad view of memory. Although psychologists and neurobiologists typically focus their analytic efforts on single behavioral consequences of Pavlovian learning experiences, it must be remembered that those experiences engage multiple behavior systems, often drastically changing the organism's commerce with its environment. Thus, although Pavlovian conditioning is often caricatured as a trivial learning process, lord only of spit and twitches, I believe Pavlovian learning is a major basis for the organization and integration of behavior. In this chapter I describe three lines of research in my laboratory, with intact adult rats, which I hope capture some of that richness in ways that are amenable to neural analogies. In the first section I discuss some traditional and nontraditional views of substitution and event representation, which emphasize perceptual processing in the memorial consequences of conditioning. Next I describe research that focuses on conditioning as an integrator of organized behavior systems. Finally I discuss recent work concerning a conditioning function that I call "occasion setting" and the formation of more complex, higher order units in conditioning.

EVENT REPRESENTATION AND MEMORY

In a prototypical Pavlovian conditioning experiment, two stimuli are presented contiguously in time and independently of the subject's behavior. Usually, one of those events (the unconditioned stimulus, US) spontaneously produces an easily measurable change in the subject's behavior (the unconditioned response, UR), and the other (the conditioned stimulus, CS) does not. Learning is inferred if pairing the CS and US generates change in the behavior during the CS (the conditioned response, CR).

In traditional theoretical accounts, Pavlovian conditioning is described as the substitution of a previously neutral stimulus into an existing reflex system, the transfer of control of an unconditioned reflex from the US to the CS. This view was encouraged by early observations suggesting that the conditioned response was a replica of the unconditioned response. Furthermore, this substitution view is amenable to neurobiological analysis: the underpinnings of learning could be charted by tracing the activation of the unconditioned reflex system upstream (e.g., Thompson, 1986) toward the receptor pathways activated by the CS, or by working downstream from the receptor surface (e.g., Cohen, 1985) until sites of plasticity are discovered.

The notion that the CS acts as a substitute elicitor of the UR was also pervasive in early psychological accounts because it is consistent with both of the two major theoretical approaches to conditioning debated in the early days of psychology, S–R and S–S. Unconditioned response–like CRs might be evoked either directly by associations of CS and UR or indirectly by the CS's activation of a "US center," which in turn elicited the UR. To the modern neurobiologist, this distinction often seems to have a mystical ring to it, because the S's, R's, and centers of the psychologist seldom bear much resemblance to recognizable neural events or systems. Clearly, describing a single "food representation" or "center" is illusory: food, or any other US, is a multimodal experience. It is hard to imagine that the rat's nervous system partitions the world to match my conceptual frame. Nevertheless, I believe discussions based on such simple notions of event representation and on distinctions between S–S and S–R links may help illuminate the neural organization of learned behavior.

In its simplest form, the S–R versus S–S distinction concerns whether a site of plastic, functional convergence of CS and US pathways is near the sensory or motor end of the US–UR reflex. Loosely speaking, how much of the US–UR machinery is engaged by the CS alone after conditioning?

Figure 4.1 is a fanciful sketch of two reflex pathways, that of a US, say food, which elicits a reflex response, say salivation, and of a CS, say tone. For the moment, we are concerned with the US pathway, because most views of Pavlovian conditioning concentrate on this particular behavior change (I will correct this oversimplification in the next section of this chapter). The pathway imagined here should be viewed as containing whatever sensory input and mediating systems are necessary to produce untrained, reflexive responding. I presume that these CS and US pathways converge at many levels and loci. For the learning theorist, the question is, what is the locus of plastic change that relates these two pathways? Does the CS acquire the ability to directly activate late portions of the US pathway, or does it act early in the US pathway?

Consider two extreme representations. The site labeled S–S reflects a changed potential for the CS to excite the first US-path unit. Essentially *all* of the US-path machinery is thus engaged by CS presentation alone. Thus the rat not only will salivate when the tone comes on, but also will taste food, feel it, and otherwise experience it in all the ways a rat would experience the food itself. In short, this path generates a hallucination of food; the tone is a perfect surrogate. Conversely, the site labeled S–R reflects a changed potential for the CS to excite the output unit that controls the UR. But the final common path between CS and US pathways includes only that unit: no other US-patch machinery is

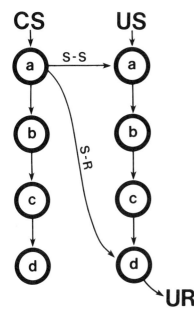

FIGURE 4.1. Simple representation of S–S and S–R associations between CS and US paths.

engaged. The rat that has gained this link because of tone–food pairing salivates when the tone is presented, but experiences nothing else of US-path activity.

It is unlikely that any significant Pavlovian CR is generated entirely by plasticity at either one of these loci, in all but the simplest systems. Rats probably do not hallucinate perfect copies of absent USs, nor are final output neurons likely to be the culprit. It is possible that *some* plasticity occurs at all levels (e.g., Cohen, 1985), but the changes most closely correlated with the emergence of CRs are likely to be a bit more central. Nevertheless, the question of how much US-path machinery is engaged by the CS remains a useful one. Considerable recent data from the laboratories of learning theorists suggest (1) there are multiple sites of plasticity along the US path, (2) the relative importance of those various sites is influenced greatly by the nature of the learning experience, and (3) in many situations, considerably more of the US-path machinery is engaged by the CS after learning than we were previously willing to admit.

Today, the performance of simple Pavlovian conditioned responses is almost universally described as mediated by internal representations of the conditioned and unconditioned stimuli: associations formed between those representations endow the CS alone with the ability to activate the representation of the US (e.g., Rescorla, 1974). For present purposes, a "US representation" refers to a path of activation of the US–UR, or a portion of it. Within the context of Figure 4.1, if a CS is said to evoke a US representation, plastic changes more like the one labeled S–S than the one labeled S–R are presumed to predominate. Thus pairing a tone with food gives the tone the ability to activate a representation of food, in the absence of food itself. Conditioned responses (CRs) then are not evoked directly by the CS (as would be the case if the site labeled S–R predominated), but rather are mediated by higher portions of the US pathway, the "US representation." This simple notion has proved useful in describing a number of features of Pavlovian conditioning, two of which I will summarize next.

Mediated Performance of Conditioned Responses

The ability of previously trained CSs to evoke CRs often depends on the current status of the US. For example, Holland (1989b) first presented hungry rats with two kinds of conditioning trials. Tone 1 (T_1) was followed by delivery of food 1 (F_1) and tone 2 (T_2) was followed by food 2 (F_2). (The two foods were wintergreen- and peppermint-flavored sucrose, selected so that the rats showed identical URs and no preferences between them.) Identical conditioned food-related behavior was established to both tones (left side of Fig. 4.2). Then, in the absence of either tone, one food was paired with a toxin (lithium chloride). Thus one former US (F_2) now served as a CS in a new Pavlovian relation. The rats rapidly formed an aversion to F_2: as a consequence of F_2–toxin pairings, F_2 no longer evoked many aspects of its previous UR, nor would it serve as an effective US for Pavlovian conditioning of a new CS. Finally, the original tone CSs were pre-

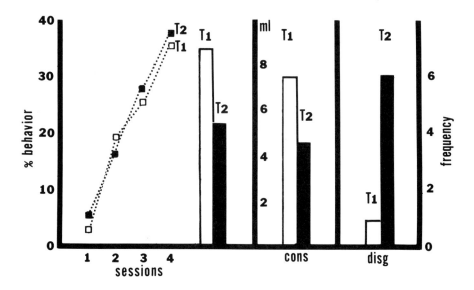

FIGURE 4.2. Results of mediated performance experiment (after Holland, 1989b). The curves in the left panel show acquisition of conditioned responding during T_1 and T_2, two tone CSs that were each paired with distinctive foods, F_1 and F_2, respectively; the bars show test responding during those tones, after F_2 was paired with a toxin. The center and right panels display data from a subsequent test session in which the rats received presentations of T_1 and T_2 while consuming plain water. The center panel shows consumption, and the right panel shows the frequence of disgust responses in that test.

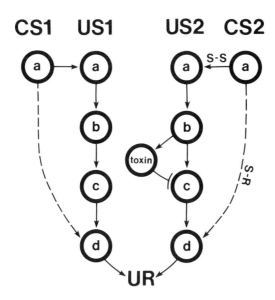

CS1 US1   US2 CS2

FIGURE 4.3. Representation of possible S–S and S–R associations established in the mediated performance experiments. ⟶= excitatory action; ⟶(= inhibitory action.

sented to the rats, in the absence of the foods or toxins. In this test, T_2, whose F_2 associate had been paired with toxin, showed a substantially reduced CR, but T_1, whose F_1 associate had not been devalued, continued to display substantial CRs (center portion of Fig. 4.2).

This outcome is consistent with the S–S view of conditioning described above, that is, a fair amount of the US-path activity is engaged by the CS. The potentiated S–S link between T_2 and F_2 pathways must be upstream from whatever link is established by F_2–toxin conditioning (Fig. 4.3). If instead the T_2–F_2 link was downstream from the F_2–toxin link (the S–R path), then the T_2 alone would not activate the F_2–toxin link, and hence would still evoke the intact CR. Furthermore, because the response evoked by US1 (and T_1) was unaffected, the F_2–toxin plasticity must have been upstream from a final common output path.

Perceptual Nature of Substitution

Apparently the information coded by these CS-evoked representations is quite detailed. In the experiment just described, the two foods were delivered to the same food cup and differed only in the flavoring added. Furthermore, the concentrations of flavorings were selected so that there were no preferences for one or the other in groups of rats or for most individual rats. Thus rats interacted with the two foods in identical ways. Consequently, the rats' very selective use of the representations of the foods makes it likely that the substitution of tones for foods is more easily labeled "perceptual" than "motor." However, it is difficult conceptually to distinguish between "stimulus" and "response" information in representations or between "sensory" and "motor" interneurons in pathways. At what point in processing do we class the response of cell assemblies as specifying properties of the organism's response rather than its sensory processing? I have made several attempts to deal with this issue at an operational–behavioral level.

Perhaps the most dramatic method of distinguishing between stimulus- and response-based mediation in these experiments involved slow-motion video monitoring of the form of the rats' consummatory responses. Grill and Norgren (1978) noted that identifiable patterns of responses, which reflect active "acceptance" and "rejection," occur to naturally occurring positive (e.g., sweet) and negative (e.g., bitter) flavors. Furthermore, Pelchat, Grill, Rozin, and Jacobs (1983) noted that pairing a formerly accepted flavor with toxin results in the rejection of that flavor in a characteristic rejection or "disgust" pattern; conversely, pairing it with shock results in passive spilling of the flavor but no acquistion of the disgust response. Pelchat et al. (1983) suggested that these outcomes indicate that flavor–toxin pairings reduce consumption by making the flavor taste bad, but flavor–shock pairings reduce consumption less directly by signaling an upcoming aversive event (see also Garcia, Kovner, & Green, 1970).

Observation of the response forms in my experiments (Holland, 1989b) supports claims that taste information can be conveyed in these CS-evoked representations. In the "mediated performance" experiment just described, I observed the form of the rats' consumption of a plain sucrose solution (which contained neither peppermint nor wintergreen), in the presence of tone 2 or tone 1, after food 2 had been devalued. During tone 2, the rats showed more characteristic disgust responses and fewer active acceptance responses than during tone 1, whose food 1 partner had not been devalued (right side of Fig. 4.2).

Note that in the first phase of the experiment, when the tones were originally paired with the flavored solutions, no disgust responses were observed during either tone or food presentations. Furthermore, control experiments (Holland, 1989b) show that tones paired with toxins do not acquire the ability to evoke disgust responses, unless those tones were previously paired with a flavored food substance. Thus the tone-associated rejection responses portrayed in Figure 4.2 were likely to be mediated by the tone's activation of perceptual processes normally evoked by the food itself.

A related experiment (Holland, 1989b) pitted the perceptual and response consequences of the evoked representations against each other. Rats first received pairings of tone 1 with sucrose (A) and tone 2 with salt (B). Both of these solutions evoked acceptance but not disgust responses; thus if consummatory responses were directly conditioned to the tones, they would be acceptance responses. Next, in the absence of the tones, the rats received pairings of a compound of A and B with toxin, but unpoisoned presentations of A and B separately. The rats learned this discrimination easily, so that they readily consumed either A and B when presented separately, but they rejected the AB compound. Finally, consumption of plain water was examined in the presence of tone 1, tone 2, and a compound of tone 1 and tone 2.

If the tones' effects on consumption were mediated by consummatory responses conditioned directly to the tones, then the compound of the two tones should evoke even greater acceptance than elicited by either tone alone. However, if the tones mediated performance by activating *perceptual* processing of the sugar and salt, then the tone 1 + tone 2 compound would activate a compound sugar + salt unit. Because in the second phase the rats had learned to reject the sugar + salt compound, they would accept *less* water and show more *rejection* responses during the compound than during either tone 1 or tone 2. This latter outcome was observed, indicating that the rats' performance was controlled more by the perceptual (flavor) features evoked by the tones than by any responses that may have been conditioned to those tones. (A companion experiment, in which in the second phase the AB compound was unpoisoned, but A and B were poisoned when presented separately, supported these conclusions: in the test, the tone 1 + tone 2 compound evoked fewer rejection responses but more acceptance responses than either tone 1 or tone 2 alone.)

Mediated Learning

Consider further the nature of the plasticity represented in the link labeled S–S in Figure 4.1. By virtue of this link, the CS acquires the ability to activate some of the upstream processing machinery of the US–UR system. How much? Is the CS's substitutability for the US limited to its response-evoking role, or does the CS-activated US-path activity bear closer resemblance to the activity produced by the US itself?

I have claimed that in some circumstances, activation of a US path or representation by a CS may not only influence the performance of learned responses, but also may permit new learning about that absent US. The basic observation I have elaborated on is that an aversion to a food substance may be acquired if a CS-activated representation of that food, rather than the food itself, is paired with toxin. For example, Holland (1981a, 1989b) paired one tone with a wintergreen-flavored food and another tone with a peppermint-flavored food. Then, in the absence of any of the foods, one of the *tones* was paired with a toxin. Consistent with the observations of Garcia and Koelling (1966), we found no evidence of the formation of associations between the *tone* and toxin, but associations apparently were formed between the absent *food* and toxin. Later tests of food consumption in the absence of the tones showed the establishment of an aversion to the food whose tone signal had been paired with toxin. That food provoked less consumption, less acceptance responding, and more disgust responses than the other food (Fig. 4.4). Apparently the occurrence of illness while the representation of one of the foods was activated by the tone was sufficient to establish an aversion to that food, even though the food was never paired with toxin or a substitute for toxin. In terms of Figure 4.3, activation of

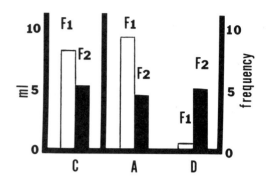

FIGURE 4.4. Responding in the consumption test of the mediated acquisition experiment (after Holland, 1989b). F_1 and F_2 were distinctive foods which had been signaled by two tones, T_1 and T_2, respectively. Before the consumption test, T_2 was paired with a toxin. The bars labeled C refer to consumption, those labeled A refer to the frequency of acceptance responses, and those labeled D refer to the frequency of disgust responses.

unit US2b by the CS allowed the establishment of the food 2–toxin link, just as if that unit had been activated by presentation of food 2 itself.

Similarly, Holland and Forbes (1982b) found that the *nonoccurrence* of illness in the presence of a CS-evoked representation of an avoided food produced partial extinction of the previously established aversion to that food. As in Holland's (1981a) experiment just described, two tones were first paired with two foods, presumably endowing each tone with the ability to activate the representation of its food partner. Each of the two foods next was paired with a toxin, to condition aversions to them. One of the tones then was presented in the absence of foods or toxin. Subsequent tests of consumption of the two foods showed a reduced aversion to the food whose tone partner had been presented in the absence of toxin in the previous phase. Apparently nonreinforcement of a CS-evoked representation of a food substance was sufficient to at least partially extinguish a previously trained aversion to that substance, just as nonreinforcement of that food itself would have done. (Note that a similar technique is often used in human antiphobic treatment: patients are taught to relax while imagining scenes assoicated with fear, with the hope that the replacement of fear by relaxation in the presence of imaginary surrogates of fearful situations will transfer to the real situations.)

Clearly, the activation of an event representation or pathway by an associate can do more than just mediate conditioned responding: the experiments just described show that both the establishment of new associations to an event and the extinction of old associations can occur in the absence of the event itself, if a previously established surrogate for that event is present during experimental manipulations. Other experiments from my laboratory have shown that evoked representations of events can substitute for those events in a variety of other condition functions. I mention three examples briefly.

Mediated Overshadowing
Typically, a stimulus, A, acquires less conditioned responding if it is reinforced in the presence of another cue (e.g., AX) than if it is reinforced alone. This interference by X of acquisition to A is pervasive (but see below) and has played an important role in the construction of recent conditioning theories (e.g., Mack-

intosh, 1975; Pearce & Hall, 1980; Rescorla & Wagner, 1972). A recent series of experiments (Holland, 1983b) showed that conditioning of a flavor aversion to a food substance can be overshadowed by a CS-evoked representation of another flavor. In three groups of rats, a tone was first endowed with the ability to evoke a representation of a flavor, X, by presenting several tone–X pairings. Then, in group A, another flavor, A, was paired with toxin; in group AX, a compound of the flavors A and X was paired with toxin, and in group AT+, a compound of the flavor A and the tone (which presumably evoked a representation of the flavor X) was paired with toxin. Finally, consumption of flavor A alone was examined. There was less aversion to A in the groups that received either the X + A compound (AX) or the tone + A compound (AT+) in conditioning. Thus conditioning of A was overshadowed by both the flavor X and its tone-evoked representation. Another comparison showed that the overshadowing in group AT+ was the consequence of the flavor representation evoked by the tone, not simply the presence of the tone: there was less aversion to A in group AT+ than in another group (AT−), which received tone + A paired with toxin in phase 2, but for which the tone did not activate a representation of flavor X, because it did not receive tone–X pairings in the first phase.

Mediated Potentiation

Although overshadowing is the typical outcome when a compound stimulus is reinforced, in some circumstances the opposite occurs. For example, although conditioning of an aversion to a *flavor* A is overshadowed when it is compounded with another flavor, X, conditioning to an *odor* A is *potentiated* when it is compounded with a flavor. That is, *more* conditioning of the A odor is observed if it is accompanied by a flavor in conditioning than if it is conditioned alone. Holland (1983b) duplicated the experiment just described, but substituted an odor A for the flavor A. In that experiment, presence of the flavor X in group AX *augmented* the aversion established to A rather than reducing it. More important, in group AT+, the aversion to the odor A was also potentiated by the presentation of the tone, which presumably evoked a representation of the flavor X. Thus, once again, the tone-evoked representation of a flavor substituted for the flavor itself: in circumstances in which the flavor X overshadowed conditioning to A, the evoked representation of X also overshadowed, but in circumstances where X potentiated conditioning to A, so did the evoked representation of X.

Mediated Occasion Setting

Finally, evoked representations of events can substitute for those events in modulating or setting the occasion for other associations, as will be described in a later section of this chapter. To anticipate a bit, cues presented in particular temporal and logical relations to other pairs of events can acquire a conditional control function that seems relatively independent of simple associative functions. Thus a cue's power to signal when a relation between two other cues is in effect is separable from its power to signal one or the other of those events.

Holland and Forbes (1982a) first endowed two visual cues with the ability to evoke representations of two flavored foods. Then the rats were trained to use those flavors to indicate when a tone would be followed by water: when a tone was preceded by one flavor, water was delivered, but when the tone was preceded by the other flavor, water was not delivered. In a final test, the tone was preceded by the visual cues but not the flavored foods. Performance to the tone after each visual cue mimicked the performance observed when the tone was preceded by the corresponding flavored foods. Thus the occasion-setting function of those flavored foods was also controlled by CS-evoked representations of those foods.

Limits on Event Representation

The previous discussion implies an interchangeability of evoked representations and their referents, in at least five functions: (1) evocation of CRs by CSs, (2) acquisition and extinction of new learning to cues, (3) interference with conditioning between other, coincident CSs and USs (overshadowing), (4) catalyzing the formation of associations between other CSs and USs (potentiation), and (5) setting the occasion for the action of other associations. But it seems unreasonable to assume that organisms do not distinguish between events and evoked representations of those events. In fact, most of my data suggest that evoked representations of events and the events themselves are not processed identically.

First, the effects produced by event surrogates are considerably smaller than those produced by the events themselves. Second, several experiments (e.g., Holland, 1981a, 1983b, 1989b) indicate that the stimulus that activates a representation is not affected by the activated representation. For example, Holland (1983b, 1989b) established an odor cue X as an evoker of a representation of a flavor cue F by presenting an FX compound. Later, a compound of odor X and another odor, Y, was paired with toxin. The aversion to Y was potentiated (relative to subjects for whom odor X had not been paired with the flavor), presumably by the flavor representation evoked by X. However, despite X's also being present during activation of the flavor representation, the aversion to X was not potentiated. In another experiment, although a flavor representation evoked by A overshadowed conditioning to another flavor, B, when an AB compound was reinforced, it did not overshadow conditioning to A. Finally, after A–X pairings, such that A evoked a representation of X, presentation of an A–B compound, under some circumstances, established B–X associations but extinguished the A–X associations (Holland, 1989b).

In all cases, presentation of X itself (rather than its evoked representation) coincident with the AB compound had similar effects on both A and B. Thus X and its evoked representation are not treated identically: the evoker of a representation is uniquely immune to modification by the representation. In some fashion, a CS's current activation of a US path apparently prevents further plasticity between those two paths at that time, except for whatever changes lead to extinction. Elsewhere (Holland, 1989b), I have described how this limitation may be diagnostic as to the nature of action of evoked representations.

Finally, despite the many instances of substitution of signals for their referents documented above, this substitution is by no means universal. The experiments described were carefully designed to demonstrate such effects, to assure activation of upstream portions of the US circuitry. Many variations in procedure can reduce the mediational effects I have described. Two variations are especially noteworthy. The first concerns the salience or associability of the evoked representation relative to that of events that are physically present. Typically, a real event, being more salient than an evoked representation of an absent event, is likely to overwhelm. My success at demonstrating a variety of mediational effects in the experiments described in this section is due in part to selection of a situation in which the real events (tones, lights, and odors) that evoke the flavor representations are themselves only poorly associable with the toxin, whereas the represented flavors are well associated (e.g., Garcia & Koelling, 1966). Elsewhere (Holland, 1985), I showed that several manipulations that increase the relative salience of other aspects of the training context (e.g., real events, response patterns) can eliminate evidence for mediational effects, even for the normally robust case of mediated performance of CRs. Apparently these manipulations encourage plastic convergence of CS and US pathways more downstream, that is, more S–R links.

Second, I have found that at least some of these mediational effects vanish if the original training designed to permit one stimulus to evoke a representation of another is prolonged (Holland, 1989b). For instance, with extended tone–food training, the tone loses the ability to substitute for that food in learning a food aversion if the tone is paired with a toxin. Although the response to the tone CS is maintained, the tone seems to lose its ability to activate a functionally effective representation of the food. This loss of plasticity with more experience has a variety of parallels in psychology (e.g., Allport, 1937; Kimble & Perlmuter, 1970) and neurobiology (e.g., Held & Hein, 1963), and implies functional differences between the effects of newly altered and extensively altered pathways. Quite simply, with repeated execution of the CS–UR complex, more downstream portions of the circuit become more highly tuned and come to predominate.

These outcomes suggest that plasticity may occur at many levels within a response system, depending on the precise nature of the conditioning experience, and the resultant behavior may have different characteristics and sensitivities to various manipulations, depending on the locus of plasticity. Although the mediational effects just described may not be a major determinant of behavior in all traditional conditioning paradigms, they have important implications for the mechanisms of conditioning and integration of behavior systems. At the very least, these mediational processes permit the integration of behavior systems that many have claimed are normally distinct, both functionally and anatomically (e.g., Garcia, Lasiter, Bermudez-Rattoni, & Deems, 1985).

MULTIPLE BEHAVIOR SYSTEMS IN PAVLOVIAN CONDITIONING

The experiments discussed in the previous section were concerned primarily with conditioned behaviors that were elicited by the US prior to conditioning. Perhaps because these behaviors are most consistent with the simplest "reflex transfer" accounts of Pavlovian conditioning, most psychological and neurobiological research has focused on them. But Pavlovian conditioning procedures usually engender more complex behavioral adaptations than a simple substitutive replica of the UR. Very early in the history of conditioning experiments it was noted that the CR often lacked obvious features of the UR; for instance, swallowing and jaw movements were typically not observed in canine salivary conditioning, although these behaviors form a prominent part of the UR (Zener, 1937). Conversely, frequently the CR included behaviors that were not part of the UR, for example, motor activity often accompanied signals for food even though that activity is typically not evoked by food delivery itself (e.g., Zener, 1937). And some CRs even involve behavior changes that seem opposite to those produced by the US. For example, although foot shock usually elicits a jump and heart rate acceleration, a signal for that shock generally evokes freezing and heart rate deceleration (e.g., DeToledo & Black, 1966; see Cohen, 1985). The occurrence of these so-called compensatory responses is especially prevalent when the US is the administration of toxic drugs. For instance, Siegel (1977) reports that although the rat's UR to morphine includes hyperthermia and hypoalgesia, the CR to signals for that US include hypothermia and hyperalgesia.

Deviations from perfect substitutability of CS and US may help illuminate conditioning mechanisms. Any "US" is likely to be a multifaceted event, generating various behaviors through many paths. The lack of some component of the UR in the CR might reflect a lack of plasticity in the circuitry involved in generating that particular response. Although that rigidity might be intrinsic to that path, it could well be that the conditioning parameters ideal for conditioning one component are not ideal for another component. For example, Kierylowicz, Soltysik, and Divac (1968) suggested that the absence of swallowing in many salivary conditioning experiments was not the consequence of a general nonplastic nature of that response, but an artifact of delivering food to a dish; swallowing was simply too temporally separated from the CS to be easily conditioned to it. They found that if food was instead delivered to the back of the mouth, robust swallowing responses occurred to the CS. Even CRs opposite to URs might be explained in this manner: many USs evoke both immediate primary responses and delayed compensatory responses that might be viewed as serving a homeostatic function (e.g., Eikelboom & Stewart, 1982). It would not be unreasonable to anticipate greater plasticity of the secondary response in some circumstances, particularly those in which anticipating and countering homeostatic disruptions confer adaptive advantage.

An especially striking influence on the nature of the behavior obtained in Pavlovian conditioning experiments is the nature of the conditioned stimulus. CS parameters such as modality, localization, duration, and CS–US interval have been reported to affect the form of a variety of conditioned responses. Although it is inconsistent with simple reflex transfer schemes and was initially regarded as a somewhat unusual outcome, I have claimed that CS determination of CR form is a basic and important feature of many conditioning paradigms (Holland, 1977, 1984).

The most systematically studied example of the influence of CSs on the form of the CR comes from my direct observations of rats' behavior anticipatory to food (summarized in Holland, 1984). Most of those experiments compared the responses evoked by various auditory and visual CSs paired with food delivery. Typically, localizable visual cues evoked first rearing on the hind legs and various attempts to contact the CS source followed by passive standing at the food magazine, but auditory cues evoked a startle response followed by short, rapid movements of the head (head jerk) and some passive standing at the food magazine.

Some of these responses, like magazine behavior, were never observed to occur during the CSs alone prior to conditioning. However, other behaviors, especially the rear and startle responses, were observed to occur to the CS prior to conditioning, although at relatively low levels. I call these behaviors "orienting responses" (ORs). If the CS was not paired with the US, then these orienting responses rapidly habituated. But if the CSs were paired with food, then the ORs increased in frequency. These increases were found to be the consequence of the Pavlovian CS–US relation, rather than the mere presentation of the US (sensitization) or operant response–reinforcer relations.

Consequently, I (Holland, 1977, 1984) distinguished between two broad classes of CR components, one determined by and appropriate to the US, and the other an enhancement of the response elicited by the CS prior to conditioning. Although both classes of response were found to be the consequence of the same Pavlovian CS–US relation, considerable evidence suggested they were often quite separable. First, the ORs occurred primarily early in the CS–US interval, and the UR-like CRs near the end. Second, if CS onset (which was the reliable generator of an OR) was made less relevant to delivery of the US than were later portions of the CS, by extending the CS–US interval or by intermixing short, nonreinforced CSs with longer, reinforced ones, the early, OR-like behaviors were substantially reduced in frequency. Third, changes in the nature of the CSs affected the nature of responding early in the CS intervals but had relatively little effect on late CS behavior, thought to be determined by the US. Conversely, changes in the nature of the unconditioned stimulus affected the nature of behavior late in the CS–US intervals but had little effect on responding during early portions of the CS, though to reflect an OR. Fourth, several experimental manipulations, such as varying US magnitude or probability (Fig. 4.5), the imposition of omission contingencies, the use of partial reinforcement contingencies, and the postconditioning devaluation of the reinforcer (to be discussed in detail later) differentially affected the putative CS- and US-generated behaviors.

The scheme outlined in Figures 4.1 and 4.3 concerned only US-based behav-

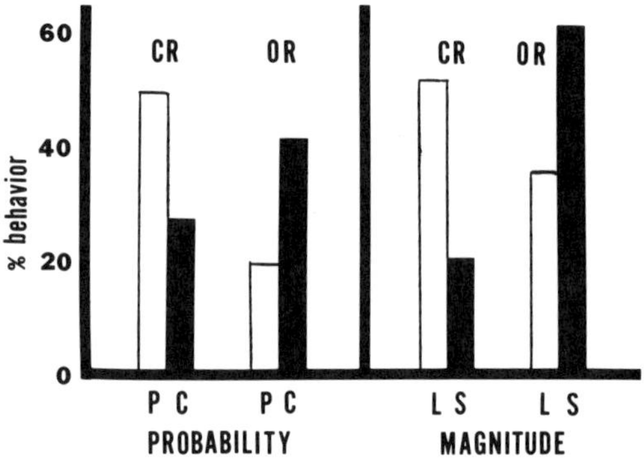

FIGURE 4.5. Effects of varying the probability (left panel) and magnitude (right panel) of reinforcement on CRs and conditioned ORs. P = partial reinforcement; C = consistent reinforcement; L = large; S = small.

iors, that is, changes that permitted the CS to engage some aspects of the US–UR machinery. The recognition of an independent CS-generated component to the CR demands an addition to those schemes. That addition distinguishes the US's role in providing the machinery for response production from its role in potentiating links: for the US-generated behavior class, the US both potentiates the link (between CS and US path) and provides the machinery for response production. But for the CS-generated behavior class, the US serves only as a potentiator for responding that is determined by another pathway. The simplest possibility would be to imagine that contiguity of CS and US potentiates some level(s) of the CS–OR path (Fig. 4.6, heavy arrow); this possibility makes obvious the independence of OR and UR components of the CR.

A more reasonable possibility is that the potentiation of the OR is mediated

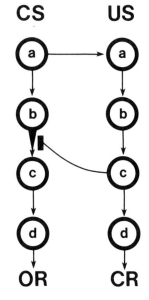

FIGURE 4.6. Representation of associations between CS and US pathways that could underlie the acquisition of CRs and conditioned ORs. The symbols are explained in the text.

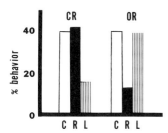

FIGURE 4.7. The frequency of CRs and conditioned ORs during the tone conditioned stimulus, after its food associated was paired with lithium chloride (bars labeled L), rotation (R), or neither event (C). (After Holland and Straub, 1979)

by activity in the US path (the modulatory link in Fig. 4.6). That is, potentiation of the CS–OR path is conditional on activity of both CS and the unit USb. Thus changes in the activation of unit USb would affect not only US-path behaviors, but also CS–OR behaviors. I suggest this latter path because the bulk of our evidence indicates that the performance of OR behaviors is also mediated in this fashion: postconditioning devaluation of the US either by pairing it with rotation (Holland & Straub, 1979; Fig. 4.7) or by satiation on that particular foodstuff (Holland, 1981b) lowered the probability of those responses as well as US-generated ones.

Holland and Straub (1979) noted that devaluation of the US by pairing it with one toxin, lithium chloride, eliminated US-based behaviors but left CS-determined behaviors unscathed (see Fig. 4.7). This outcome suggests that devaluation by food–LiCl pairing either modulated activity of the US pathway at some point after that pathway potentiates CS-path activity (shown in Fig. 4.8) or affected a parallel pathway that mediates the UR-like CR component but does

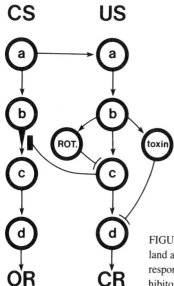

FIGURE 4.8. Representation of associations established in Holland and Straub's (1979) experiment. OR = conditioned orienting response; ROT = rotation; ——▶ = excitatory action; ——(= inhibitory action; ——■ = facilitory action.

not potentiate CS–OR relations. It further points out that whether a given site of plasticity is labeled S–R or S–S by the psychologist depends on the methods and responses used to assess mediation: with OR-like CRs, tone–food plasticity at site USa would be labeled S–S if food was devalued by association with rotation but S–R if food was devalued by pairings with toxin.

Other evidence also supports the view that different CRs evoked by various CSs nonetheless have a common mediator within the US pathway. Briefly, the data show that despite their different CRs, these CSs are functionally interchangeable in conditioning experiments. For example, Holland (1977) found that pretraining a CS that evoked one response enabled that CS to block conditioning of a very different response to another CS when the pretrained and new CSs were reinforced in compound. Because considerable data suggest that the pretrained stimulus blocks conditioning involving only the US with which it was pretrained, the occurrence of blocking despite different CRs suggests the various CSs are associated with a common US. Similarly, the power of a CS to serve as a reinforcer for second-order conditioning to another cue seems unrelated to the precise response that it evokes: Holland (1977) noted similar forms of responding to an auditory cue, whether it was paired with another auditory cue that evoked the same conditioned behaviors or with a visual CS that evoked entirely different behaviors. Furthermore, the reinforcing powers of two CSs sum when those CSs are combined, regardless of whether the CRs they evoke are similar or dissimilar. Thus considerable commonality of learning must exist, despite the different CRs.

Specificity of CS- and US-Path Changes

The plasticities described in the last two sections have all been specific to a CS–US pair. That is, conditioning operations were said to potentiate particular links between a CS and a US path, the associations of the learning theorist. The changes were not general enhancements or inhibitions of CS or US pathway activity. For example, the enhanced orienting response to a visual stimulus paired with food depends on specific learning: it is not enough that the US path be activated (say, by another cue that had been previously paired with food) while a stimulus is presented (Holland, 1977, 1981b).

Most modern learning theorists claim that conditioning operations also may modulate the effectiveness of a CS and/or US pathway in general. For example, many hypothesize that conditioning operations modulate processing of the CS in some way, such as enhancing attention to it. This enhanced attention to the CS might be described as a potentiation of one or more links within the CS path, which in turn could serve to enhance the OR (alpha-conditioning), as well as any responses it controls by virtue of links with the US path. This modulation in attention to the CS, while perhaps established concomitantly with CS–US associations, is independent of that link (much like the heavy arrow in Fig. 4.6). Consequently, action of that CS is modulated, regardless of changes in the US.

For example, that CS might be more effective as a CS even if it were retrained with another US.

Other theorists (e.g., Rescorla & Wagner, 1972; Wagner, 1981) have suggested that conditioning operations modulate activity of the US path in general, as well as establishing particular associations. For example, a frequent claim is that "expected" USs are less effective than surprising ones, in terms of their reinforcing power, response-generating capacity, and endurance in memory. In terms of the pathway jargon, if the US pathway is already active, by virtue either of immediately prior presentation of that US or by presentation of a CS that is capable of activating that path because of past associations, then presentation of that US will have less effect than if that path was not already active (Wagner, 1981). Thus a US that is anticipated because it was preceded by a previously paired CS is unlikely to be an effective reinforcer for any cue that may occur contiguously. This phenomenon, called blocking (Kamin, 1968), has been demonstrated hundreds of times, even in simple systems.

Another example of hypothesized modulation of the US path comes from the study of conditioned inhibition. Consider a procedure in which a CS, A, is paired with the US, and a compound of A and another stimulus, B, is nonreinforced. Rats rapidly learn the discrimination, responding on A alone trials and not on AB trials. Rescorla and Holland (1977) suggested that B acquired the power to inhibit the action of the US path. If so, then B should inhibit the CR to any CS whose responding was mediated by that US path, but not the CR to CSs whose responding was mediated by some other US. Rescorla and Holland found those outcomes.

Other Behavior Systems

I have emphasized distinctions between CS and US path behaviors, mainly because I have investigated them extensively behaviorally and because they seem amenable to the type of analysis I propose here. It should be recognized that this dichotomy is just the tip of the iceberg. Historically, different classes of conditioned behavior (e.g., emotional vs. skeletal) have been posited as having separate conditioning loci (e.g., Rescorla & Solomon, 1967; Thompson, 1986). In addition, it seems likely that the circuits of the US paths are well integrated, so that the use of any particular US will engender not only the precise response evoked by that particular event, but also a more complex set of naturally occurring behavior patterns appropriate to that US.

For instance, feeding is a complex activity containing many separate, sequentially organized action patterns such as individual foraging, social approach and food sharing, investigation, predation, food handling, hoarding, and ingestion or rejection. Conditioning may occur at many levels and points within a behavior system; the precise conditioned behaviors observed might depend on the nature of the cues used and their resemblance to cues naturally used in the feeding situation. In the language of Tolman (1932), the CR is more appropriate to the *expectancy* of food engendered by the CS than to food per se. For example, the use of short CSs would be likely to encourage behavior appropriate to imminent food, such as mouthing and search of the food cup, but longer CSs would encourage more early chain behaviors, like searching. Those CSs, by virtue of their timing, tap into different portions of natural feeding sequences. The form of the CR would be further filtered and tuned by other features of the cues. For example, the use of static cues like tones and lights might encourage investigation and consummatory responses, but using small moving objects as CSs might encourage predatory activity, and use of conspecifics as cues might lead to social food-sharing activities. Experiments conducted in my laboratory (Holland, 1984) and, more extensively, by Timberlake (1983) support these claims. In essence, Pavlovian conditioning often acts as a mechanism of modulating naturally organized behavior patterns.

Of course at this point I have left far behind the plausibility of neurobiological analysis. But more feasible investigations of simpler interacting systems, for example CS- and US-generated behaviors, may provide a reasonable prototype of the more complex interactions that comprise adaptive behavior.

HIGHER ORDER UNITS

In the previous sections I have discussed very simple conditioning arrangements, which usually involved only one CS and one US. In contrast, most theoretical and empirical investigation of Pavlovian conditioning has concerned compound CSs (e.g., AB). Nevertheless, most of that work focused on associations between each individual event and the US, or more recently (e.g., Rescorla, 1985a), on associations between the elements (A and B). This work thus concerns the same event–event relations I discussed earlier.

Interest has been growing in other potential conditioning functions that might be involved when compound cues are used, especially in solving conditional discriminations in which the meaning of one cue depends on the value of another cue. In this section I briefly discuss two such functions, occasion setting and configuring. They are of special interest to the topic of this book because they are directly related to some of the more articulate memory distinctions in animal learning.

Occasion Setting

One of the simpler conditional discriminations is the feature positive discrimination, in which a compound stimulus (XA) is reinforced, but one of its elements (A) is separately nonreinforced. If X and A are presented simultaneously on compound trials, X comes to evoke a CR based on its association with the US, and A controls little or no responding. However, if the onset of X precedes that of A, X acquires the ability to modulate the action of an association that is formed between A and the US. Thus X "sets the occasion" for responding to A (Holland, 1983a). After serial training, X gates or enables the A–US link, permitting A to activate the US path, whereas after simultaneous training, X directly activates the US path and A does not.

The results of several kinds of experiments support this distinction. First, Ross and Holland (1981) found that the form of the CR differed in serial (S → A$^+$, A$^-$) and simultaneous (XA$^+$, A$^-$) feature positive discriminations. With simultaneous compounds, the form of the CR was determined by X, as would be anticipated if the CR were the consequence of X–US associations. But with serial compounds, A determined the nature of the CR, consistent with the view that X acted by modulating the effectiveness of an A–US association.

Second, several manipulations differentially affect the acquisition and extinction of these occasion-setting and simple associative functions. For example, increasing the interval or inserting a stimulus-free trace between X and the US reduces the strength of X's association with the US but (up to a point) increases its ability to set the occasion for responding based on the A–US association (Holland, 1986a; Ross & Holland, 1981). Similarly, Ross (1983) and Ross and LoLordo (1986) found that A → US pairings prior to feature-positive discrimination training blocked the acquisition of X–US associations but not X's ability to modulate responding based on A–US associations. Similarly, Ross (1983) found that enhancing X–US associations by prior X–US training interfered with X's acquisition of occasion setting (see Rescorla, 1986b). Finally, nonreinforced presentations of X alone quickly abolish its ability to elicit CRs by virtue of its simple association with the US (or A) but have relatively little effect on X's ability to set the occasion for responding to A (Rescorla, 1986a).

Third, cues trained in serial and simultaneous discriminations acquire different properties. For instance, Ross and LoLordo (1987) found that an X that was previously trained in a serial discrimination blocked the acquisition of operant stimulus control to another cue when a compound of that cue and X were trained as a discriminative stimulus, but an X trained in a simultaneous discrimination had no such blocking effect. Finally, Holland (1986b) found that whereas the simple associative powers of an X trained in a simultaneous discrimination were manifest regardless of whether it was accompanied by the original A cue or some other cue, the occasion-setting powers of an X trained in a serial discrimination were greatly diminished if X was combined with cues other than A.

These observations, together with analogous ones from feature-*negative* discriminations, in which an XA compound is nonreinforced while A is separately reinforced, suggest that simple associative and occasion-setting functions are quite dissociable. Interestingly, these functions may be anatomically distinct as well. Ross, Orr, Holland, and Berger (1984) trained rats on serial-feature positive discriminations of the form light → trace → tone → food; tone → no food, which endowed the light with the ability to set the occasion for responding to the tone and with the ability to evoke CRs based on direct light–US associations and on within-compound light–tone associations. Additionally, the same rats received training on a nonconditional discrimination between a reinforced clicker and a nonreinforced noise.

Rats that received bilateral hippocampectomy prior to training were unable to acquire the serial feature-positive discrimination (occasion setting), and rats that were trained intact and then hippocampectomized lost the ability to perform that discrimination (Fig. 4.9). Conversely, relative to unoperated controls, hippocampectomy completely spared learning and performance of CRs based on the light–food association and on the clicker–noise discrimination, and it had no more deleterious effect on CRs based on the light–tone association than had lesions of the neocortex overlaying hippocampus (which was also destroyed in hippocampectomized rats). Thus the behavioral–functional independence of simple associative and occasion-setting powers of CSs was complemented by a degree of anatomical independence.

The nature of the behavioral deficit observed in these experiments deserves further attention. First, it was not due to a simple short-term memory deficit—an inability to learn across a trace interval—because both the light–food and light–tone learning, which required bridging the same trace interval, were unaffected. Second, the occasion-setting deficit cannot be attributed merely to its being a more difficult task, because there was little difference in the performance levels of the conditional (serial feature positive) and nonconditional discriminations. Furthermore, Orr and I (unpublished) subsequently found that hippocampectomy had no effect on the acquisition of a difficult nonconditional discrimination (between two tones of similar pitches) but prevented the acquisition of a much easier (for unoperated controls) conditional discrimination.

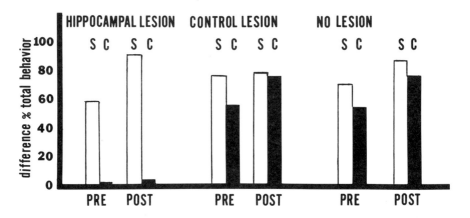

FIGURE 4.9.   Effects of hippocampal lesions on performance in conditional (closed bars, labeled C) or simple (open bars, labeled S) discriminations. The bars labeled PRE refer to performance during the last 12 training sessions when the lesions were made prior to training, and those labeled POST refer to performance during the last 12 retraining sessions when the lesions were made after training.

Finally, hippocampectomy had relatively little impact on performance during the serial light → trace → tone compound: the rats acquired the CRs appropriate to that compound in a practically normal fashion. The deficit came in their being unable to withhold responding during the nonreinforced tone-alone presentations. Note, however, that there was no global deficit in inhibition: the rats' ability to withhold responding to the nonreinforced cue in the nonconditional discrimination was unimpaired. This data pattern implies that hippocampal systems do not involve only processing of the compound, for example, forming of a higher order light + tone configuration. If these systems involved only processing of the compound, then hippocampectomy after training would have been expected to abolish responding to the compound.

Our findings are compatible with a variety of theoretical languages that have been used to describe hippocampal memory function (see Ross et al., 1984). Common to most of these languages is the notion that the simple pairings of CSs and USs engage a nonhippocampal memory system that stores only information about the strength of that association, but that certain more complex problems engage a hippocampal memory system that makes use of some other kind of information or process. One possibility that appeals to me is that hippocampus acts as a selector (e.g., Teyler & DiScenna, 1985) which disambiguates cues that have multiple histories. That is, the tone may have been represented as both reinforced and nonreinforced, and the light served to select the reinforced path. Supporting this claim is recent evidence (Holland, 1986b; Lamarre & Holland, 1987; Rescorla, 1985b) that shows particular sorts of ambiguity in the treatment of the target (tone in the previous example) to be critical to the occurrence of occasion setting, as opposed to simple association.

This view of hippocampus as modulator or selector is a very Jacksonian one: the main purpose of higher (or at least synaptically distant) structures like hippocampus is to improve the precision of processes that can be performed elsewhere. It implies that the memory for the conditional discrimination, despite requiring intact hippocampal circuitry to be acquired or displayed, is probably not really localized there. Although hippocampal systems may enable formation of separate representations for reinforced and nonreinforced trials, which may or may not importantly involve hippocampal circuitry itself, essential memory processing goes on in other portions of the perceptual–motor paths, as always.

Configurations

The simplest strategy for solving the feature-positive discriminations just described (XA$^+$, A$^-$) is to associate X and the US. A more complex strategy is to use X to signal when A is reinforced, which I called occasion setting (above). In a sense, the occasion-setting strategy for solving those discriminations involves the construction of an A–US unit, which in turn is signaled or selected by another cue, X. A third way to solve the problem is to treat the compound as a single unit or configuration, light + tone, which is discriminated from the tone alone. Considerable evidence suggests that rats use the first strategy when

X and A are presented simultaneously but use the second when X precedes A on compound trials. There is no evidence that rats ever use the configurational strategy to solve this problem.

However, consider a discrimination in which an XA compound is reinforced, but neither X nor A alone is reinforced. This positive-patterning discrimination cannot be mastered with the simple associative strategy. If X precedes A on compound trials, rats use the occasion-setting strategy described earlier and find the task no more difficult than the feature-positive discrimination (Holland, 1989a). But if X and A are presented simultaneously, the positive-patterning discrimination is far more difficult than the feature-positive discrimination. Considerable evidence indicates that to solve the former discrimination, rats associate a light + tone configuration with the US (Holland & Block, 1983; Rescorla, 1972). Although the rats may simply attend to a weak feature unique to that compound (Rescorla, 1972), it is tempting to suggest that they may actively form a higher order XA unit or superfeature, which is then associated with the US (Razran, 1971). Either way, this strategy is quite different from the occasion-setting strategy in that no special "selector" function seems to accrue to the cues involved. Furthermore, I (Holland, 1989a) have found that several manipulations that make the solution of simultaneous patterned discriminations easier (and by implication, encourage configuring), such as increasing X–A similarity, make the solution of serial patterned discriminations more difficult (and hence discourage occasion setting).

Studies of configurating in learning and memory (Lamb & Riley, 1981) share much with the study of perception. My guess is that the sort of higher level unit formed in the experiments just described is perceptual in nature, an elaboration of early path activity, whereas the unit formed in the occasion-setting experiments is an elaboration of later stream activity. Thus, although the serial and simultaneous positive patterning discriminations are logically equivalent conditional discriminations, I would anticipate important hippocampal involvement in solving the former, but not the latter.

CONCLUSIONS

What do these data have to do with "forms of memory"? It could be argued that they distinguish at least three pairs of subsystems. In the first section I distinguished between S–S and S–R links, which some psychologists (e.g., Dickinson, 1980) have characterized as declarative ("knowing what") and procedural ("knowing how"). Then I contrasted CS–OR and CS–UR paths to conditioned behavior, and finally I distinguished simple associative and occasion-setting functions.

In each case I showed considerable evidence for the independence of subsystems. That evidence was in the form of functional dissociations of the performance indicators of those memory skills. Several variables affected performance based on S–S but not behavior based on S–R links, enhanced CS–OR responding but reduced CS–UR responding, or vice-versa, or differentially affected simple associative and occasion-setting functions of CSs. Just these types of dissociations have led others to propose the existence of multiple independent memory systems.

However, not everyone agrees that such data patterns demand major memory system distinctions. For example, Roediger (1984) argued for the insufficiency of dissociation outcomes in inferring independent memory systems by claiming that some task demands may enourage the use of one subset of processes (say, A and B) from a memory system, whereas another task may demand the use of a different subset of processes (say, B and C) from the same memory system. But should this be viewed as a single memory system, two separate systems that share a subsystem, or three separate systems that occasionally work together, depending on the demands of the moment? To a large extent, the adequacy of any methodology in inferring multiple memory systems depends on how "memory systems" are viewed.

Tulving (1985) argued that *stochastic* rather than *functional* independence of two memory task measures provides better evidence for independence of two memory systems. Briefly, if a given memory task engages two completely separate memory systems, then the product (measure) of one system should be uncorrelated with that of the other. Thus if one views recall and recognition as involving separate memory systems, then the probability of recalling an item that was recognized should be identical to the probability of recalling an item that was not recognized. Statistically, the probability that an item is both recognized and recalled should be equal to the product of the overall probabilities of recall and recognition. There is no necessary logical connection between stochastic and functional independence; Tulving (1985) described how it is perfectly possible to find one with no evidence of the other.

Although stochastic independence may be sufficient to infer separate forms of memory, it is probably misleading to consider it necessary. First, consider the problem of measurement. Imagine two memory systems that follow completely different rules, respond to every manipulation in opposite ways, and are localized in completely different parts of the nervous system. The output of memory system 1 is the performance of behavior 1 and the output of system 2 is behavior 2. If a given task taps both systems, then we will find stochastic *dependence* in our memory task to the extent that behaviors 1 and 2 compete at the output level. Although the 2 *measures* are dependent, it may be unreasonable to claim that the *memories* are. Second, is it reasonable to demand, as did Roediger (1984), that two memory systems share *no* common path or process in order to describe them as "separate systems"? One could just as easily claim that one system is separate from another if at least one path or process is unique to one of them. The more practical truth must lie somewhere between these extremes.

Again, the problem reduces to disagreement about what is meant by a memory system. One resort is to turn the tables on the psychologist and define them in terms of neural processes or localization. Even psychologists often take this approach (e.g., Sherry & Schacter, 1987). But this cannot be the only answer. To the psychologist who is interested in how memory works, the knowledge of neural localization is not particularly valuable, unless systems in different loci follow different rules and systems with similar loci follow similar rules. That would be convenient, but it is not logically necessary. Moreover, at our current level of localizing memory function, there is no reason why several different processes cannot occur at the same locus. We are comfortable distinguishing unit plasticity that is the consequence of intrinsic presynaptic or postsynaptic changes, or changes in a modulator, which then act on that unit presynaptically or postsynaptically. It may not be absurd to think that these various types of plasticity at more or less the same locus might underlie different memory functions (e.g., Hawkins & Kandel, 1984).

Fortunately, there may be a way out. Evolution tends to be conservative. Once a "memory system" emerges as a solution to a problem of adaptation, it is likely to come to serve other functions and solve other problems, too—even if that system might not be the best imaginable solution to any of the other problems. Memory may reflect a sort of adaptive compromise among the needs of a variety of behavioral systems that require plasticity with experience. Only when that compromise is incompatible with a major demand of some behavioral system is a new memory system likely to evolve. Sherry and Schacter (1987) have described many popular memory system distinctions in terms of their functional incompatibility, suggesting that separate learning systems are most profitably sought by considering the purposes served by those systems. Perhaps we should follow evolution's lead and be conservative in postulating separate memory systems.

REFERENCES

Allport, G. W. (1937). *Personality: A psychological interpretation.* New York: Holt.

Cohen, D. H. (1985). Some organizational principles of a vertebrate conditioning pathway: Is memory a distributed property? In N. M. Weinberger, J. L. McGaugh, & G. Lynch, (Eds.), *Memory systems of the brain* (pp. 27–48). New York: Guilford.

DeToldeo, L., & Blach, A. H. (1966). Heart rate: Changes during conditioned suppression in rats. *Science, 152,* 1404–1406.

Dickinson, A. (1980). *Contemporary animal learning theory.* Cambridge: Cambridge University Press.

Eikelboom, R., & Stewart, J. (1982). Conditioning of drug-induced physiological responses. *Psychological Review, 89,* 507–528.

Garcia, J., & Koelling, R. A. (1966). Relation of cue to consequence in avoidance learning. *Psychonomic Science, 4,* 123–124.

Garcia, J., Kovner, R., & Green, K. S. (1970). Cue properties versus palatability of flavors in avoidance learning. *Psychonomic Science, 20,* 313–314.

Garcia, J., Lasiter, P. S., Bermudez-Rattoni, F., & Deems, D. A. (1985). A general theory of aversion learning. *Annals of the New York Academy of Sciences, 443,* 8–21.

Grill, H. J., & Norgren, R. (1978). The taste reactivity test: I. Mimetic responses to gustatory stimuli in neurologically normal rats. *Brain Research, 143,* 263–279.

Hawkins, R. D., & Kandel, E. R. (1984). Is there a cell-biologist alphabet for simple forms of learning? *Psychological Review, 91,* 375–391.

Held, R., & Hein, A. (1963). Movement-produced stimulation in the development of visually-guided behavior. *Journal of Comparative and Physiological Psychology, 56,* 872–876.

Holland, P. C. (1977). Conditioned stimulus as a determinant of the form of the Pavlovian conditioned response. *Journal of Experimental Psychology: Animal Behavior Processes, 3,* 77–104.

Holland, P. C. (1981a). Acquisition of representation-mediated conditioned food aversions. *Learning and Motivation, 12,* 1–18.

Holland, P. C. (1981b). The effects of satiation after first- and second-order appetitive conditioning. *Pavlovian Journal of Biological Science, 16,* 18–24.

Holland, P. C. (1983a). Occasion-setting in Pavlovian feature positive discriminations. In M. L. Commons, R. J. Herrnstein, & A. R. Wagner (Eds.), *Quantitative analyses of behavior: Discrimination processes* (Vol. 4, pp. 183–206). New York: Ballinger.

Holland, P. C. (1983b). Representation-mediated overshadowing and potentiation of conditioned aversions. *Journal of Experimental Psychology: Animal Behavior Processes, 9,* 1–13.

Holland, P. C. (1984). The origins of Pavlovian conditioned behavior. In G. Bower (Ed.), *The psychology of learning and motivation* (Vol. 18, pp. 129–173). Englewood Cliffs, N.J.: Prentice-Hall.

Holland, P. C. (1985). Element pretraining influences the content of appetitive serial compound conditioning in rats. *Journal of Experimental Psychology: Animal Behavior Processes, 11,* 367–387.

Holland, P. C. (1986a). Temporal determinants of occasion setting in feature positive discriminations. *Animal Learning and Behavior, 14,* 111–120.

Holland, P. C. (1986b). Transfer after serial feature positive discrimination training. *Learning and Motivation, 17,* 243–268.

Holland, P. C. (1989a). Acquisition and transfer of conditional discrimination performance. *Journal of Experimental Psychology: Animal Behavior Processes, 15,* 154–165.

Holland, P. C. (1989b). *Event representation in Pavlovian conditioning: Image and action.* Manuscript submitted for publication.

Holland, P. C., & Block, H. (1983). Evidence for a unique cue in positive patterning. *Bulletin of the Psychonomic Society, 21,* 297–300.

Holland, P. C., & Forbes, D. T. (1982a). Control of conditional discrimination performance by CS-evoked event representations. *Animal Learning and Behavior, 10,* 249–256.

Holland, P. C., & Forbes, D. T. (1982b). Representation-mediated extinction of flavor aversions. *Learning and Motivation, 13,* 454–471.

Holland, P. C., & Straub, J. J. (1979). Differential effects of two ways of devaluing the unconditioned stimulus after Pavlovian appetitive conditioning. *Journal of Experimental Psychology: Animal Behavior Processes, 5,* 65–78.

Kamin, L. J. (1968). Attention-like processes in classical conditioning. In M. R. Jones (Ed.), *Miami symposium on the prediction of behavior: Aversive stimulation* (pp. 9–32). Coral Gables, Fla.: University of Miami Press.

Kierylowicz, H., Soltysik, S., & Divac, I. (1968). Conditioned reflexes reinforced by direct and indirect food presentation. *Acta Biologica Experimentalis, 28,* 1–10.

Kimble, G. A., & Perlmuter, L. C. (1970). The problem of volition. *Psychological Review, 77,* 361–384.

Lamarre, J., & Holland, P. C. (1987). Acquisition and transfer of serial feature negative discriminations. *Learning and Motivation. 18,* 319–342.

Lamb, M. R., & Riley, D. A. (1981). Effects of element arrangement on the processing of compound stimuli in pigeons *(Columba livia). Journal of Experimental Psychology: Animal Behavior Processes, 7,* 45–58.

Mackintosh, N. J. (1975). A theory of attention: Variations in the associability of stimuli with reinforcement. *Psychological Review, 82,* 276–298.

Pearce, J. M., & Hall, G. (1980). A model for Pavlovian learning: Variations in the effectiveness of conditioned but not of unconditioned stimuli. *Psychological Review, 106,* 532–552.

Pelchat, M., Grill, H. J., Rozin, P., & Jacobs, J. (1983). Quality of acquired responses to tastes by *rattus norvegicus* depends on type of associated discomfort. *Comparative Psychology and Behavior, 97,* 140–153.

Razran, G. H. S. (1971). *Mind in evolution.* Boston: Houghton Mifflin.

Rescorla, R. A. (1972). "Configural" conditioning in discrete-trial bar pressing. *Journal of Comparative and Physiological Psychology, 79,* 307–317.

Rescorla, R. A. (1974). A model of Pavlovian conditioning. In V. S. Rusinov (Ed.), *Mechanisms of formation and inhibition of conditional reflex* (pp. 25–39). Moscow: Academy of Sciences of the USSR.

Rescorla, R. A. (1985a). Associative learning: Some consequences of contiguity. In N. M. Weinberger, J. L. McGaugh, & G. Lynch (Eds.), *Memory systems of the brain* (pp. 211–230). New York: Guilford.

Rescorla, R. A. (1985b). Inhibition and facilitation. In R. R. Miller & N. E. Spear (Eds.), *Information processing in animals: Conditioned inhibition* (pp. 299–326). Hillsdale, N.J.: Erlbaum.

Rescorla, R. A. (1986a). Extinction of facilitation. *Journal of Experimental Psychology: Animal Behavior Processes, 12,* 16–24.

Rescorla, R. A. (1986b). Facilitation and excitation. *Journal of Experimental Psychology: Animal Behavior Processes, 12,* 325–332.

Rescorla, R. A., & Holland, P. C. (1977). Associations in Pavlovian conditioned inhibition. *Learning and Motivation, 8,* 429–447.

Rescorla, R. A., & Solomon, R. L. (1967). Two process learning theory: Relationships between classical conditioning and instrumental learning. *Psychological Review, 74,* 151–182.

Rescorla, R. A., & Wagner, A. R. (1972). A theory of Pavlovian conditioning: Variations in the effectiveness of reinforcement and nonreinforcement. In A. H. Black & W. F. Prokasy (Eds.), *Classical conditioning* (Vol. 2, pp. 64–99). New York: Appleton-Century-Crofts.

Riley, A. L., Jacobs, W. J., & LoLordo, V. M. (1976). Drug exposure and the acquisition and retention of a taste aversion. *Journal of Comparative and Physiological Psychology, 90,* 799–807.

Roediger, H. L. III (1984). Does current evidence from dissociation experiments favor the episodic/semantic distinction? *Behavioral and Brain Sciences, 7,* 252–254.

Ross, R. T. (1983). Relationships between the determinants of performance in serial feature positive discriminations. *Journal of Experimental Psychology: Animal Behavior Processes, 9,* 349–373.

Ross, R. T., & Holland, P. C. (1981). Conditioning of simultaneous and serial feature-positive discriminations. *Animal Learning and Behavior, 9,* 293–303.

Ross, R. T., & LoLordo, V. M. (1986). Blocking during serial feature-positive discriminations: Associative versus occasion setting functions. *Journal of Experimental Psychology: Animal Behavior Processes, 12,* 315–324.

Ross, R. T., & LoLordo, V. M. (1987). Evaluation of the relation between Pavlovian occasion setting and instrumental discriminative stimuli: A blocking analysis. *Journal of Experimental Psychology: Animal Behavior Processes, 13,* 3–16.

Ross, R. T., Orr, W. B., Holland, P. C., & Berger, T. W. (1984). Hippocampectomy disrupts acquisition and retention of learned conditional responding. *Behavioral Neuroscience, 98,* 211–225.

Sherry, D. F., & Schacter, D. L. (1987). The evolution of multiple memory systems. *Psychological Review, 94,* 439–454.

Siegel, S. (1977). Morphine tolerance acquisition as an associative process. *Journal of Experimental Psychology: Animal Behavior Processes, 3,* 1–13.

Teyler, T. J., & DiScenna, P. (1985). The role of hippocampus in memory: A hypothesis. *Neuroscience and Biobehavioral Reviews, 9,* 377–389.

Thompson, R. F. (1986). The neurobiology of learning and memory. *Science, 233,* 941–947.

Timberlake, W. (1983). The functional organization of appetitive behavior: Behavior systems and learning. In M. D. Zeiler & P. Harzem (Eds.), *Advances in the analysis of behavior: Vol. 3. Biological factors in learning* (pp. 177–221). Chichester: Wiley.

Tolman, E. C. (1932). *Purposive behavior in animals and men.* New York: Appleton-Century.

Tulving, E. (1985). How many memory systems are there? *American Psychologist, 40,* 385–398.

Wagner, A. R. (1981). SOP: A model of automatic memory processing in animal behavior. In N. E. Spear & R. R. Miller (Eds.), *Information processing in animals: Memory mechanisms* (pp. 5–47). Hillsdale, N.J.: Erlbaum.

Zellner, D. A., Berridge, K. C., Grill, H. J., & Ternes, J. W. (1985). Rats learn to like the taste of morphine. *Behavioral Neuroscience, 99,* 290–300.

Zener, K. (1937). The significance of behavior accompanying conditioned salivary secretion for theories of the conditioned response. *American Journal of Psychology, 50,* 384–403.

5

Functional Forms of Human Memory

MARCIA K. JOHNSON

Several recent theories of memory can be classed as "functional subsystems" approaches. They share the ideas that human memory is composed of distinguishable subsystems that serve different behavioral and cognitive functions, operate according to different laws, and are represented by different neural structures or mechanisms. These subsystems may develop at different rates from infancy to adulthood, and they may be differentially susceptible to disruption from alcohol and other drugs, aging, disease, or injury (e.g., Cohen, 1984; Johnson, 1983; Squire, 1982; Tulving, 1983; Warrington & Weiskrantz, 1982).

Although the field is still struggling to characterize these subsystems, progress does not depend on consensus; many schemes have been proposed that have generated valuable ideas and research. I haven't space here to discuss various viewpoints in detail, but one way they differ is in the aspects of the meaning of "function" they seem to emphasize by the way subsystems are labeled. Terms such as episodic versus semantic memory (Cermak, 1984; Schacter & Tulving, 1982; Tulving, 1983), procedural versus declarative memory (Cohen & Squire, 1980), and memories versus habits (Mishkin, Malamut, & Bachevalier, 1984) emphasize the purpose/result/consequence meaning of function. Terms such as horizontal versus vertical processes (Wickelgren, 1979), mediated versus stimulus–response learning (Warrington & Weiskrantz, 1982), and sensory versus perceptual versus reflective subsystems (Johnson, 1983) emphasize the activity/process meaning of function. Of course, most investigators who have tackled the problem of defining subsystems have considered both aspects of function—purpose and process—to some degree, but the terms we use reflect certain tacit assumptions, I think.

In any event, one major goal of a psychological analysis of memory is to account for memory in terms of purposes such as skill learning, autobiographical recall, generalization of concepts, and learned emotional reactions. It seems unlikely, however, that the processes that serve these goals are uniquely dedicated to particular purposes of this sort. For example, some of the same types of memory processes might, under some circumstances, contribute to skill learning, autobiographical recall, generalization of concepts, and learned emotional reactions. In fact, as processes were added (and/or modified) during evolution, purposes probably multiplied. Thus the framework I describe in this chapter assumes as a point of departure that the "functional forms" of human memory (i.e., subsystems) yet to be specified are sets of processes that contribute in different combinations to the many purposes memory serves.

A MULTIPLE-ENTRY MODULAR MEMORY SYSTEM

The framework that I have found useful for thinking about memory is called a multiple-entry modular memory system (MEM) (Johnson, 1983). I propose that memory is composed of at least three interacting but distinguishable subsystems: the sensory system, the perceptual system, and the reflection system (Fig. 5.1). Each subsystem is really a set of processes; thinking in terms of subsystems allows us to group processes that have something in common and to highlight apparent differences in processes that may imply interesting directions for research.

The sensory and perceptual subsystems record the consequences of perceptual processing. They differ in the type of perceptual information to which they are most sensitive.[1] The sensory system records the type of information that typically is not in itself the major object of perception but that operates as perceptual

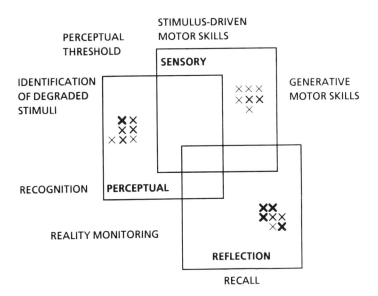

FIGURE 5.1. A particular event creates entries in three subsystems of memory: sensory, perceptual, and reflection. The x's indicate activation, the heavier the x's, the greater the likelihood that the activation will recruit attention. Various memory tasks are listed near the subsystem(s) that they are particularly likely to draw upon. (From Johnson, 1983, by permission)

cues. The sensory system develops associations involving such aspects of perception as brightness, localization, and direction of movement. The sensory record is important in many skills, such as developing hand–eye coordination, learning to adjust one's posture to changes in external cues, improving performance in tracking tasks, and other largely stimulus-driven tasks. The perceptual subsystem records phenomenally experienced perceptual events, that is, external objects in relation to one another. The reflection system records the active thinking, judging, and comparing that we do. It records our attempts to organize and control what happens to us, and our commentary on events. Thus it records memories that are internally generated.

In Figure 5.1 the subsystems are depicted as overlapping. If you look at the figure for a few moments, it will begin to reverse like a Necker cube; each subsystem may appear in the front, middle, or back. This visually represents the interactive quality of the entire system. No subsystem is primary, and the order in which processes are engaged is not fixed. As Kolers (1975) suggested, entries in memory are the records of the specific processes that created them. Activation (indicated by ×'s in Fig. 5.1) indicates that processing is taking place. The heavier ×'s indicate that we are aware of only a subset of activated information at any particular time. Nevertheless, activation, not awareness, is the necessary and sufficient condition for changing memory.

Most experiences will generate entries in all subsystems. For instance, in a complex activity like playing tennis, various components are probably largely mediated by different subsystems. Learning to get to the right place at the right time involves sensory information that itself is not the object of perception, especially visual information about trajectories such as the rate of change in the size of the ball as a function of time. Learning to respond to configurational aspects in the stimulus array is a perceptual function, for example, learning to see relations among an opponent's position on the court, posture, and racket orientation that signal what shot she is likely to make. Reflection is critically involved in learning to understand an opponent's strategy, or to plan or initiate one of your own. The memory for playing tennis is not a single type of representation in a unitary memory system, but is multiply represented in various subsystems of memory. Furthermore, most experiences have this same complex character and are thus multiply represented.

I do not think of MEM as finished, but as a general framework for proceeding. It may be necessary to add subsystems, and those already proposed need to be specified more precisely (for example, several ideas for clarifying some of what is involved in reflection are suggested in the section on recall below). One possibility is that subsystems should be defined in terms of relations that certain neural networks are prepared (through either evolution or past experience) to handle. For example, certain stimulus information may more easily be associated with body adjustments than with a complex plan. On the other hand, centrally generated representations or plans may more easily serve as cues for the revival of other ideas than as cues for certain body adjustments. If so, in MEM, the question of the interaction of subsystems might be framed in terms of whether and how sensory information contributes to the activation of reflections and whether and how self-generated information such as plans affect actions (such as eye movements) that are predisposed to respond to external cues.

The MEM framework helps organize a number of empirical findings from normal human subjects. For example, memory can be measured in various ways: with recall tests, recognition tests, or tests that show the effect of experience in indirect ways (or "implicitly"; Schacter, 1987b), such as improved ability to identify a stimulus under degraded perceptual conditions. In normal human subjects, these various measures are often not correlated or necessarily affected in the same way by experimental manipulations (e.g., Jacoby & Dallas, 1981; Tulving, 1983; see Schacter, 1987b for a recent review and Spear, 1984 for a discussion of related issues). This lack of correlation among measures can be understood if we assume that recall draws heavily on the reflection system, recognition draws on the perceptual system, and perceptual-threshold tasks like perceptual identification depend mainly on the sensory system. In Figure 5.1, tasks are listed near the subsystems that are most implicated, but there is no "pure" one-to-one correspondence between tasks and subsystems.

This model can also be applied to amnesia.[2] Quite a bit of evidence is consistent with the idea that anterograde amnesia results from a deficit primarily in the reflection subsystem, with the sensory and perceptual memory subsystems relatively intact (for reviews see Parkin, 1982; Cermak, 1982; Hirst, 1982). For example, amnesics show dramatic deficits in recall tasks. At the same time, they show relatively normal performance in certain perceptually based tasks such as learning mirror drawing (Milner, 1966), learning to read mirror text (Cohen & Squire, 1980), and perceptual identification of previously exposed words (Cermak, Talbot, Chandler, & Wolbarst, 1985). In the MEM framework, the more an activity requires reflection—that is, the more it requires self-generated cues—the more difficult it should be for amnesics to master. The more perceptual support for an activity there is (i.e., the more it is externally guided), the easier it should be for amnesics to learn.

Current research in areas such as skill learning (e.g., Nissen & Bullemer, 1987) and priming (e.g., Graf, Squire, & Mandler, 1984; Schacter, 1987b) is clarifying our picture of some of the memory functions that appear to be preserved in anterograde amnesia (e.g., development of sensory–motor associations and perceptual analysis processes, activation of semantic concepts). Here I focus on amnesic performance in tasks that are relevant to understanding memory functions that are not preserved. This chapter applies the MEM framework to the analysis of amnesia in three areas of research: recognition memory, acquisition of affective responses, and free recall. These areas are particularly interesting because amnesia's most profound consequence is loss of memory for recent personal experience and often what makes a memory seem personal is that it is recognized as familiar from a particular context or source, evokes affective responses, and can be revived or reconstructed voluntarily. Thus understanding processes involved in recognition, memory for affect, and recall eventually should help us better understand the loss of personal memory that is so characteristic of amnesia.

RECOGNITION

One specific prediction generated from MEM is that amnesics should show less disruption in recognition than in recall, because unlike recall, recognition presumably does not always require reflection but can be based on perceptual records alone (e.g., Jacoby, 1982; Mandler, 1980). Direct support for this idea comes from several experiments. In one study (Hirst et al., 1986) we tested two groups of amnesics, patients with Korsakoff's syndrome (a memory disorder associated with thiamine deficiency and chronic alcoholism) and a group of nonalcoholic amnesics of mixed etiology (e.g., hypoxic ischemia, anterior communicating artery aneurysm). Each amnesic group was compared to an appropriate age- and education-matched control group. The subjects studied word lists and we equated the performance of amnesics and controls on forced-choice recognition by giving the amnesics more time to study the words—amnesics took 8 sec per item of study time to reach the same level of recognition performance as normals given only 0.5 sec per item. Then we looked at recall for the same lists. Because the same patterns of results were obtained for the two amnesic groups, they have been combined in Table 5.1A. As you can see, even though their recognition performance was equal to that of controls, amnesics still showed a marked decrement in their ability to recall the words.

We extended these results in subsequent experiments with the mixed-etiology amnesics. In one experiment (Hirst, Johnson, Phelps, & Volpe, 1988, experiment 1) amnesics and normals both had 8 sec to study each item, but we equated amnesic and normal recognition by lengthening the retention interval for the normal subjects. That is, the recognition performance of normals tested after a 1-day delay was about the same as that of amnesics tested immediately. Again,

TABLE 5.1   Mean Proportion Correct Recognition and Recall for Three Experiments

Group	Time	n	Recognition	Recall
A. Amnesics	(8 sec)	13	.78	.07
Controls	(0.5 sec)	13	.77	.25
B. Amnesics	(30-sec delay)	6	.85	.06
Controls	(1-day delay)	6	.86	.22
C. Amnesics	(2 × 5 sec)	6	.85	.07
Controls	(1 × 0.5 sec)	6	.77	.16

Source: Data from (A) Hirst, Johnson, Kim, Phelps, Risse, and Volpe (1986; blocked, categorized lists) and (B) and (C) Hirst, Johnson, Phelps, and Volpe (1988, experiments 1 and 2; unrelated words).

with recognition equated, amnesics were at a substantial disadvantage in recall (Table 5.1B). In another experiment (Hirst et al., 1988, experiment 2) the list was presented to the amnesics twice at a 5 sec rate and only once for 0.5 sec to normals. Under these conditions the amnesics actually scored significantly better on recognition than the normals. But even with this recognition advantage, amnesics scored much poorer on the recall test (Table 5.1C).

Although these experiments show that amnesic recognition is less disrupted than recall, the amnesics still had a substantial recognition deficit that could be overcome only with long or repeated exposures. One explanation is that word stimuli are relatively "impoverished" perceptually. In addition, words are extremely familiar and probably do not create discriminable memory records without some reflection (e.g., Eysenck, 1979; Jacoby & Craik, 1979). It is possible that if we could make the perceptual qualities of the stimulus more important, the amnesics would more closely approximate normal performance. This in fact sometimes seems to be the case when the stimuli are unfamiliar pictures rather than words.

In one experiment we showed Korsakoffs and controls pictures of abstract "paintings" that we had made up (Johnson & Kim, 1985). Subjects saw each item 1, 5, or 10 times; then they were given a forced-choice recognition test in which they had to discriminate the more familiar picture from a new distractor and rate their confidence in their choice. Korsakoff patients were mildly, but not significantly, impaired in recognition memory (for both forced choice and choice weighted by confidence) (Table 5.2A). Furthermore, we retested subjects 20 days later, and even after 20 days, Korsakoff patients' recognition performance for

TABLE 5.2 Recognition Scores for "Paintings" after 5-Minute and 20-Day Retention Intervals

	Number of Exposures		
Test	1	5	10
A. 5-minute delay			
Mean proportion correct			
Korsakoff ($n = 9$)	.67	.81	1.00
Control ($n = 9$)	.78	.94	1.00
Choice weighted by confidence[a]			
Korsakoff	4.03	4.72	5.33
Control	4.31	5.31	5.64
B. 20-day delay			
Mean proportion correct			
Korsakoff	.56	.54	.78
Control	.53	.71	.86
Choice weighted by confidence			
Korsakoff	3.65	3.82	4.46
Control	3.60	4.19	4.72

[a]Correct choice: 6 = very sure; 5 = quite sure; 4 = guessing. Incorrect choice: 3 = guessing; 2 = quite sure; 1 = very sure.
Source: From Johnson and Kim (1985).

pictures seen 10 times was a remarkably good 78%, compared with 86% for controls (Table 5.2B).

To put these findings in perspective, we compared them with previously reported studies of picture recognition in Korsakoff patients. Figure 5.2 shows the relative performance of Korsakoff and control subjects who were tested under comparable conditions, where controls were below maximum performance (not at ceiling). It includes 11 data points from six different experiments including ours using abstract paintings (Johnson & Kim, 1985) and other experiments using faces, miscellaneous magazine pictures, magazine covers, and patterns (Biber, Butters, Rosen, Gertsman, & Mattis, 1981; Cutting, 1981; Huppert & Piercy, 1976, 1977; Talland, 1965). If Korsakoffs and normals performed exactly alike, the points would all be on a 45° line. In some of the conditions, the amnesics showed a significant deficit; in others the amnesics did not differ significantly from normals. More important, the correlation between the performance of Korsakoff patients and that of normals is quite clear ($r = .80$). Items or conditions that were difficult for controls were difficult for Korsakoffs; items or conditions that were easy for controls were easy for Korsakoffs (also see Mayes, Meudell, & Neary, 1980). This general pattern supports the idea that picture recognition involves some memory processes that are relatively intact in amnesia.

A dissertation by Weinstein (1987) helps clarify the conditions under which we might expect to find comparable recognition for amnesics and controls, and those conditions under which amnesics might show a deficit. All subjects saw a series of pictures that were line drawings of familiar objects, each colored in a single color. The type of orienting task was varied. Half of each group were given a perceptual task in which they were directed to keep track of the number of black objects. This task is perceptual because it requires subjects to attend to only a physical feature of each object, its color. The other half of the subjects were given a reflective task; they were to decide whether each object was presented in a common color or a novel color. For example, a *yellow lemon* would

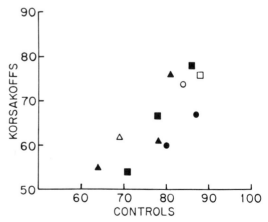

FIGURE 5.2. Relative performance of Korsakoff patients and control subjects on picture recognition. Data are from the following studies: Biber et al., 1981 (▲); Cutting, 1981 (△); Huppert and Piercy, 1976 (○); Huppert and Piercy, 1977 (●); Talland, 1965 (□); Johnson and Kim, 1985 (■). (Reprinted from Johnson and Kim, 1985, by permission)

TABLE 5.3   Mean Proportion Correct for Yes/No Picture Recognition

Distraction Condition	Perceptual Orienting Task		Reflective Orienting Task	
	Amnesic ($n = 12$)	Control ($n = 12$)	Amnesic ($n = 12$)	Control ($n = 12$)
A. New–novel	.69	.76	.76	.90
B. New–common	.51	.79	.80	.93
C. Old–common	.44	.68	.58	.87

Source: From Weinstein (1987).

be common; a *purple camel* would be novel. This task is reflective in that it requires subjects to consider the ongoing perceptual product and information activated about the object from general knowledge and then to compare the information from these two sources and make a decision. After all the pictures were presented, subjects were given a Yes/No recognition task, consisting of novel-colored objects from the acquisition list mixed with new novel colored objects.

The results are shown in Table 5.3A, which combines Korsakoffs and nonalcoholic amnesics, who showed the same patterns. After the perceptual task, recognition was not significantly different for amnesics and controls. After the reflective task, the controls were significantly better than the amnesics. These results suggest that if controls and amnesics process information perceptually, their recognition performance will be similar. If they process information reflectively, either controls engage in more embellished reflection or they are better able to reinstate memory for this reflection at the time of the test, or (most likely) both.

Normals and amnesics appeared to be equally good at using perceptual records for discriminating familiar old pictures from unfamiliar new pictures. Perhaps this was because no conflicting familiarity response was evoked by the distractor items. If the test involved some ambiguity about the source of familiarity, the importance of reflective processes should show up (e.g., Johnson, 1988; Johnson & Raye, 1981; Lindsay & Johnson, 1987). Thus Weinstein (1987) tested these same subjects on two other picture series in which the recognition decisions should have required reflection. In these conditions the acquisition series were of the same type as before (involving, of course, new pictures). But the distractors in the second condition were new objects in common colors and the distractors in the third condition were old objects from the acquisition list that had previously appeared in novel colors but now appeared in common colors. In both these cases we expected the distractors to evoke some sort of familiarity response (based on either semantic knowledge or semantic knowledge plus recent experience). Discriminating the targets from the distractors under these conditions should be more difficult because familiarity alone should not be a sufficient cue. Thus the benefit from reflective activity should be greater.

The results for these more difficult distractor conditions are shown in Table

5.3B and C). When the test involved familiar distractors, the amnesics performed considerably worse than the controls even in the perceptual orienting task condition. These results are consistent with the idea that reflection helps specify the source of a familiarity response and that amnesics perform more poorly with increasing reflective demands.

To summarize these experiments on word and picture recognition, the fact that the amnesics' recall deficit is greater than we would expect from their recognition performance indicates that regardless of what processes are disrupted in amnesia, they are more important in recall tasks than in recognition tasks.[3] We think the disrupted processes are controlled, self-generated mental activities of the sort I have been calling reflection. The fact that amnesic recognition can actually equal normal recognition when the recognition task is largely perceptual, and that amnesics begin to show marked deficits as recognition requires more reflection, makes the point even more strongly. A sense of familiarity does not necessarily depend on reflection, but further specifying the source of the familiarity does (Huppert & Piercy, 1978; Schacter, Harbluk, & McLachlan, 1984).

AFFECT

There has not been much work on amnesics' acquisition of affective reactions, but scattered reports suggest that amnesics do acquire affective responses (e.g., Claparede, 1911, cited in Baddeley, 1982), although some suggest that they do not (Redington, Volpe, & Gazzaniga, 1984). As with recognition, a closer analysis of the problem suggests that we might be able to characterize the conditions under which amnesics will and will not acquire affective responses.

According to the MEM model, emotion may originate with experiences that are perceptual or with experiences that are more self-generated or reflective. For example, after a traffic accident, the squeal of brakes may be associated in the perceptual system with fear. Frustration or anger may be another part of the affective response associated in the reflection system with thoughts after the accident about its consequences (e.g., missed appointments, lost work time, the inconvenience of getting the car repaired). Later, hearing the squeal of brakes may directly revive some components of the total affective response (e.g., the fear); the revival of other components (e.g., the frustration) will be more dependent on recalling earlier reflective activity.

If this characterization of emotion is correct, amnesics should still be able to develop affective responses—emotions, preferences, etc.—in situations that do not depend on reflection but in which the affect is tied to perceptual features of a situation. In one experiment exploring this idea (Johnson, Kim, & Risse, 1985, experiment 1), Korsakoff and control subjects heard unfamiliar Korean melodies. Then these melodies were mixed with a number of new melodies and the subjects were asked to rate how much they liked each one. We chose this situation because we reasoned that the affective response to melodies is largely based on perceptual characteristics of the melody; if so, the preferences of amnesics should be affected by the same variables as the preferences of normals. Research by Zajonc (1980) and others has shown that normal subjects often prefer stimuli they have previously experienced, and this is the result we obtained. The control subjects liked the old melodies better than the new melodies. The interesting new finding was that the Korsakoff subjects also gave higher ratings to the previously heard melodies; furthermore, the magnitude of the effect was the same as for normals (Table 5.4A). On the other hand, even though the amnesics preferred the old melodies to new ones, on a recognition test they showed the usual deficit in ability to say what they had and had not heard before (Table 5.4B).

These results suggest that affective reactions develop normally in amnesics if the situation is largely perceptual. In a second experiment (Johnson et al., 1985, experiment 2) we used a situation that we thought would be much more likely to involve reflection. The subjects were the same as in the melody experiment. They were shown pictures of two young men, Bill and John, and were asked to give their impression of each by rating him on several characteristics, such as honesty, politeness, and intelligence. Then subjects heard some facts about Bill and some facts about John. John was depicted as a "good guy" (he helped his father, got a Navy commendation for saving someone's life, etc.), and Bill was depicted as a "bad guy" (he stole things, broke someone's arm in a fight, etc.). After an interval, the subjects were shown the pictures and were asked about their impressions again.

The subjects heard the biographical information a total of three times over 3 or 4 days. We brought them back 20 days later and asked for their impressions again. The results are shown in Figure 5.3; the higher the score, the more positively the man in the picture was rated on such traits as honesty, politeness, and intelligence. Look first at the control subjects (squares and triangles). The pictures were rated first before the subjects heard any biographical information, and, as you would expect, Bill and John were rated about equally. After the control subjects heard the biographical information for the first time, the ratings changed dramatically with the good guy rated more favorably and the bad guy less favorably. Ratings did not change much with repetitions of the biographical information, and the effect of the biographical information persisted over the 20-day retention interval (day 3 in Fig. 5.3). Now look at the Korsakoff patients

TABLE 5.4   Preference Ratings and Recognition Scores for Melodies

Group	A. Preference Ratings[a]		B. Proportion Correct Recognition
	Old	New	
Amnesic (n = 9)	4.10	3.74	.59
Control (n = 9)	3.77	3.46	.83

[a]Higher ratings indicate more preferred.
Source: From Johnson, Kim, and Risse (1985, experiment 1).

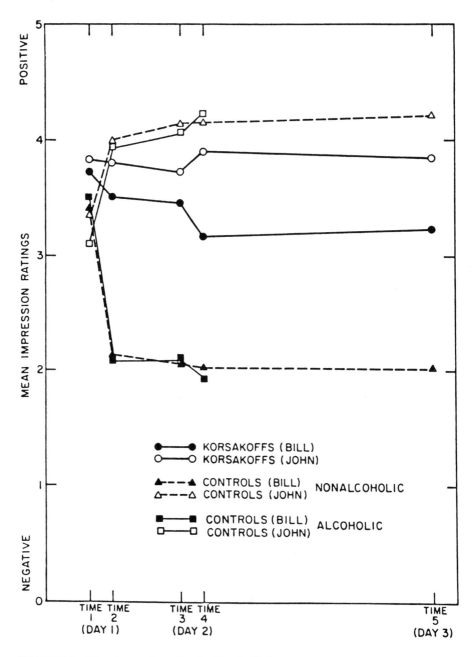

FIGURE 5.3.   Mean impression ratings for Korsakoffs ($N = 9$), nonalcoholic controls ($N = 9$), and alcoholic controls ($N = 6$). (From Johnson, Kim, and Risse, 1985, experiment 2)

(circles). Again, the ratings for Bill and John started out the same and diverged significantly. Even after a 20-day retention interval, the amnesics gave the good guy higher ratings than the bad guy. After 20 days, the control subjects could recall about 35% of the biographical information, whereas the Korsakoffs recalled virtually nothing. Therefore, although the Korsakoffs could not recall the biographical information, it still affected their judgments about which of the two men was nicer.

In the Bill and John study, Korsakoff patients clearly developed less extreme impressions than did controls. In contrast, these same Korsakoff patients showed the same development of preference for melodies as controls did. Differences in the results of the two studies are interpretable within the MEM framework. Compared to developing preferences for melodies, when we develop preferences for people there is much more room for reflection to operate. The MEM framework assumes that some affective responses are tied to the perceptual features of the pictures of the two men, whereas other affective responses are tied to the reflective activity the subjects engaged in while hearing the biographical information (e.g., comparing the men to other people they have known, evaluating the severity of misdeeds). Later, reinstating perceptual cues from the pictures should revive some affective components, but other aspects of the total affective response should depend on reinstating previous reflection. Normal subjects could cue themselves by recalling specific biographical details and should therefore have a more embellished affective response.

In summary, our two experiments on affect indicate that Korsakoff patients retain the capacity for developing affective reactions. But the degree to which we can expect amnesics to retain affective responses in any particular case depends on the relative involvement of different memory subsystems in supporting affective responses of nonamnesic subjects.

RECALL

The most salient and central symptom of amnesia is profoundly poor free recall (e.g., Butters & Cermak, 1980; Milner, Corkin, & Teuber, 1968). Precisely because amnesic recall is so poor, it is difficult to study systematically. By considering the various mental activities required by recall, however, we should be able to break the problem down into tractable component parts. This will also help further clarify the concept of reflection.

Basic Reflective Subprocesses

Even in its simplest form, normal recall clearly depends on a number of basic reflective subprocesses, the most important of which have to do with establishing relations among elements to be recalled (e.g., Bower, 1970; Mandler, 1967; Tulving, 1962). Consider a hypothetical organizational problem involving a free recall list that includes the words *pig, dog, weed,* and *dinner* (Fig. 5.4A). Each

A.

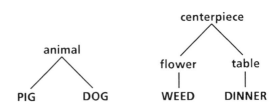

B.

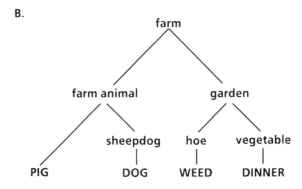

FIGURE 5.4.   Hypothetical activation patterns and noted relations for four items (pig, dog, weed, dinner) from a free recall list. (A) Initial activation and noted relations. (B) Activation and noted relations after a shift in perspective.

word activates some set of relations based on prior experience and current context. One primary reflective function is *noting* the relations that are given in this current activation pattern. For example, a subject might note that *pig* and *dog* are both *animals,* and that *flower* (which is activated by *weed*) can be used as a *centerpiece* on a *table* (which is activated by *dinner*). This noting activity would establish two small units.

Another critical reflective function is *shifting* activation to other information in order to change what is given. The change is accomplished by changing perspective or shifting attention from the currently activated aspects of a stimulus to other potentially useful aspects (see Fig. 5.4B). Suppose that for our hypothetical subject, attention is shifted from the idea of *animals* to the fact that *pigs* and *dogs* are found on *farms.* At the same time, suppose the subject thinks about aspects of *weeds* and *dinner* that in turn suggest the idea of *garden. Garden* and *farm animals* are both related through *farm.* Now the subject has a single interrelated set of relations including the four items.

A third reflective process is *refreshing.* Clearly, various ideas and relations must remain active during *shifting* and *noting* until a stable or cohesive set of relations has been noted. Keeping them active requires some sort of continuous scan of current activation in order to keep it refreshed.

A fourth reflective function is delayed *reactivation* of information that has disappeared from consciousness. Through internally generated remindings, sets of relations become more cohesive.

To simplify, I have illustrated these subprocesses applied to learning and remembering a word list, but all these basic reflective activities are central in processing more complex, naturally occurring events.

Layers of Reflection

Reflective processes differ not only in type, but also along a continuum of "planfulness," which may affect the characteristics of these basic reflective activities. At the minimum level of planfulness, basic reflective activities may consist largely of allowing the activation consequences of successive events to settle and noting whatever cohesive sets of relations emerge.[4] Even such relatively passive mental activity receives some direction from ongoing goals or agendas (e.g., the goal to read words aloud). Agendas vary in the degree of deliberation they require to execute and monitor. Thus some agendas call up well-learned perceptual and reflective schemata that may organize component processes relatively automatically, while others bring basic subprocesses under strategic control in order to organize them to meet new, unusual, or complex demands.

Figure 5.5 shows how we might label reflective processes differently, depending on the degree of deliberation or planfulness involved. The cube represents basic reflective processes that occur spontaneously or under control of relatively simple agendas on the bottom and reflective processes under control of more strategic planning on the top. Look first at the lower front corner. *Shifting* is a change in perspective as a consequence of overlapping spreading activation patterns. *Initiating* is a change in perspective via strategically controlled activities (such as listing all the properties you can think of for two objects that are to be related). *Refreshing* is activation prolonged by simple attention; *rehearsal* is activation prolonged by systematic, strategically controlled recycling. *Reactivating* refers to the revival of inactive information via spontaneous or accidental mental events that provide a reminder; *retrieval* refers to reviving information through conscious attempts to get back to it. *Noting* involves seeing relations that are relatively direct, and *discovering* involves seeing relations that are less direct. Thus there are at least two layers of internal control, or layers of reflection involved in learning and remembering. The idea that these two layers correspond to two functional subsystems of reflection, R-1 and R-2, is developed elsewhere (Johnson, in press; Johnson & Hirst, in press). (Furthermore, some mental activities could be thought of as combinations of these component processes. For example, the combination of *initiating* and *discovering,* represented along the top edge of the cube, would produce "elaboration" [e.g., Stein & Bransford,

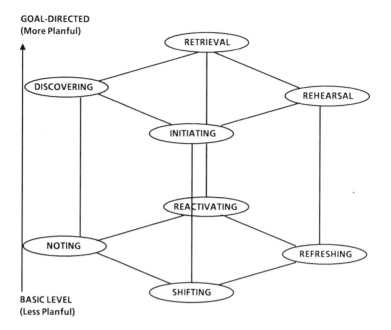

LAYERS OF REFLECTION

FIGURE 5.5.   Reflective processes differ in degree of "planfulness." Basic reflective processes are represented at the bottom corners of the cube; corresponding but more strategic, goal-directed reflective functions are represented at the top corners of the cube.

1979]). To understand amnesia, we need to specify exactly which reflective sub-processes are disrupted and which are not, and among those that can vary in strategic control, which layer of control is disrupted.

Amnesia and Reflective Subprocesses

Amnesia could cause problems with all reflective subprocesses or with only some of them. What is our best guess about amnesia's effect on these basic reflective subprocesses? Several lines of evidence suggest that *noting* given relations is intact. First, amnesics understand ordinary conversation. Also, amnesics do fairly well on easy pairs on the Wechsler Memory Scale (hot–cold). Despite early evidence to the contrary (Cermak & Butters, 1972), it appears that amnesics spontaneously categorize items from taxonomic categories (McDowell, 1979). What we need is more detailed or analytic information about this noting func-tion—for example, what kinds of relationships can be noted, and under what conditions?

A recent study from our lab (Johnson, Hirst, Phelps, & Volpe, unpublished data) illustrates one potential approach. Nonalcoholic amnesics and normal controls were presented with some difficult-to-understand sentences (e.g., Birnbaum, Johnson, Hartley, & Taylor, 1980; Johnson, Doll, Bransford, & Lapinski, 1974). Half the sentences were preceded by an appropriate context (e.g., *Bagpipes: The notes went sour when the seams split*) and half were preceded by an inappropriate context (e.g., *New car: The house turned to water when the fire got too hot*). As each sentence was presented, subjects were asked to rate how much sense it made. The points over ACQ (for acquisition) in Figure 5.6 show the mean ratings; higher ratings reflect greater comprehension. As you can see, both amnesics and controls showed a large context effect.

Comprehension ratings were also taken later for the sentences alone (without the contexts) at three retention intervals, 2 min, 1½ hr, and 1 week; these ratings are also shown in Figure 5.6. Notice that the effect of having heard a relevant context is relatively long-lasting for amnesics. This is an example of new learn-

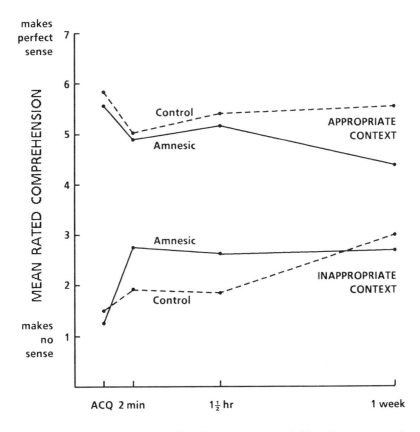

FIGURE 5.6. Mean comprehension ratings for sentences preceded by either an appropriate or inappropriate context at acquisition (ACQ) and later (2 min, 1½ hr, 1 week) presented without contexts (amnesic N = 4; control N = 4). (Johnson, Hirst, Phelps, and Volpe, unpublished data)

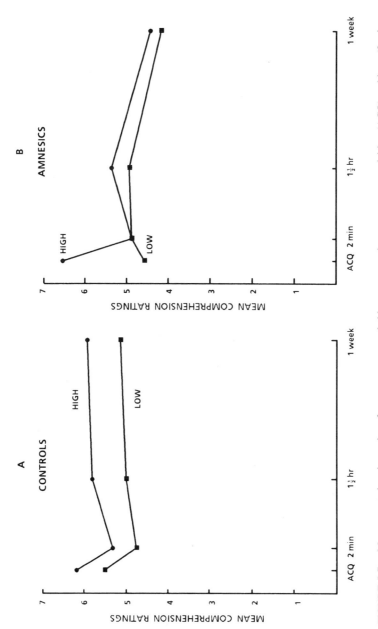

FIGURE 5.7.   Mean comprehension ratings for sentences preceded by an appropriate context at acquisition (ACQ) and later (2 min, 1½ hr, 1 week) presented without contexts. Ratings are shown separately for high- and low-related context–sentence pairs and for controls (A) and amnesics (B). (Johnson, Hirst, Phelps, and Volpe, unpublished data)

ing that cannot simply be attributed to short-term priming (see McAndrews, Glisky, & Schacter, 1987, for a similar finding).

We also looked at comprehension ratings separately for sentences in which the context and sentence were highly related and for sentences in which the context–sentence relation was low. Figure 5.7A shows the comprehension ratings for the control subjects; these verify the ratings of the subjects who gave us the normative data for high and low. In contrast to the controls, the amnesics showed a relatedness-by-delay interaction; the initial advantage of highly related items disappeared over the retention interval (Figure 5.7B).

At the 2-min, 1½-hr, and 1-week retention intervals (when sentences were presented without any context), we also asked subjects to tell us what they thought each sentence was about. Table 5.5 shows the mean number of appropriate contexts given in this context-generation task, collapsed across retention interval. There was a subject-by-relatedness interaction; the difference between amnesics and controls was greater on low than on highly related items. The less obvious the relation between the context and sentence was, the more difficulty amnesics had in later describing what the sentence was about (see also Warrington & Weiskrantz, 1982). The initial comprehension ratings taken as the context–sentence pairs were first presented showed a similar (though not significant) pattern.[5]

One reasonable hypothesis supported by the results of our comprehension study is that amnesics are able to note relations that are a relatively direct consequence of activation patterns set up by incoming stimuli. The more distant the relation—the more seeing, or discovering, a connection depends on shifting attention from initially activated but not useful relations to new possibilities—the more problems the amnesic may have.

At the one-week retention interval, we also gave subjects a recognition test on the sentences presented without contexts. Amnesics' recognition of these sentences, although clearly worse than normals, was quite good after a week (Table 5.6). More important, amnesics recognized more of the low-related sentences than the high-related sentences. This recognition advantage of the low-related sentences is interesting because it indicates that amnesics based their recognition judgments on information somewhat different from that used for their compre-

TABLE 5.5 Mean Number of Contexts Given for Sentences Initially Presented with an Appropriate Context (averaged over 2-min, 1½-hr, and 2-week retention intervals)

Group	Relation Between Context and Sentence	
	High	Low
Amnesic ($n = 4$)	2.33	2.00
Control ($n = 4$)	2.83	3.25

Source: From Johnson, Hirst, Phelps, and Volpe (unpublished data).

TABLE 5.6   Mean Proportion Correct Yes/No Recognition (1-week delay)

Group	Appropriate Context		Inappropriate Context		
	High	Low	High	Low	New Items
Amnesic (n = 4)	.75	1.00	.69	.88	.72
Control (n = 4)	.94	1.00	1.00	1.00	1.00

Source: From Johnson, Hirst, Phelps, and Volpe (unpublished data).

hension judgments and their attempts to describe what the sentences were about.

One way contexts help comprehension is by activating a schema that is used in interpreting further information and in retrieving it later (e.g., Bransford & Johnson, 1973; Schank & Abelson, 1977). Thus our context study indicates that amnesics can use schemas. Another piece of evidence that amnesics can apply schematic knowledge to incoming information comes from an experiment conducted by Phelps (Phelps, Hirst, Johnson, & Volpe, 1988). Mixed-etiology amnesics and controls were asked to remember two stories. All subjects heard a general story that involved a topic with which most people are familiar (a shopping trip). In addition, each amnesic and his or her control heard a story tailored to the individual interests of each amnesic. For example, one amnesic knew a lot about basketball, so he (and his control, who was not particularly interested in basketball) received a story about a basketball game. As Figure 5.8 shows, the controls recalled a larger percentage of the general story than the subject-specific stories. In contrast, the amnesics recalled a larger percentage of the subject-specific stories than the general story. Thus, although for normal subjects the subject-specific stories were more difficult, they were relatively easy for amnesics because the amnesics were able to draw on their special interest in and knowledge of these areas to aid recall.[6] It would be valuable to have more specific information about the types of schemas that amnesics can and cannot use.[7]

We also do not know much about the subprocess of *refreshing* activated information, but verbal rehearsal seems to be relatively intact. Available evidence from short-term memory experiments with amnesics suggests that when they are not distracted, amnesics are relatively good at *rehearsing* currently activated verbal information (but perhaps not nonverbal information; Milner, 1966). Later recall, however, depends on more than rehearsal (e.g., Glenberg, Smith, & Green, 1977). *Noting* and, if necessary, *shifting* must take place as well. Amnesics may have more trouble than control subjects simultaneously engaging in these various subprocesses (which may require coordinating layers of reflective processes). Thus not only should amnesics show greater disruption when unrelated distraction is introduced, as in typical STM experiments (Cermak, Butters,

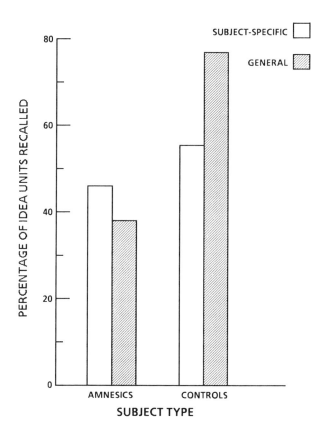

FIGURE 5.8.   Mean percentage of idea units recalled from a story about a shopping trip (general) and stories tailored to the interest of amnesics (subject-specific) (amnesic $N = 6$; control $N = 6$). (Data from Phelps, Hirst, Johnson, & Volpe, 1988, experiment 1)

& Goodglass, 1971; Kinsbourne & Wood, 1975), but they should also show greater disruption when additional *task-relevant* demands such as *noting* and *initiating* are introduced. For example, in one experiment (Warrington, 1982) subjects were quickly read three words, distracted for 15 seconds, and then tested for recall. Whereas amnesics performed as well as normals if the words were unrelated, they showed a deficit on related-word trials (e.g., drink–coffee–cold).

Clearly, amnesics are impaired on delayed strategic *retrieval* of information that has dropped out of consciousness. But what should be emphasized is the critical role that such delayed reactivation plays in normal memory (Johnson, 1987; Levin et al., 1985; Ribot, 1882/1977). Without subsequent rehearsals, many autobiographical memories do not remain clear or vivid (Suengas & Johnson, 1988). Some investigators suggest that a consolidationlike process in which memories gradually become more resistant to disruption takes place over years (Squire, 1982; Wickelgren, 1979). Whether or not such long-lasting processes are initiated when a memory is first established, it seems clear that the accessibility of memories is related to their subsequent reactivation (also see Squire, 1986, p. 1616) and that the loss of the consequences of reactivation contributes to the amnesic deficit.

TYPES AND DEGREES OF AMNESIA

Investigators have tried to isolate memory deficits from other cognitive deficits, but this is easier said than done (see, for example, discussions by Baddeley, 1982; Kinsbourne & Wood, 1982; Moscovitch, 1982; Warrington, 1982). In practice, isolating memory amounts to either (1) defining amnesia as deficits on certain simple word, picture, and prose recall and recognition tasks (along with clinically diagnosed impaired memory for recent personal events), and considering normal performance on these tasks but disrupted performance on more complex memory tasks to be due to secondary cognitive deficits, or (2) defining amnesia as whatever is disrupted by lesions confined to certain areas of the temporal lobes and diencephalon and attributing memory deficits from lesions in other areas (e.g., prefrontal cortex) to secondary cognitive deficits. Both alternatives imply that the major objective is to understand the "core amnesia" thus defined. From this "core amnesia" point of view, many reflective processes would be considered secondary cognitive processes.

Focusing on "core amnesia," although one reasonable strategy, is based on a perhaps too simple view of memory (also see Morton, 1985). Many cognitive psychologists would argue against the idea that memory can be isolated from other cognitive processes such as attention, comprehension, thinking, planning, and problem solving.[8] Memory is the result of many processes, from those engaged by "simple" perception to those engaged by highly organized plans and schemas. In fact, remembering itself can be thought of as a skill (e.g., Ericsson, Chase, & Faloon, 1980) or a type of problem solving. Thus the idea of "core amnesia" may be misleading. Rather, there may be many types and degrees of amnesia, depending on which combination of memory subprocesses is required for particular memory tasks, and on which memory processes are disrupted.[9] But the fact that few differences among amnesics as a function of etiology have been reported (e.g., Corkin et al., 1985) suggests that reflection is a highly integrated system.

If we adopt a relatively complex view of memory, we should be more likely to attempt to integrate the results from a wider range of patterns of memory deficits, and this (in combination with ongoing efforts in cognition to analyze normal memory functioning) could be quite informative. One goal might be to refine and embellish a preliminary categorization scheme for reflective processes such as the following:

		Strategic Reflective Subprocesses	
		Intact	Disrupted
Basic Reflective Subprocesses	Intact	Normal memory	Deficits in complex information and sequences
	Disrupted	"Core amnesia"	Severe amnesia

According to the scheme, even if certain strategic reflective processes were intact, major disruption in one or more basic reflective processes would produce profound deficits in even the easiest memory tasks ("core amnesia"). If strategic reflective processes were disrupted but basic reflective processes were intact, the patient might show considerable memory for some things but have difficulty with others requiring more sophisticated reflective processing (e.g., complex information, sequences, or temporal orderings). Disruption of both levels of reflection—basic subprocesses and those under more strategic control—would produce the most severe amnesia. It is likely that different types of reflective subprocesses depend on different neurological structures and thus different lesion sites should produce amnesias differing in type or severity. For example, certain temporal and diencephalic lesions may disturb basic reflective subprocesses and certain frontal lesions may affect strategic reflective planning subprocesses (Goldman-Rakic, 1987; Milner & Petrides, 1984; Schacter, 1987a; Squire, 1987; Warrington & Weiskrantz, 1982). This categorization is undoubtedly too simple, but it illustrates the approach of assuming memory depends on a rich repertoire of processes and exploring the relation between specific reflective subprocesses and memory, including the effects of various lesions on these specific subprocesses.

CONCLUSIONS

A fundamental idea embodied in MEM is that it is useful to consider as separate classes those processes initiated and maintained by external stimuli and those initiated and maintained by internally directed reflective processes (e.g., Johnson & Raye, 1981). This idea can help in understanding findings from amnesia and in fact has also figured in recent analyses of prefrontal cortex function (Goldman-Rakic, 1987) and aging effects in memory (Craik, 1986).

Available evidence about preserved learning abilities in amnesics indicates that the deficit is much more specific than was once thought. In terms of MEM, the sensory and perceptual systems appear to be largely intact, whereas the reflective system is disrupted. Furthermore, the reflective system may be only partially disrupted. (I have concentrated on disruptions in reflective functions because these seem to underlie the amnesias that have been most salient in the cognitive literature, but according to the MEM framework there could be memory deficits associated with disruptions in the sensory and the perceptual subsystems as well.)

Clearly, amnesics are affected by events in important ways in spite of their profound memory deficit. Their comprehension of the meaning of stimuli may change, as indicated by comprehension ratings, context generation, and affective responses. They may experience a feeling of familiarity and, under some conditions, show good recognition after long intervals. If appropriately cued, they may show surprising levels of recall and be able to use prior knowledge to aid new learning.

These facts are not consistent with the idea that amnesics show no new "episodic" learning but can only reinforce or "prime" what is in "semantic memory" already (Cermak, 1986). These results are also not easily accounted for by the procedural–declarative distinction (Cohen & Squire, 1980). Ideas that seem closer to describing amnesic deficits have been around for some time: that amnesia reflects a "premature closure of function" (Talland, 1965), failure of consolidation (Milner, 1966; Squire, 1982), disruption of vertical processes (Wickelgren, 1979) or mediated learning (Warrington & Weiskrantz, 1982), an encoding deficit (Butters & Cermak, 1980; Cermak, 1979), a deficit in initial learning (Huppert & Piercy, 1982), or a contextual encoding deficit (Hirst, 1982). These ideas, although somewhat vague or unsatisfactory for various reasons, all focus attention on the fact that amnesic processing is somehow attenuated. Such attenuated processing would disrupt both acquisition and retrieval.

MEM provides one potentially useful framework for further clarifying the nature of amnesic processing. Within this framework, what amnesics seem to have lost is internally guided access to more information than is directly activated by external stimuli. If more information is not needed, as in certain perceptual/motor tasks, priming tasks, understanding ordinary conversation, and recognition of novel stimuli, then amnesics do quite well. But if further reflection is required, an amnesic is at a severe disadvantage. Situations in which further information (and thus reflection) is required include recognition tests in which familiarity alone is not a sufficient cue but in which the source of the familiarity must be specified, the reinstatement of certain types of affect, and, of course, free recall of events. I have also suggested that progress in understanding the role of reflection in amnesia might be made by further decomposing reflection into component subprocesses and then attempting to match these subprocesses with neurological findings (e.g., specific lesion sites).

Acknowledgments

This chapter was prepared while I was a fellow at the Center for Advanced Study in the Behavioral Sciences. I am grateful for financial support provided by the John D. and Catherine T. MacArthur Foundation, Princeton University, and National Science Foundation Grant BNS-8510633. I would also like to acknowledge the excellent assistance of Sharon Ray, Deanna Knickerbocker, Kathleen Much, and Rosanne Torre (members of the CASBS staff) in preparing the manuscript, and the comments from Bill Hirst, Amy Weinstein, Liz Phelps, and Shahin Hashtroudi on an earlier draft of this chapter. Special thanks to Bill Hirst for our many spirited discussions about memory and amnesia.

Notes

1. Sensory and perceptual subsystems are called P-1 and P-2, respectively, in subsequent papers (Johnson, in press; Johnson & Hirst, in press).

2. In this chapter I do not discuss retrograde amnesia (impaired memory for events occurring before the onset of amnesia), but focus on anterograde amnesia (impaired learning and memory for events and information occurring after the onset of amnesia).

3. Recall and recognition are sometimes treated as measures of "declarative" memory that should be equally disrupted by amnesia (e.g., Squire, 1982). Our comparison of recall and recognition in amnesics indicates that this is not always the case and, at the least, requires that the concept of declarative memory be further analyzed into component subprocesses that may be differentially disrupted.

4. These basic reflective subprocesses are typically fast-acting and perhaps they are largely controlled by variations in activation level in the memory system (e.g., Johnson, 1983). For example, amnesic deficits could be produced by turning down the amount of potential activation level contributed by experience (McClelland, 1985), by reducing the probability that a given level of activation will recruit attention (Johnson, 1983), or by attenuating the spread of activation.

5. With a greater range of difficulty level (or simply more subjects), comprehension ratings (as well as later context generation) would very likely show an increasing deficit for amnesics as difficulty is increased. Comprehension ratings are an example of a task that taps reflective processes without requiring the subject to remember new information (see also Cermak, Reale, & Baker, 1978). Such tasks should help clarify amnesic deficits in reflective processes.

6. Although the focus here is on amnesics' ability to use meaningful schemas, it should be noted that amnesics also showed a marked improvement in recall of unrelated words when the experimenter embedded the words in a bizarre story with high imagery value and gave amnesics spaced practice and cues when needed (Kovner, Mattis, & Goldmeier, 1983).

7. In Phelps et al. (1988) the relevant prior knowledge was presumably acquired before the onset of amnesia. A second experiment (Phelps et al., experiment 2), however, demonstrated that under certain conditions amnesics can also use information acquired after the onset of amnesia to help in learning new information. (Thus they did not show the "hyperspecific" learning reported by Glisky, Schacter, & Tulving, 1986. Also see Hirst, Phelps, Johnson, & Volpe, 1988, and Shimamura & Squire, 1988, for other reports of "flexible" memory in amnesics.)

8. Memory is also often presumed to be independent of something called "intellectual capacity" and thus intelligence is said to be intact in pure amnesia uncomplicated by other problems. But memory is critically involved in most intellectual tasks, from seeing previously unnoted relationships to solving extremely complex problems. Standard IQ tests are probably not the most sensitive way to look for deficits in intellectual functioning that may result from disruption of reflective processes.

9. It has in fact been suggested that there are two types of amnesia: bitemporal (patient H.M. and ECT patients) and diencephalic (patient N.A. and Korsakoff patients) (Squire, 1982). Although it is consistent with the present view of memory that "these two brain regions contribute in different ways to normal memory functions" (Squire, 1982, p. 246), current evidence is quite weak (Corkin, Cohen, Sullivan, Clegg, & Rosen, 1985). The case rests largely on studies of forgetting rates in picture recognition (Huppert & Piercy, 1979b, Squire, 1981b), and one central finding did not replicate (Freed, Corkin, & Cohen, 1984). More sensitive tests, however, developed to discriminate among the various reflective subprocesses outlined here, might be useful in discriminating bitemporal and diencephalic amnesics.

REFERENCES

Baddeley, A. (1982). Amnesia: A minimal model and an interpretation. In L. S. Cermak (Ed.), *Human memory and amnesia* (pp. 305–336). Hillsdale, N.J.: Erlbaum.

Biber, C., Butters, N., Rosen, J., Gertsman, L., & Mattis, S. (1981). Encoding strategies and recognition of faces by alcoholic Korsakoff and other brain-damaged patients. *Journal of Clinical Neuropsychology, 3,* 315–330.

Birnbaum, I. M., Johnson, M. K., Hartley, J. T., & Taylor, T. H. (1980). Alcohol and elaborative schemas for sentences. *Journal of Experimental Psychology: Human Learning and Memory, 6,* 293–300.

Bower, G. H. (1970). Organizational factors in memory. *Cognitive Psychology, 1,* 18–46.

Bransford, J. D., & Johnson, M. K. (1973). Considerations of some problems of comprehension. In W. Chase (Ed.), *Visual information processing.* New York: Academic Press.

Butters, N., & Cermak, L. S. (1980). *Alcoholic Korsakoff's syndrome: An information-processing approach to amnesia.* New York: Academic Press.

Cermak, L. S. (1979). Amnesic patients' level of processing. In L. S. Cermak & F. I. M. Craik (Eds.), *Levels of processing in human memory* (pp. 119–139). Hillsdale, N.J.: Erlbaum.

Cermak, L. S. (1982). *Human memory and amnesia.* Hillsdale, N.J.: Erlbaum.

Cermak, L. S. (1984). The episodic-semantic distinction in amnesia. In L. R. Squire & N. Butters (Eds.), *Neuropsychology of memory* (pp. 55–62). New York: Guilford.

Cermak, L. S. (1986). Amnesia as a processing deficit. In G. Goldstein & R. E. Tarter (Eds.), *Advances in clinical neuropsychology* (Vol. 3, pp. 265–290). New York: Plenum.

Cermak, L. S., & Butters, N. (1972). The role of interference and encoding in the short-term memory deficits of Korsakoff patients. *Neuropsychologia, 10,* 89–95.

Cermak, L. S., Butters, N., & Goodglass, H. (1971). The extent of memory loss in Korsakoff patients. *Neuropsychologia, 9,* 307–315.

Cermak, L. S., Reale, L., & Baker, E. (1978). Alcoholic Korsakoff patients' retrieval from semantic memory. *Brain and Language, 5,* 215–226.

Cermak, L. S., Talbot, N., Chandler, K., & Wolbarst, L. (1985). The perceptual priming phenomenon in amnesia. *Neuropsychologia, 23,* 615–622.

Cohen, N. J. (1984). Preserved learning capacity in amnesia: Evidence for multiple memory systems. In L. R. Squire & N. Butters (Eds.), *Neuropsychology of memory* (pp. 83–103). New York: Guilford.

Cohen, N. J., & Squire, L. R. (1980). Preserved learning and retention of pattern analyzing skill in amnesia: Dissociation of knowing how and knowing that. *Science, 210,* 207–209.

Corkin, S., Cohen, N. J., Sullivan, E. V., Clegg, R. A., & Rosen, T. J. (1985). Analyses of global memory impairments of different etiologies. *Annals of the New York Academy of Sciences, 444,* 10–40.

Craik, F. I. M. (1986). A functional account of age differences in memory. In F. Klix & H. Hagendorf (Eds.), *Human memory and cognitive capabilities* (pp. 409–422). Amsterdam: North-Holland.

Cutting, J. (1981). Response bias in Korsakoff's syndrome. *Cortex, 17,* 107–112.

Ericsson, K. A., Chase, W. G., & Faloon, S. (1980). Acquisition of a memory skill. *Science, 208,* 1181–1182.

Eysenck, M. W. (1979). Depth, elaboration, and distinctiveness. (1979). In L. S. Cermak & F. I. M. Craik (Eds.), *Levels of processing and human memory.* Hillsdale, N.J.: Erlbaum.

Freed, D. M., Corkin, S., & Cohen, N. J. (1984). Rate of forgetting in H.M.: A reanalysis. *Society for Neuroscience Abstracts, 10,* 383.

Glenberg, A., Smith, S. M., & Green, C. (1977). Type I rehearsal: Maintenance and more. *Journal of Verbal Learning and Verbal Behavior, 16,* 339–352.

Glisky, E. L., Schacter, D. L., & Tulving, E. (1986). Computer learning by memory-impaired patients: Acquisition and retention of complex knowledge. *Neuropsychologia, 24,* 313–328.

Goldman-Rakic, P. S. (1987). Circuitry of primate prefrontal cortex and the regulation of behavior by representational memory. In F. Plum (Ed.), *Handbook of physiology: Sec. 1. The nervous system: Vol. 5. Higher functions of the brain* (pp. 373–417). Bethesda, Md.: American Physiological Society.

Graf, P., Squire, L. R., & Mandler, G. (1984). The information that amnesic patients do not forget. *Journal of Experimental Psychology: Learning, Memory, and Cognition, 10,* 164–178.

Hirst, W. (1982). The amnesic syndrome: Descriptions and explanations. *Psychological Bulletin, 91,* 435–460.

Hirst, W., Johnson, M. K., Kim, J. K., Phelps, E. A., Risse, G., & Volpe, B. (1986). Recognition and recall in amnesics. *Journal of Experimental Psychology: Learning, Memory, and Cognition, 12,* 445–451.

Hirst, W., Johnson, M. K., Phelps, E. A., & Volpe, B. T. (1988). More on recall and recognition in amnesia. *Journal of Experimental Psychology: Learning, Memory, and Cognition, 14,* 758–762.

Hirst, W., Phelps, E. A., Johnson, M. K., & Volpe, B. T. (1988). Amnesia and second language learning. *Brain and Cognition, 8,* 105–116.

Huppert, F. A., & Piercy, M. (1976). Recognition memory in amnesic patients: Effects of temporal context and familiarity of material. *Cortex, 12,* 3–20.

Huppert, F. A., & Piercy, M. (1977). Recognition memory in amnesic patients: A defect of acquisition? *Neuropsychologia, 15,* 643–652.

Huppert, F. A., & Piercy, M. (1978). The role of trace strength in recency and frequency judgments by amnesic and control subjects. *Quarterly Journal of Experimental Psychology, 30,* 347–354.

Huppert, F. A., & Piercy, M. (1979a). Dissociation between learning and remembering in organic amnesia. *Nature, 275,* 317–318.

Huppert, F. A., & Piercy, M. (1979b). Normal and abnormal forgetting in amnesia: Effect of locus of lesion. *Cortex, 15,* 385–390.

Huppert, F. A. & Piercy, M. (1982). In search of the functional locus of amnesic syndromes. In L. S. Cermak (Ed.), *Human memory and amnesia* (pp. 123–137). Hillsdale, N.J.: Erlbaum.

Jacoby, L. L. (1982). Knowing and remembering: Some parallels in the behavior of Korsakoff patients and normals. In L. S. Cermak (Ed.), *Human memory and amnesia* (pp. 97–112). Hillsdale, N.J.: Erlbaum.

Jacoby, L. L., & Craik, F. I. M. (1979). Effects of elaboration of processing at encoding and retrieval: Trace distinctiveness and recovery of initial context. In L. S. Cermak & F. I. M. Craik (Eds.), *Levels of processing and human memory.* Hillsdale, N.J.: Erlbaum.

Jacoby, L. L., & Dallas, M. (1981). On the relationship between autobiographical memory and perceptual learning. *Journal of Experimental Psychology: General, 110,* 306–340.

Johnson, M. K. (1983). A multiple-entry, modular memory system. In G. H. Bower (Ed.), *The psychology of learning and motivation: Advances in research and theory* (Vol. 17, pp. 81–123). New York: Academic Press.

Johnson, M. K. (1987, February). The origin of memories. Paper presented at the annual meeting of the Lake Ontario Visionary Establishment, Niagara Falls, N.Y.

Johnson, M. K. (1988). Discriminating the origin of information. In T. F. Oltmanns & B. A. Maher (Eds.), *Delusional beliefs: Interdisciplinary perspectives* (pp. 34–65). New York: Wiley.

Johnson, M. K. (in press). Reality monitoring: Evidence from confabulation in organic brain disease patients. In G. Prigatano & D. L. Schacter (Eds.), *Awareness of deficit after brain injury.* New York: Oxford University Press.

Johnson, M. K., Doll, T. J., Bransford, J. D., & Lapinski, R. H. (1974). Context effects in sentence memory. *Journal of Experimental Psychology, 103,* 358–360.

Johnson, M. K., & Hirst, W. (in press). Processing subsystems of memory. In R. G. Lister & H. J. Weingartner, *Perspectives in cognitive neuroscience.* New York: Oxford University Press.

Johnson, M. K., Hirst, W., Phelps, E. A., & Volpe, B. T. Context, comprehension and amnesia (unpublished data).

Johnson, M. K., & Kim, J. K. (1985). Recognition of pictures by alcoholic Korsakoff patients. *Bulletin of the Psychonomic Society, 23,* 456–458.

Johnson, M. K., Kim, J. K., & Risse, G. (1985). Do alcoholic Korsakoff's syndrome patients acquire affective reactions? *Journal of Experimental Psychology: Learning, Memory, and Cognition, 11,* 22–36.

Johnson, M. K., & Raye, C. L. (1981). Reality monitoring. *Psychological Review, 88,* 67–85.

Kinsbourne, M., & Wood, F. (1975). Short-term memory processes and the amnesic syndrome. In D. Deutsch & J. A. Deutsch (Eds.), *Short-term memory* (pp. 258–291). New York: Academic Press.

Kinsbourne, M., & Wood, F. (1982). Theoretical considerations regarding the episodic-semantic memory distinction. In L. S. Cermak (Ed.), *Human memory and amnesia* (pp. 195–217). Hillsdale, N.J.: Erlbaum.

Kolers, P. A. (1975). Specificity of operations in sentence recognition. *Cognitive Psychology, 7,* 289–306.

Kovner, R., Mattis, S., & Goldmeier, E. (1983). A technique for promoting robust free recall in chronic organic amnesia. *Journal of Clinical Neuropsychology, 5,* 65–71.

Levin, H. S., High, W. M., Meyers, C. A., Von Laufen, A., Hayden, M. E., & Eisenberg, H. M. (1985). Impairment of remote memory after closed head injury. *Journal of Neurology, Neurosurgery, and Psychiatry, 48,* 556–563.

Lindsay, D. S., & Johnson, M. K. (1987). Reality monitoring and suggestibility: Children's ability to discriminate among memories from different sources. In S. J. Ceci, M. P. Toglia, & D. F. Ross (Eds.), *Children's eyewitness memory* (pp. 92–121). New York: Springer-Verlag.

Mandler, G. (1967). Organization and memory. In K. W. Spence & J. T. Spence (Eds.), *The psychology of learning and motivation* (Vol. 1, pp. 327–372). New York: Academic Press.

Mandler, G. (1980). Recognizing: The judgment of previous occurrence. *Psychological Review, 87,* 252–271.

Mayes, A., Meudell, P., & Neary, D. (1980). Do amnesics adopt inefficient encoding strategies with faces and random shapes? *Neuropsychologia, 18,* 527–540.

McAndrews, M. P., Glisky, E. L., & Schacter, D. L. (1987). When priming persists: Long-lasting implicit memory for a single episode in amnesic patients. *Neuropsychologia, 25,* 497–506.

McClelland, J. L. (1985). Distributed models of cognitive processes: Applications to learning and memory. In D. S. Olton, E. Gamzu, & S. Corkin (Eds.), *Memory dysfunctions: An integration of animal and human research from preclinical and clinical perspectives* (Annals of the New York Academy of Sciences, Vol. 444). New York: New York Academy of Sciences.

McDowell, J. (1979). Effects of encoding instructions and retrieval cuing on recall of Korsakoff patients. *Memory and Cognition, 7,* 232–239.

Milner, B. (1966). Amnesia following operation on the temporal lobes. In C. W. M. Whitty & O. L. Zangwill (Eds.), *Amnesia* (pp. 109–133). London: Butterworths.

Milner, B., Corkin, S., & Teuber, H. L. (1968). Further analysis of the hippocampal amnesic syndrome: 14 year follow-up study of H.M. *Neuropsychologia, 6,* 215–234.

Milner, B., & Petrides, M. (1984, November). Behavioural effects of frontal-lobe lesions in mar *Transactions in Neuroscience,* 403–407.

Mishkin, M., Malamut, B., & Bachevalier, J. (1984). Memories and habits: Two neural systems. In G. Lynch, J. L. McGaugh, & N. M. Weinberger (Eds.), *Neurobiology of learning and memory* (pp. 65–77). New York: Guilford.

Morton, J. (1985). The problem with amnesia: The problem with human memory. *Cognitive Neuropsychology, 2,* 281–290.

Moscovitch, M. (1982). Multiple dissociations of function in amnesia. In L. S. Cermak (Ed.), *Human memory and amnesia* (pp. 337–370). Hillsdale, N.J.: Erlbaum.

Moscovitch, M., Winocur, G., & McLachlan, D. (1986). Memory as assessed by recognition and reading time in normal and memory-impaired people with Alzheimer's disease and other neurological disorders. *Journal of Experimental Psychology: General, 115,* 331–347.

Nissen, M. J., & Bullemer, P. (1987). Attentional requirements of learning: Evidence from performance measures. *Cognitive Psychology, 19,* 1–32.

Parkin, A. J. (1982). Residual learning capability in organic amnesia. *Cortex, 18,* 417–440.

Parkinson, S. R. (1979). The amnesic Korsakoff syndrome: A study of selective and divided attention. *Neuropsychologia, 17,* 67–75.

Phelps, E. A., Hirst, W., Johnson, M. K., & Volpe, B. T. (1988). *Amnesia and recall: Building on prior knowledge.* Unpublished manuscript.

Redington, K., Volpe, B. T., & Gazzaniga, M. S. (1984). Failure of preference formation in amnesia. *Neurology, 34,* 536–638.

Ribot, T. A. (1977). Diseases of memory: An essay in positive psychology. In D. N. Robinson (Ed.), *Significant contributions to the history of psychology 1750–1920.* Washington, D.C.: University Publications of America. (Original work published 1882)

Schacter, D. L. (1987a). Memory, amnesia, and frontal lobe dysfunction. *Psychobiology, 15,* 21–36.

Schacter, D. L. (1987b). Implicit memory: History and current status. *Journal of Experimental Psychology: Learning, Memory, and Cognition, 13,* 501–518.

Schacter, D. L., Harbluk, J. L., & McLachlan, D. R. (1984). Retrieval without recollection: An experimental analysis of source amnesia. *Journal of Verbal Learning and Verbal Behavior, 23,* 593–611.

Schacter, D. L., & Tulving, E. (1982). Memory, amnesia, and the episodic/semantic distinction. In R. L. Isaacson & N. E. Spear (Eds.), *The expression of knowledge* (pp. 33–65). New York: Plenum.

Schank, R., & Abelson, R. (1977). *Scripts, plans, goals and understanding.* Hillside, N.J.: Erlbaum.

Shimamura, A. P., & Squire, L. R. (1988). Long-term memory in amnesia: Cued recall, recognition memory, and confidence ratings. *Journal of Experimental Psychology: Learning, Memory, and Cognition, 14,* 763–770.

Spear, N. E. (1984). Behaviours that indicate memory: Levels of expression. *Canadian Journal of Psychology, 38,* 348–367.

Squire, L. R. (1981a). *Memory and brain.* New York: Oxford University Press.

Squire, L. R. (1981b). Two forms of human amnesia: An analysis of forgetting. *Journal of Neuroscience, 1,* 635–640.

Squire, L. R. (1982). The neuropsychology of human memory. *Annual Review of Neuroscience, 5,* 241–273.

Squire, L. R. (1986). Mechanisms of memory. *Science, 232,* 1612–1619.

Squire, L. R. (1987, November). *Neural substrates of memory in humans and non-human primates.* Paper presented at the annual meeting of the Psychonomic Society, Seattle.

Squire, L. R., & Shimamura, A. P. (1986). Characterizing amnesic patients for neurobehavioral study. *Behavioral Neuroscience, 100,* 866–877.

Stein, B. S., & Bransford, J. D. (1979). Constraints on effective elaboration: Effects of precision and subject generation. *Journal of Verbal Learning and Verbal Behavior, 18,* 769–777.

Suengas, A. G., & Johnson, M. K. (1988). Qualitative effects of rehearsal on memories for perceived and imagined complex events. *Journal of Experimental Psychology: General, 117,* 377–389.

Talland, G. A. (1965). *Deranged memory.* New York: Academic Press.

Tulving, E. (1962). Subjective organization in free recall of "unrelated" words. *Psychological Review, 69,* 344–354.

Tulving, E. (1983). *Elements of episodic memory.* New York: Oxford University Press.

Warrington, E. K. (1982). The double dissociation of short- and long-term memory deficits. In L. S. Cermak (Ed.), *Human memory and amnesia* (pp. 61–76). Hillsdale, N.J.: Erlbaum.

Warrington, E. K., & Weiskrantz, L. (1982). Amnesia: A disconnection syndrome? *Neuropsychologia, 20,* 233–248.

Weinstein, A. (1987). *Preserved recognition memory in amnesia.* Unpublished doctoral dissertation, State University of New York at Stony Brook.

Wickelgren, W. A. (1979). Chunking and consolidation: A theoretical synthesis of semantic networks, configuring in conditioning, S–R versus cognitive learning, normal forgetting, the amnesic syndrome, and the hippocampal arousal system. *Psychological Review, 86,* 44–60.

Zajonc, R. B. (1980). Feeling and thinking: Preferences need no inferences, *American Psychologist, 35,* 151–175.

COMMENTARIES AND
ALTERNATIVE PERSPECTIVES

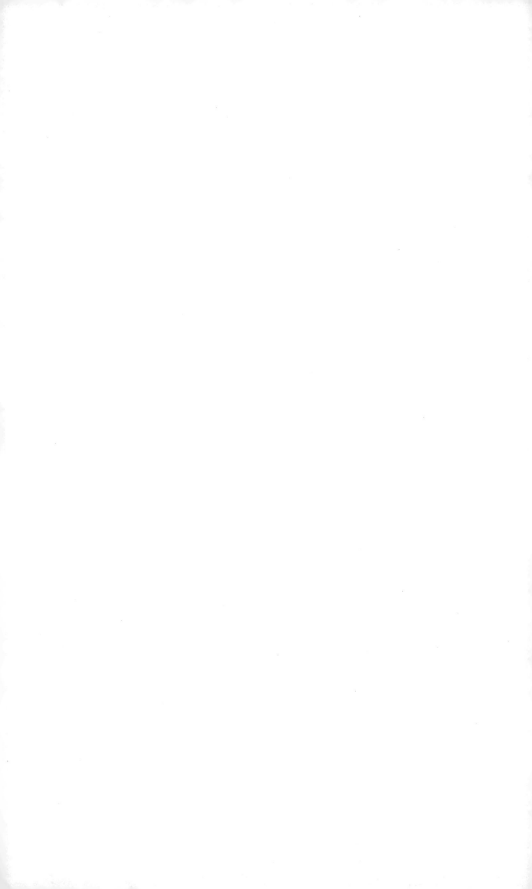

6

Neuromnemonics: Forms and Contents

NORMAN M. WEINBERGER

"Forms of memory" encompasses a broad and heterogeneous set of problems and approaches. The preceding chapters provide an indication of the extensive dimensions of current research.

Carew and his co-authors are concerned with different forms of memory within the domain of the neurophysiology of habituation, sensitization, and dishabituation in a marine gastropod mollusk. Holland also deals with forms of memory from the viewpoint of conditioning, but he does so within the framework of behavioral analyses alone; the conditioning paradigms used with rats are considerably more complex than those employed by Carew. Johnson focuses on three mnemonic processes in normal and amnesic humans, using tasks quite different from those involved in conditioning as well as stimulus material unique to human animals, that is, language-based stimuli. Morris emphasizes the importance of the network within which a mechanism of plasticity is embedded; he argues that although there may be a "cell alphabet" of *plasticity,* there is not yet an alphabet of *learning.*

In this short commentary I will try to point out some agreements and disagreements among the authors and emphasize some issues they do not cover. Specifically, I will deal with some aspects of the contents of memories, in distinction to forms, types, or processes of *neuromnemonics.* Future directions toward achieving closer relations between studies of memory in humans and other animals will also be considered briefly.

FORMS OF MEMORY

There is not uniform agreement concerning how one delineates forms of memory. The criteria to determine if there are multiple forms of memory focus on dissociations of one sort or another. Three chapters seem to consider dissociations as both necessary and sufficient criteria for the establishment of different forms, across species and learning situations; in one, judgment is reserved.

Carew and his colleagues argue that habituation, sensitization, and dishabituation are three different forms of memory because they appear sequentially during ontogenesis in a gastropod mollusk.

For Johnson, there are three sets of memory subsystems or processes: sensory, perceptual, and reflective. These are established by behavioral manipulations in normal and amnesic adults by the use of various tasks that a priori tap these various processes. Amnesics appear to be impaired most in the use of the reflective subsystem. Whether one refers to forms or subsystems, the thrust of Johnson's formulation is that of tripartite processing of stored experience.

Although Morris does not explicitly address the criteria for forms, his analysis of the theoretical position of Kandel implicitly accepts the division of some forms of learning into sensitization, pseudoconditioning on the one hand and alpha- and beta-conditioning on the other hand. His emphasis is on relationships between the former and the latter. Within the present context, this qualitative distinction is in the spirit of different forms of memory.

Holland provides evidence for independence between three pairs of subsystems: S–S versus S–R, CS–OR versus CS–UR pathways, and simple associative versus occasion-setting functions. Nonetheless, and unlike the other authors, Holland is reluctant to conclude that these constitute different forms of memory, suggesting that reification requires an explication of "functional incompatibility" within the context of the separate purposes served by each reputed system (Sherry & Schacter, 1987).

Like Holland, I am uncomfortable in having forms of memory proliferate with every demonstrable dissociation. The multiplication of types, particularly in the absence of adequate criteria, may not be particularly illuminating. This is especially so when reification entails little more than a restatement of operational definitions. My reservations concern the criteria, particularly the importance of dissociations. In brief, a dissociation may be a necessary criterion, but it does not seem to be a sufficient criterion.

For example, dissociations could occur if two behavioral manifestations of a single underlying process have different thresholds. Regarding this point, I am reminded of one of the major reasons for extensive use of the nictitating membrane-conditioned response in the rabbit: it is reputed to exhibit no response to a CS prior to pairing with airpuff to the cornea or shock to the orbit, so that the conditioned response is a beta rather than an alpha type—a new response rather than an elaboration of an existing response. These observations are valid at the behavioral level, but they do not permit conclusions at the neural level. Thus Cegavske (1974) reported that although an acoustic stimulus, to be used as the CS, did not produce neuromuscular responses, it did evoke neuronal discharges in the final common path, the nucleus of the VIth cranial nerve. In other words, there was an alpha response at the level of the motor neurons but a beta CR at the level of behavioral detection of conditioning. Moreover, while the behavioral detection of learning at the nictitating membrane exhibits no sensitization or pseudoconditioning, Cegavske, Patterson, and Thompson (1979) reported evidence for these processes in the VIth cranial nucleus. In short, the use of a dissociation as a *necessary* criterion for establishing separate forms or processes of learning and memory should be viewed with extreme caution if not considerable skepticism.

From another viewpoint, one may ask about the extent to which dissociations imply more than a lack of identity. If they do, what are they? If not, then is it fundamentally different to speak of forms of memory versus forms of limbs, forms of locomotion, forms of goal-attainment, and so on? In short, we must take care not to allow the common language terms, or "folk psychology language," to assume a role of importance that they do not merit.

At least two approaches might be helpful. First, one might look to other sciences—such as biological taxonomy and systematics—for methodologies for categorizing forms of memory (e.g., Tulving, 1985). This possibility immediately raises the question of the extent to which various forms of memory are related, as opposed to emphasizing dissociations that foster (but do not demand) simpler yes or no answers. This interrelatedness is certainly a very real concern of all of the authors.

Second, one might look to a logical analysis and a thorough explication of the various meanings of "forms" of memory. This includes the distinction of Morris—that a single cellular basis for information storage could be expressed as different forms of memory, depending on the network within which it is embedded. In this case, one could argue for a single form of memory at a cellular level but various forms of memory at a network level.

Both approaches are likely to result in a somewhat more precise and helpful formulation of forms than we now have.

INVOLVEMENT OF SENSORY SYSTEMS

There seems to be a surprisingly high degree of agreement concerning the fact that sensory systems are intimately involved in the storage of information. Thus for Carew and his co-authors the primary sensory neurons of *Aplysia* are actual sites of learning-induced plasticity. Morris accepts these findings. Holland concludes that associative conditioning can engage the CS "early" in the chain that ultimately leads to CRs. His conclusion is based on evidence that the CS can acquire the sensory properties of the US. Johnson's evidence supports the dynamic involvement of sensory and perceptual systems in learning and memory, in addition to the reflective processes to which most attention has been given.

This high degree of agreement is noteworthy in view of a tradition in which sensory systems have been viewed as of little or no importance in the dynamics of learning and memory (e.g., Fuster, 1984). One major reason for the reluctance to accord sensory systems the dynamic, learning-involved properties that have been repeatedly and exhaustively established since the mid-1940s (see Weinberger & Diamond, 1987, for a review of auditory cortex and learning) seems to center on a paradox. There seems to be a fundamental conflict between having sensory system neurons subject to two types of influence: the physical parameters of stimuli as transduced by a sheet of sensory epithelium, and the "psychological parameters" or acquired meaning of stimuli (Weinberger & Diamond, 1988). Neurons subject to both influences would provide ambiguous "reports"; for example, increased discharge might indicate increased stimulus intensity, increased psychological salience, or both.

We have provided both data and conceptual support for a solution to this paradox in the auditory system (Ryugo & Weinberger, 1978; Weinberger, 1980, 1982, 1984). Briefly, parallel subcortical paths may deal separately with the physical and psychological aspects of sound. The two paths (lemniscal and lemniscal–adjunct, respectively) coalesce in auditory cortex where in fact neuronal discharges represent their combined influence in pyramidal neurons. Strictly speaking, perception is the result.

This issue seems to have received little attention in the neurobiology of learning and memory. Thus the inherent ambiguity described above must be present in any organism in which learning alters primary sensory neurons, as in *Aplysia* or primary sensory receptors, as in *Hermissenda* (Alkon, 1986). It is not clear how or if this ambiguity is resolved in such organisms. A fundamental change in the role of sensory systems in learning may have evolved for vertebrates, more complex invertebrates, or both.

As to the engagement of the CS early in the sensory network that processes the US, Holland has provided evidence that the CS may actually "take on" some characteristics of the US. One might expect neurons in the CS path to acquire some of the properties of the US. That this may take place at the level of the magnocellular medial geniculate nucleus in the auditory system is suggested by a series of studies by LeDoux and associates. The circuit for conditioned fear to sound apparently goes from the lemniscal–adjunct auditory thalamus to the amygdala (LeDoux, Sakaguchi, & Reis, 1983; LeDoux, Sakaguchi, Iwata, & Reis, 1986; Iwata, LeDoux, Meeley, Arneric, & Reis, 1986). Thus while the story of brain and learning/memory is still incomplete, it would seem that sensory system plasticity will be a part of the large picture.

CONTENTS OF MEMORIES

There is another side to memory in addition to its forms: its contents. Inferences about what is learned—more specifically, what is stored and retrievable—are based on behavioral tests. Detailed characterization of such contents of memory, in distinction to the processes involved in storage and retrieval, usually requires precise tests following the learning experience in question. Failures to detect evidence of learning are a function of the sensitivity of the test, including the type of question posed by the experimenter. A full account of what was learned is seldom attempted because of the dauntingly large number of behavioral tests required. Reasonably, behavioral tests focus on the particular topic of the experimenter's interests, that is, the purpose of the experiment. For example, unless specifically tested for, the extent of contextual dependence is generally unknown.

As an example, Morris cites the oft-ignored report of Wagner (1978) indicating that habituation can be context dependent.

Neurobiological approaches to memory offer the potential for determining *all* of the information stored and the possible postlearning alterations, transformations, and even loss of the contents of storage. Since all behaviors are expressions of neurobiological structure and function, the neurobiological measures are potentially more sensitive and direct than are behavioral data. Currently used behavioral measures have not only the advantage of a reasonably well established methodology, but provide integrated output from the nervous system. Neurobiological measures could concentrate on the "trees" while missing the behavioral "forest."

Nonetheless, it should be admitted that both behavioral and neurobiological research on memory is largely the study of processes and forms rather than the study of the contents of memories. A notable attempt to use neurophysiology to read out content is the corpus of research by E. Roy John (e.g., 1967). This research attempted to use the frequency of flashes as "tracers" for memory content (see also John, 1980). Regardless of the ultimate status of this body of work, it seems clear that few neurobiologists have since trod that path.

To the extent that experiments on the content of memory continue to be disregarded because of technical problems, it is likely that theoretical formulations and their tests will also ignore issues relating to memories themselves. From this viewpoint, agreement about forms of memory and about the cellular and network bases of memory storage processes, in the absence of formulations about the nature of what is actually stored, will still leave us with a highly unsatisfactory account of memory. When neurobiological knowledge of the contents of memory can be used to accurately predict specific memory-dependent behavior, not limited to the contractions of a limited set of muscles, then we may achieve a comprehensive understanding of memory.

The agreement among the four chapters regarding the involvement of sensory systems in learning and memory suggests, as John argued, the possibility of "reading out" something about content, particularly within sensory systems. Through work by my colleagues and me on learning in the auditory system, something is now known about the "content" of the auditory cortex plasticity. It is not expressed as a general change in responsiveness to acoustic stimuli. Rather, the learning-dependent plasticity that rapidly develops in auditory cortex is highly specific to the frequency of the tone used as the conditioned stimulus (Diamond & Weinberger, 1986). The same type of findings have been obtained for habituation; the decrement in response is specific to the repeated frequency (Condon & Weinberger, in preparation; Westenberg & Weinberger, 1976). These types of data, in which changes in a stimulus dimension are induced by learning, may provide a basis for reading out content, to the extent that the change in representation of the CS, as part of the domain of acoustic frequency, for example, can be revealed. It seems feasible to extend these studies to humans because tonotopic organization has been found in human auditory cortex using noninvasive magnetoencephalography (MEG, Romani et al., 1982).

FUTURE DIRECTIONS

That a major gap exists between understanding of human and animal memory should come as no surprise. Carew and co-authors, Holland, Johnson, and Morris do not address the problem explicitly, but they illustrate the situation by emphasizing habituation and classical conditioning tasks with animals versus the types of tasks Johnson uses with humans. At the same time, some tasks seem to have a lot in common. Examples are found in the chapters by Holland and Johnson involving context, stimulus devaluation, and the use of complex tone sequences.

Regarding the first point, Holland's discussion of "occasion setting" in rats seems to be closely related to studies of context in humans. From a formal point of view, both involve control or modulation of relationships between events by designated cues—conditional learning. In the case of humans, the context is often more complex than in the rat experiments, such as place versus a flashing cue light. Nonetheless, the conditional control of associations can be explored in parallel in both types of subject.

Stimulus devaluation is widely used in animal experiments but not in humans. However, Johnson presented an intriguing example of stimulus devaluation ("John is good; Bill is bad"). She concluded that stimulus devaluation is an effective means of dissecting memory processes.

Because of the heavy reliance on language in studies of human memory, there is an insurmountable gap between human and animal research. However, there are alternatives between presenting animals with isolated stimuli in conditioning experiments and presenting humans with linguistic material. I refer here to music as stimulus. The processing of information and its storage may be quite different for individual stimuli and for stimulus sequences that are extended in time. Certainly some aspects of language involve such extended sequences. Furthermore, there are both human (e.g., Warren, 1982) and animal (e.g., D'Amato, in press) studies of memory for acoustic sequences. Since single neurons in auditory cortex are sensitive to the structure of sequences (Weinberger & McKenna, 1988), it seems of interest to (1) use highly similar experimental designs for humans and animals and (2) extend neurophysiological approaches to human auditory cortex.

CONCLUSIONS

This is an exciting time for memory research and for the prospects of achieving an understanding at the cellular level through behavioral insights into the acquisition and storage of information. As more data accumulate, it becomes increasingly urgent that the conceptual frameworks be developed and that more vigorous formulations of key concepts be achieved.

REFERENCES

Alkon, D. L. (1986). Persistent calcium-mediated changes of identified membrane currents as a cause of associative learning. In D. L. Alkon & J. Farley (Eds.), *Primary neural substrates of learning and behavioral change* (pp. 291–325). New York: Cambridge University Press.

Cegavske, C. F. (1974). *An approach to the neural substrates of classically conditioned rabbit nictitating membrane response.* Unpublished doctoral dissertation, University of California, Irvine.

Cegavske, C. F., Patterson, M. M., & Thompson, R. F. (1979). Neuronal unit activity in the abducens nucleus during classical conditioning of the nictitating membrane response in the rabbit. *Journal of Comparative and Physiological Psychology, 93,* 595–609.

Condon, C., & Weinberger, N. M. (in preparation). Habituation in auditory cortex of guinea pig: Frequency-specific decrements in receptive fields.

D'Amato, M. R. (1988). A search for tonal pattern perception in Cebus monkeys: Why monkeys can't hum a tune. *Music Perception, 5,* 453–480.

Diamond, D. M., & Weinberger, N. M. (1986). Classical conditioning rapidly induces specific changes in frequency receptive fields of single neurons in secondary and ventral ectosylvian auditory cortical fields. *Brain Research, 372,* 357–360.

Fuster, J. M. (1984). The cortical substrate of memory. In L. R. Squire & N. Butters (Eds.), *Neuropsychology of memory* (pp. 279–286). New York: Guilford.

Iwata, J., LeDoux, J. E., Meeley, M. P. Arneric, S., & Reis, D. J. (1986). Intrinsic neurons in the amygdaloid field projected by the medial geniculate body mediated emotional responses conditioned to acoustic stimuli. *Brain Research, 383,* 195–214.

John, E. R. (1967). *Mechanisms of memory.* New York: Academic Press.

John, E. R. (1980). A neurophysiological model of purposive behavior. In R. F. Thompson, L. H. Hicks, & V. B. Shvykov (Eds.), *Neural mechanisms of goal-directed behavior and learning* (pp. 93–115). New York: Academic Press.

LeDoux, J. E., Sakaguchi, A., Iwata, J., & Reis, D. J. (1986). Interruption of projections from the medial geniculate body to an archi-neostriatal field disrupts the classical conditioning of emotional response to acoustic stimuli. *Neuroscience, 17,* 615–627.

LeDoux, J. E., Sakaguchi, A., & Reis, D. J. (1983). Subcortical efferent projection of the medial geniculate nucleus mediated emotional responses conditioned to acoustic stimuli. *Journal of Neuroscience, 4,* 683–698.

Romani, G. L., Williamson, S. J., Kaufman, L., & Brenner, D. (1982). Characterization of the human auditory cortex by the neuromagnetic method. *Experimental Brain Research, 47,* 381–393.

Ryugo, D. K., & Weinberger, N. M. (1978). Differential plasticity of morphologically distinct neuron populations in the medial geniculate body of the cat during classical conditioning. *Behavioral Biology, 22,* 275–301.

Sherry, D. F., & Schacter, D. L. (1987). The evolution of multiple memory systems. *Psychological Review, 94,* 439–454.

Tulving, E. (1985). On the classical problem of learning and memory. In L. G. Nilsson & T. Archer (Eds.), *Perspectives on learning and memory* (pp. 67–95). Hillsdale, N.J.: Erlbaum.

Wagner, A. R. (1978). Expectancies and the priming of STM. In S. H. Hulse, H. Fowler, & W. K. Honig (Eds.), *Cognitive processes in animal behavior.* Hillsdale, N.J.: Erlbaum.

Warren, R. M. (1982). *Auditory perception. A new synthesis.* New York: Pergamon Press.

Weinberger, N. M. (1980). Neurophysiological studies of learning in association with the pupillary dilation conditioned reflex. In R. F. Thompson, L. H. Hicks, & V. B. Shvyrkov (Eds.), *Neural mechanisms of goal-directed behavior and learning* (pp. 241–261). New York: Academic Press.

Weinberger, N. M. (1982). Sensory plasticity and learning: The magnocellular medial geniculate nucleus of the auditory system. In C. D. Woody (Ed.), *Conditioning: Representation of involved neural function* (pp. 697–710). New York: Plenum.

Weinberger, N. M. (1984). The neurophysiology of learning: A view from the sensory side. In L. Squire & N. Butters (Eds.), *The neuropsychology of memory* (pp. 489–503). New York: Guilford.

Weinberger, N. M., & Diamond, D. M. (1987). Physiological plasticity in auditory cortex: Rapid induction by learning. *Progress in Neurobiology, 29,* 1–55.

Weinberger, N. M., & Diamond, D. M. (1988). Dynamic modulation of the auditory system by associative learning. In G. M. Edelman, W. E. Gall, & W. M. Cowan (Eds.), *Auditory function: The neurobiological bases of hearing* (pp. 485–512). New York: Wiley.

Weinberger, N. M., & McKenna, T. M. (1988). Sensitivity of single neurons in auditory cortex to frequency contour: Toward a neurophysiology of music perception. *Music Perception, 5,* 355–389.

Westenberg, I. S., & Weinberger, N. M. (1976). Evoked potential decrements in auditory cortex, II: Critical test for habituation. *Electroencephalography and Clinical Neurophysiology, 40,* 356–369.

7

Time and Memory

ROBERT W. DOTY

While memory preserves times past, a record that will instruct an organism's future, time also enters the mnemonic process in many other guises. A critical aspect is how long the mnemonic trace will endure, a time stretching from seconds to a lifetime. Vastly shorter, yet meaningfully measurable to some degree, is the time it takes to retrieve a memory.

The time between the occurrence of two successive events is also important. This temporal relation will determine whether, and in what direction, an enduring association will be formed between the events, as in the rules found applicable in forming conditioned reflexes. In terms of expectations from neurophysiology (e.g., Auyeung, May, Goh, & Sastry, 1987; Larson & Lynch, 1986), the direction of this association is paradoxical, for in the formation of a conditioned reflex it is the response to the first occurring event, the conditional stimulus, that becomes altered, whereas the response to the subsequent, unconditional stimulus is stable. I have termed this the "temporal paradox" of conditioning (Doty, 1979). This relation prevails for the usual type of Pavlovian conditioning, even in bees (Menzel, 1983), as well as when assayed with electrical excitation of randomly chosen points in mammalian neocortex (Doty & Giurgea, 1961) or, with entirely different parameters, for establishing long-term potentiation in the hippocampus with stimulus relations similar to those in conditioning (Levy & Steward, 1983). The temporal paradox is thus an underlying principle in the formation of such associations.

A more subtle temporal feature of mnemonic phenomena is the distinction that memories for events carry a relative "date," so that their sequence as well as their identity can be retrieved, whereas memories for "rules" or "habits" need no such tag, nor do they usually bear one. This is by now a familiar dichotomy (e.g., Mishkin, Malamut, & Bachevalier, 1984; Squire & Cohen, 1984; Thomas, 1984) and, as discussed below, there is strong reason to suppose that it is the hippocampus which somehow attaches the "date" to memory for unique events.

To varying degrees these themes of time and memory run through what follows; more important, they provide a number of opportunities for understanding the nature of mnemonic processes.

SLUGS AND SLUGGISHNESS

As Morris (Chapter 3, this volume) points out, there is a remarkable similarity in the optimum times for initiation of associative effects in mammals and the sea slug, *Aplysia*—something of the order of 500 msec in each case. Similarly, Carew and colleagues (Chapter 2, this volume) used interstimulus intervals of 1, 5, and 10 sec in a study of habituation in the slug, times wholly familiar from many comparable studies on mammals. Why, it must be asked, is the slug not sluggish in this regard? The answer is probably that the determinants are physical processes rather than chemical reactions in each case and therefore, given the comparable sizes of the critical elements (neurons, their terminals, and the intercellular spaces), are relatively independent of the temperature differences between the mammal and the slug (see, e.g., Höber, 1945).

The slug, too, is rather facile in the time it takes to recover from the perturbation of its synapses achieved by habituation, at least if the series of stimuli is not repeated. Again, the time course of recovery may reflect what is basically a diffusional process, complicated by sequestration, transport, or ionically controlled availability of transmitter. In other words, retention of this marginally mnemonic effect fits the earlier classification (Doty, 1979) as being "ionic" rather than "macromolecular."

The term macromolecular was introduced to indicate the probability that mnemonic processes that result in an essentially permanent trace and display the temporal paradox ultimately will involve more than a shuffling of ionic concentrations or permeabilities. A restructuring of synaptic–postsynaptic relations at a complex chemical level is implied by a macromolecular form of memory. This was originally visualized as being analogous to an immunochemical bonding, a concept that may still have merit. However, it now appears that although macromolecular changes occur locally at sites of altered synaptic function in a mnemonic context (e.g., Alkon, 1986; Hawkins, Clark, & Kandel, 1987; Hu et al., 1987; Lynch, 1986; Lynch & Baudry, 1984; Montarolo et al., 1986), they are unlikely to be permanent.

The rather ephemeral nature of these mnemonic effects may well be related to the metabolic half-life of the relevant macromolecules. Indeed, this severe problem is difficult to attack and hence often ignored in endeavors to understand how conditioned reflexes or human memory endures in the face of continual turnover in the chemical constituents at the presumed site of storage. The maximal half-life of neuronal proteins seems to lie in the order of a few weeks, most being much shorter (Dunlop, 1983; Margolis & Margolis, 1983). It is thus logical to suppose that this metabolic instability is counteracted by instructions at the nuclear level, modulating transcription of the genome to provide a continuing supply of the chemical constituents needed to maintain the mnemonically altered structure. Thus, although the effect is macromolecular, the essential feature of enduring memory may be that it is "transnuclear."

This was Halstead's original thesis (e.g., 1951): neuronal memory should utilize the already perfected processes of genetic memory. This concept fostered the examination of memory in relation to disruption of protein synthesis that has continued for three decades. The timing in such experiments, however, may go awry, for it is possible that the presumably chemical signal, which must pass from terminal or dendrite into the nucleus, is for some time inaccessible to manipulation during its transport. Kesner, McDonough, and I (1970) subjected cats to an aversive experience, followed 4 sec later by an electroconvulsive seizure. When tested 24 hr later, they were amnesic for the experience; but if 5 to 15 days later they received a second experience again followed in 4 sec by a seizure, the aversive experience was remembered. In other words, within 4 sec after the experience enough of a "trace" has been formed and become inaccessible to disruption by seizure activity that two such experiences formed a robust memory.

That synaptic processes can induce modulation of enzyme synthesis is now well documented for sympathetic ganglia (Thoenen, Otten, & Schwab, 1979) and the adrenal medulla (Guidotti & Costa, 1977). Furthermore, Thoenen and his colleagues showed that presynaptic terminals can imbibe chemical moieties, such as nerve growth factor, and transport them retrogradely to the nucleus where they alter protein production. Thus a mechanism can be perceived whereby both presynaptic and postsynaptic elements could mutually exchange some chemical constituent, provided that the timing of events in these two elements is appropriate (the "temporal paradox"?). Attaining the nucleus by microtubular transport, this signal might then permanently alter genetic transcription to produce whatever chemistry it may be that renders effective and permanent the connections of one neuron selectively to another.

Should it be true that memory as well as the regulation of neuronal interconnectivity is dependent on imbibition and subsequent transport of some chemical moiety to the cell nucleus, there to effect a modulation of the genome, then it is understandable why both vertebrate and invertebrate nervous systems (e.g., Kuffler, 1967; Landolt, 1965) are protected by a glial barrier from inadvertent macromolecular contamination. Unlike the immune system, whose function requires genomic response to newly present molecular species, function of the nervous system would, in the present speculation, be severely disrupted by random exposure to irrelevant molecules; it thus remains "immunologically privileged," shielded by the blood–brain barrier.

It must be noted that no permanent alteration, of either genomic output or mnemonic result of transnuclear effects, has yet been observed. The durations, so far, are measured in days or hours (Alkon, 1986; Guidotti & Costa, 1977; Hu et al., 1987; Montarolo et al., 1986; Thoenen et al., 1979). This might, of course, mean that the idea is merely fanciful, and that establishing permanent, mnemonically relevant synaptic alterations does not involve the hypothesized transnuclear mechanism. On the other hand, the systems amenable to test are not necessarily those in which a permanent change might be manifested or expected. There is, indeed, some question as to whether with their shorter life span and changing neuronal configurations (e.g., Carew et al., Chapter 2, this volume) invertebrates need or would benefit from permanently altered neural responses consequent to ephemeral environmental events.

SNARSKY'S PROBLEM

Not long after he began analyzing the nature of the "psychic secretions" he had observed from salivary glands of dogs, Pavlov set his student Snarsky to studying the effect of different materials, what we now call the unconditional stimuli, upon this secretion. Snarsky used three stimuli: sand, stones, and dry food, placed in the animal's mouth. He soon found that the dog produced a different type of salivation merely to the sight of these items (Pawlow, 1904). How was this to be explained? Pavlov asked, rhetorically, "Must one in order to understand these new phenomena immerse oneself in the *mental state* of the animal, endeavor to imagine its sensations, ideas, feelings, and desires similar to our own?" (Doty, 1987). This was the type of interpretation that Snarsky offered; but Pavlov, following his mentor Heidenhain, vehemently opted for limiting himself to what he considered to be the physiology.

Almost a century later Snarsky's approach is still alive and well in psychology. Holland (Chapter 4, this volume) concedes that "rats probably do not hallucinate *perfect* copies of absent USs" (italics added), yet his endeavors seem largely directed to the possiblity that they might summon up some form of mental image, for example, a "representation of food" activated by a tone. Holland, of course, is not alone in schematizing what may go on in the "black box" of the rat's mind, leaving, as he says, the plausibility of neurobiological analysis far behind. This is the stock in trade of cognitive science, discovering the rules without the neurons. The philosopher Searle (1984) astutely noted this penchant of psychologists for discerning "rules." He questions whether the rules can reveal the mechanism, for, as he says, "You don't need to suppose that there are any rules on top of the neurophysiological structures" (p. 51).

HIPPOCAMPUS AND THE STRING OF TIME

One of the common features acquired in the evolution of higher motile organisms is the ability to maintain orientation with respect to places of forage or safety. This is as true of the sand crab venturing along various radii away from its hole as of the fox patrolling the likely hunting spots of its territorial domain. Among the most remarkable and best studied examples of this orientational memory is that for vision in insects. In his meticulous and fascinating review Wehner (1981) lists some 140 species and about 200 references on this topic (see also Cartwright & Collett, 1983; Menzel, 1983).

Wasps and bees are particularly precise in this regard, ranging over a kilometer or more, yet returning within a few centimeters to the nest or hive. Among the essential features of this performance are, first, the recording of the sequence of landmarks encountered on the outward path, and then, second, the ability to navigate by these guides as they are encountered in reverse order during the return flight. In other words, there must be a "start recording" marker at the onset of the flight, differentiating those movements in time from those made previously; and there must then be a faithful registration of the sequence of the visual patterns encountered from that moment until the beginning of the return flight.

Like the sand crab, fossorial mammals must maintain an unerring orientation as to their position relative to the safety of their den, and larger mammals, including primitive humans, range over great distances without becoming "lost." There are two clues that the hippocampus plays a critical role in this ability. First is the fact that, in the rat, there is a clear candidate for a "now record" marker, the onset of theta rhythm whenever the rat begins to move itself through space (e.g., Vanderwolf & Leung, 1983). It is of particular interest that this rhythm is substantially controlled by pontine neurons (see Vertes, 1986), a site from which vestibular influences might readily be introduced. The relevance of vestibular input can be perceived from the experiments of Beritashvili, showing that the human deaf who lack the labyrinthine system are unable to reproduce blindly a path over which they have been led, whereas the deaf who lack only cochlear function are able to do so (Béritachvili, 1963).

The second clue comes from O'Keefe's discovery (see O'Keefe, 1983), now so rigorously defined by Ranck and his colleagues (e.g., Muller, Kubie, & Ranck, 1987), that many single units in the hippocampus of the rat reflect the animal's spatial location in their rate of discharge. It is also now clear that the rat needs its hippocampus to record its past positions in space (Morris, 1983, and Chapter 3, this volume; O'Keefe, 1983; Olton, 1983).

The well-studied case of H.M. (see Corkin, 1984) defined the nature of the deficit in man following bilateral loss of amygdala, hippocampus, and much of temporal cortex. The observations of Penfield and Mathieson (1974) and of Zola-Morgan, Squire, and Amaral (1986), however, suggest that most of the deficit arises from the hippocampal loss alone. Yet there is a slight problem here: first, the comparable syndrome in macaques seems also to require removal of amygdala as well as hippocampus (Mishkin, 1978; Murray & Mishkin, 1983); but, second, if H.M. is tested in the same manner as the macaques, he displays no deficit (Freed, Corkin, & Cohen, 1987).

Despite such discrepancies, there is still general agreement that the hippocampus is intimately involved in the recording and/or the retrieval of human memory for events, although it is a challenge experimentally to disentangle the recording from the retrieving. Furthermore, all normal human beings can testify that the sequence of events is a common and often essential part of their mnemonic record. Thus it can be hypothesized that in humans and other mammals the hippocampus subserves a phylogenetically ancient function, similar to that required by many flying insect species: upon a "start" signal, for example, as movement through space begins, its function is to tag each sensorial frame for subsequent identification of its position in the sequence. Indeed, this very procedure, an imaginary walk, was the principal method used by Luria's (1968) prodigious mnemonist in tagging items for subsequent retrieval. Compared with that in rodents, the "start" signal in primates may be relatively continuous, originating in the massive neocortical input to the hippocampus (Rosene & Van Hoesen, 1987) rather than or in addition to brain stem input associated with movement. This might explain the relative paucity (Crowne & Radcliffe, 1975; Isokawa-Akesson, Wilson, & Babb, 1987) of theta rhythm in primates or preservation of normal human mentality despite congenital absence of the fornix (Nathan & Smith, 1950).

It remains to be noted that although the hippocampus seems essential to the recording of memory for events, it is very unlikely to be the site of storage. This can be deduced, first, from the fact that hippocampal loss does not eliminate access to most previously established memories (e.g., Zola-Morgan et al., 1986) and, second, from the sheer magnitude of the cortical neuronal circuitry available for retaining a near infinity of memories, compared with the mere 10 million pyramidal cells bilaterally in CA1 whose loss so dramatically perturbs their recording. We have recently been able, somewhat fortuitously, to affirm the "near infinity of memory" even for macaques. An animal that had had exposure to a series of images for about 30 sec each was able, 6 or more months later, to distinguish these from highly comparable images intermingled with the earlier set (Ringo & Doty, 1985); this is similar to H.M., who can also perform such recognition of images at a 6-month interval (Freed & Corkin, 1985), even though missing hippocampus and amygdala.

The problem of mnemonic retrieval is indeed perplexing, be it such recognition or recall. For instance, mentally normal individuals suddenly afflicted with transient global amnesia lose contact with a significant, and continuous, portion of their past and are simultaneously unable to retain a record of present events: they display both retrograde and anterograde amnesia (see, e.g., Kushner & Hauser, 1985; Patten, 1971). The condition commonly clears within a matter of hours thus dramatically evidencing the separation between established memories, which remain intact, and the mechanisms for forming and retrieving them. Although the etiology of this bizarre confusion remains uncertain, speculation and suggestive evidence focuses on the hippocampal area.

Such "bidirectional" amnesia may be permanent if there is massive loss of limbic stuctures (Damasio, Eslinger, Damasio, Van Hoesen, & Cornell, 1985). More interesting, however, is the situation in which it can be demonstrated that retrieval per se is perturbed. This can be achieved to varying degrees by electrical stimulation of the hippocampus or associated structures in rats (e.g., Collier, Quirk, & Routtenberg, 1987), macaques (e.g., Overman & Doty, 1979), and humans (e.g., Halgren, Wilson, & Stapleton, 1985), the latter proving specifically an effect on retrieval per se.

One of the more fascinating and mysterious facts about retrieval of memories is that following various forms of cerebral trauma the distant past may remain available while more recent memories are inaccessible (e.g., Russell, 1959; Squire & Cohen, 1979). There is thus some temporal gradient in vulnerability, not of the memories but of their retrieval. This is again seen in humans with electrical stimulation of the hippocampal area, the distance back from time present whose retrieval is perturbed and the duration of the effect both being proportional to the intensity of the stimulation (Bickford, Mulder, Dodge, Svien, & Rome, 1958). In rare enigmatic cases access to a span of memory dating back from time present as much as 40 years may be suddenly and permanently lost (Andrews, Poser, & Kessler, 1982).

The remarkable thing in all these examples is the relative precision of the temporal dividing line between retrievable and irretrievable memories, and the near continuity of the inaccessible span. Penfield and Mathieson (1974), in their two autopsied cases of temporal lobectomy, noted that the date of irretrievable memories extended farther back in time for the patient having the more posteriorly extending hippocampal excision; they postulated that memories, or their mechanism of retrieval, might gradually migrate in time, with serial order preserved, along the extent of the hippocampus. Given current knowledge, such a mechanism is difficult to imagine, but the numerous instances of date-specific temporally continuous spans of irretrievability suggest a chronotopic mapping of times past somewhere within the nervous system. Perhaps the hippocampus is a microminiature quipu, continually knotting the present and stringing it anatomically into the past.

MACAQUE, MAN, AND CEREBRAL DUALITY

One of the major riddles of memory, seldom posed, is how or whether the two cerebral hemispheres are united in the mnemonic process: Are memories redundant, stored in each hemisphere, or, as proposed by Doty, Negrão, and Yamaga (1973), are they unilateral and available to the other hemisphere via the forebrain commissures? That one hemisphere via the forebrain commissures can gain access to memories established exclusively in the other has recently been affirmed (Kucharski & Hall, 1987). The relevance of these interhemispheric questions to Johnson's presentation (Chapter 5, this volume) lies in two facts. First, each hemisphere has somewhat different processing strategies, for example, for visual information (see Zaidel, 1987). Thus the "functional forms" of memory will have to differ even between the hemispheres.

The second issue concerns retrieval and "amnesia." Cronin-Golomb (1986) demonstrated that even in the absence of the forebrain commissures one hemisphere can gain a certain degree of access to information in the other via tenuous clues as to the affective tone generated by this information and communicated bilaterally. The situation is perhaps unique as a pure case of failure of retrieval, the one hemisphere clearly knowing while the other lacks access to all details. "Amnesia" is complete, a given hemisphere being unable to designate what is or was viewed by the other, yet the ignorant hemisphere can garner clues from the innumerably subtle shades of emotional tone generated by items that the other hemisphere perceives.

Now, is not the amnesic patient preserving some appropriate emotional evaluation of a given face, while all details as to the origin of this emotional response remain unavailable, just what Johnson describes? The point here is not that amnesia ordinarily arises from failure of interhemispheric communication, but that mechanisms, as Searle (1984) says, cannot be discerned from rules. Introspection—be it Snarsky (see above) "explaining" forms of salivation in his dogs or Johnson "noting," "shifting," "refreshing," and the like—describes the problem but does not usefully clarify it.

There is certainly a need for clarification, since amnesia does have many forms. As noted, H.M. without amygdala and hippocampus can nevertheless recognize visual material almost as well as normal macaques (Freed et al., 1987). Yet even macaques with comparable neurological loss are able somehow not only to master almost as well as normal animals the acquisition of 20 concurrent visual discriminations when presented with one trial per day, but they "learn how to learn" such discriminations as well (Murray, 1987). What, then, of the vaunted role of the hippocampus (and amygdala?) in memory?

There are at least two intertwined factors here: the role of language and the role of the hippocampus. When the former factor is essentially unavailable in tagging visual images, mnemonic performance of macaques overlaps that of humans (Doty, Ringo, & Lewine, 1988; Ringo, Lewine, & Doty, 1986). In comparing the mnemonic performance of patients such as H.M. and macaques with similar neurological loss, it would seem essential that tests be used in which human ability is at the same level as that of macaques—without the linguistic advantage.

It is now abundantly clear that many things are remembered in the absence of the hippocampus, yet is seems to serve some special role in making memory traces available for conscious analysis, Johnson's "reflection" if you will. Perhaps this is achieved by its role in "dating" each trace—preserving its temporal sequence—so that it may subsequently be identified for retrieval. The amygdala, in turn, might similarly provide an emotional "tag" to each trace. Some tantalizingly suggestive evidence for the latter is provided by the experiments of Meyer and his colleagues (see Meyer, 1984), where amnesia following electroconvulsive shock occurs for motivationally rather than temporally related "memories."

Again, an understanding of retrieval is essential to understanding memory. Sternberg (1966) invented an ingenious means of measuring the time it takes to retrieve a memory, admittedly one of recent vintage. He presented subjects with, say, one to six target items, and subsequently required them to respond as rapidly as possible to distinguish whether a presented item (probe) was or was not a member of the target set. The results were remarkably clear: there was a nearly linear relation between number of target items and accrued time to respond. Each item added roughly 30 msec to the reaction time, and since all other times—perception, movement, and so on—should be independent of set size, this 30 msec should be the time it takes to search and retrieve an additional item from memory.

Sands and Wright (1982) were able to train a macaque to perform this task, and they found a similar monotonic relation between reaction time and number of target items. We repeated this, using the identical material on macaques and humans (Lewine, unpublished data; Lewine, Doty, Provencal, & Astur, 1987). While maintaining the same level of accuracy, intact macaques require only 5 to 11 msec per added target, compared with 17 to 31 msec for the human subjects. In other words, macaques can search their memory three times faster than can man. The most parsimonious explanation would seem to be simple neurophysiology: the macaque brain being only one tenth the volume of that in humans, the relevant conduction paths and times must be significantly shorter. The possibility does remain, however, that the human mnemonic search includes a qualitatively different step, perhaps further verification prior to decision.

This paradigm takes on added interest when the task can be apportioned selectively between the two hemispheres (Lewine & Doty, work in progress). This is made possible by transection of the optic chiasm. Three macaques have been observed thus far, two with only the splenium of the corpus callosum and one with only the anterior commissure remaining of the forebrain commissures. The relation between reaction time and number of target items is unaltered in these animals; it is about 6 msec per added item. The error rate is slightly higher (5–10%) when the target information is given to one hemisphere and the probe stimuli (target and nontarget items) are presented to the other for response than when target and probe go to the same hemisphere. In other words, accuracy is slightly degraded when performance depends on commissural as opposed to intrahemispheric paths. However, there is no systematic difference in reaction time for interhemispheric versus intrahemispheric performance.

When target items are apportioned between the hemispheres, the splenium is wholly effective in unifying the mnemonic performance, so that, for instance, if three target items are given to one hemisphere and three to the other, both the error rate and the reaction time reflect the total of six items. However, with the anterior commissure in such circumstance, while the error rate is the same as if the six targets have all been given to one hemisphere, the reaction time is appropriate for the presence of only three items *if an only if the probe presented matches a target given the responding hemisphere:* otherwise here too the time reflects six items.

From these and other data it appears that unilateral input of a target forms a bilateral engram, unifying the hemispheres completely in the case of the splenium and nearly so for the anterior commissure. In each case the number of errors is correlated with the total number of target items, regardless of how target presentation and probing are distributed between the hemispheres. Nor is there any indication of the delay that might be expected were it necessary to link a probe presented to one hemisphere with target information stored in the other.

With the anterior commissure, however, it seems that one hemisphere can or does distinguish targets which it has received from those given to the other. In such a case, if each hemisphere is given three targets, the reaction time is appropriate for three if the probe is a member of the target set given to the hemisphere viewing the probe, whereas if the probe is not a member of that set, the reaction time is the same as if all six items were in a single hemisphere.

The absence of an added delay when target and probe are presented interhemispherically rather than intrahemispherically is strong evidence that the target information has been distributed bilaterally, especially with the splenium (and contrary to the prediction of Doty et al., 1973). Although it is possible that the time for interhemispheric transmission might be on the order of only a few milliseconds, the known anatomy and physiology of callosal fibers strongly suggest that the time should be much longer. Indeed, for humans, if the slower axons were involved and a conduction path of 200 mm were traversed, a one-way interhemispheric passage could easily run 200 msec or more (Swadlow, Geschwind, & Waxman, 1979). Perhaps this is the origin of the inherent slowness in the human search through the inventory of remembered targets, 20 to 30 msec per item versus 6 msec for macaques. Humans, with pronounced hemispheric specialization, must verify the engrams in each hemisphere, whereas the macaque, lacking such specialization, can rest content with the bilaterality of its target engrams.

CONCLUSIONS

Time is relevant to memory not only as (1) the duration of the mnemonic change, which may be permanent and lifelong, but also in (2) the temporal relation between two stimuli to form an association between them, (3) the relative precision of the period elided in retrograde amnesia, however produced, and (4) the time required to retrieve an item from memory. It is proposed that, in the face of continual metabolic replacement, (1) is achieved by a transport of material in and out of the cell nucleus to activate a particular genetic code, and that this feature is relevant to the phenomena in (2) which, in terms of classical neurophysiology, are temporally paradoxical.

It is also suggested that the hippocampus is the mammalian embodiment of a phylogenetically ancient mechanism for recording the sequence of events, and that the sequential "tag" that it provides is of prime importance in the process of retrieval.

Sternberg's serial probe recognition task was used to study (4) above. It was found that for recognition of a series of targets each additional item in the mnemonic inventory added 17 to 31 msec to the reaction time for individual human subjects, whereas for macaques the corresponding figures were 5 to 11 msec. In other words, macaques can "search" their mnemonic store about three times faster than can man. Judged by times accrued in the Sternberg paradigm in various experiments with "split-brain" macaques, it seems that the splenium of the corpus callosum as well as the anterior commissure produce bilateral engrams of the target items.

Acknowledgments

Preparation of these comments and original work reported here was supported by a Javits Award, NS20052, from the National Institute of Neurological and Communicative Disorders and Stroke, National Institutes of Health. I am particularly indebted to Jeffrey D. Lewine for permission to cite unpublished work from his forthcoming doctoral dissertation, and to him and James L. Ringo for consistently stimulating discussions of the phenomena of memory.

REFERENCES

Alkon, D. L. (1986). Changes of membrane currents and calcium-dependent phosphorylation during associative learning. In D. L. Alkon & C. D. Woody (Eds.), *Neural mechanisms of conditioning* (pp. 1–18). New York: Plenum.

Andrews, E., Poser, C. M., & Kessler, M. (1982). Retrograde amnesia for forty years. *Cortex, 18*, 441–458.

Auyeung, A., May, P. B. Y., Goh, J. W., & Sastry, B. R. (1987). Temporal requirements of associative short-term potentiation in CA_1 neurons of rat hippocampus. *Neuroscience Letters, 79*, 117–122.

Béritachvili, I. S. (1963). Les mécanismes nerveux de l'orientation spatiale chez l'homme. *Neuropsychologia, 1*, 233–249.

Bickford, R. G., Mulder, D. W., Dodge, H. W. Jr., Svien, H. J., & Rome, H. P. (1958). Changes in memory functions produced by electrical stimulation of the temporal lobe in man. In H. C. Solomon, S. Cobb, & W. Penfield (Eds.), *The brain and human behavior* (pp. 227–243). (Research Publications Association for Research in Nervous and Mental Disease, Vol. 30). Baltimore: Williams & Wilkins.

Cartwright, B. A., & Collett, T. S. (1983). Landmark learning in bees. Experiments and models. *Journal of Comparative Physiology-A, 151*, 521–543.

Collier, T. J., Quirk, G. J., & Routtenberg, A. (1987). Separable roles of hippocampal granule cells in forgetting and pyramidal cells in remembering spatial information. *Brain Research, 409*, 316–328.

Corkin, S. (1984). Lasting consequences of bilateral medial temporal lobectomy: Clinical course and experimental findings in H.M. *Seminars in Neurology, 4*, 249–259.

Cronin-Golomb, A. (1986). Subcortical transfer of cognitive information in subjects with complete forebrain commissurotomy. *Cortex, 22*, 499–519.

Crowne, D. P., & Radcliffe, D. D. (1975). Some characteristics and functional relations of the electrical activity of the primate hippocampus and a hypothesis of hippocampal function. In R. L. Isaacson & K. H. Pribram (Eds.), *The hippocampus: Vol. 2. Neurophysiology and behavior* (pp. 185–206). New York: Plenum.

Damasio, A. R., Eslinger, P. J., Damasio, H., Van Hoesen, G. W., & Cornell, S. (1985). Multimodal amnesic syndrome following bilateral temporal and basal forebrain damage. *Archives of Neurology, 42*, 252–259.

Doty, R. W. (1979). Neurons and memory: Some clues. In M. A. B. Brazier (Ed.), *Brain mechanisms in memory and learning: From the single neuron to man* (pp. 53–63). (International Brain Research Organization Monograph Series, Vol. 4). New York: Raven.

Doty, R. W. (1987). W. Horsley Gantt: Physiologist, Pavlovian. In F. J. McGuigan & T. A. Ban (Eds.), *Critical issues in psychology, psychiatry, and physiology. A memorial to W. Horsley Gantt* (pp. 343–356). New York: Gordon & Breach.

Doty, R. W., & Giurgea, C. (1961). Conditioned reflexes established by coupling electrical excitation of two cortical areas. In A. Fessard, R. W. Gerard, & J. Konorski (Eds.), *Brain mechanisms and learning* (pp. 133–151). Oxford: Blackwell.

Doty, R. W., Negrão, N., & Yamaga, K. (1973). The unilateral engram. *Acta Neurobiologiae Experimentalis, 33,* 711–728.

Doty, R. W., Ringo, J. L., & Lewine, J. D. (1988). Humanlike characteristics of visual mnemonic system in macaques. In C. D. Woody, D. L. Alkon, & J. L. McGaugh (Eds.), *Cellular mechanisms of conditioning and behavioral plasticity* (pp. 313–328). New York: Plenum.

Dunlop, D. S. (1983). Protein turnover in brain. Synthesis and degradation. In A. Lajtha (Ed.), *Handbook of neurochemistry (2nd ed.): Vol. 5. Metabolic turnover in the nervous system* (pp. 25–63). New York: Plenum.

Freed, D. M., & Corkin, S. (1985). Rates of forgetting in H.M.: Six-month recognition. *Society for Neuroscience Abstracts, 11,* 458.

Freed, D. M., Corkin, S., & Cohen, N. J. (1987). Forgetting in H.M.: A second look. *Neuropsychologia, 25,* 461–471.

Guidotti, A., & Costa, E. (1977). Trans-synaptic regulation of tyrosine 3-mono-oxygenase biosynthesis in rat adrenal medulla. *Biochemical Pharmacology, 26,* 817–823.

Halgren, E., Wilson, C. L., & Stapleton, J. M. (1985). Human medial temporal-lobe stimulation disrupts both formation and retrieval of recent memories. *Brain and Cognition, 4,* 287–295.

Halstead, W. C. (1951). Brain and intelligence. In L. A. Jeffress (Ed.), *Cerebral mechanisms in behavior. The Hixon Symposium* (pp. 244–288). New York: Wiley.

Hawkins, R. D., Clark, G. A., & Kandel, E. R. (1987). Cell biological studies of learning in simple vertebrate and invertebrate systems. In F. Plum (Ed.), *Handbook of physiology: Sec 1. The nervous system: Vol. 5. Higher functions of the brain* (pp. 25–83). Bethesda, Md.: American Physiological Society.

Höber, R. (1945). *Physical chemistry of cells and tissues.* Philadelphia: Blakiston.

Hu, G.-Y., Hvalby, O., Walaas, S. I., Albert, K. A., Skjeflo, P., Andersen, P., & Greengard, P. (1987). Protein kinase C injection into hippocampal pyramidal cells elicits features of long term potentiation. *Nature, 328,* 426–429.

Isokawa-Akesson, M., Wilson, C. L., & Babb, T. L. (1987). Diversity of periodic pattern of firing in human hippocampal neurons. *Experimental Neurology, 98,* 137–151.

Kesner, R. P., McDonough, J. J. Jr., & Doty, R. W. (1970). Diminished amnestic effect of a second electroconvulsive seizure. *Experimental Neurology, 27,* 527–533.

Kucharski, D., & Hall, W. G. (1987). New routes to early memories. *Science, 238,* 786–788.

Kuffler, S. W. (1967). The Ferrier lecture: Neuroglial cells: Physiological properties and a potassium mediated effect of neuronal activity on the glial membrane potential. *Proceedings of the Royal Society of London (Biology), 168,* 1–21.

Kushner, M. J., & Hauser, W. A. (1985). Transient global amnesia: A case-control study. *Annals of Neurology, 18,* 684–691.

Landolt, A. M. (1965). Elektronenmikroskopische Untersuchungen an der Perikaryenschicht der Corpora pedunculata der Waldameise *(Formica lugubris Zett.)* mit besonderer Berücksichtigung der Neuron-Glia-Beziehung. *Zeitschrift für Zellforschung, 66,* 701–736.

Larson, J., & Lynch, G. (1986). Induction of synaptic potentiation in hippocampus by patterned stimulation involves two events. *Science, 232,* 985–988.

Levy, W. B., & Steward, O. (1983). Temporal contiguity requirements for long-term associative potentiation/depression in the hippocampus. *Neuroscience, 8,* 791–797.

Lewine, J. D., Doty, R. W., Provencal, S., & Astur, R. (1987). Monkey beats man in efficiency of mnemonic retrieval. *Society for Neuroscience Abstracts, 13,* 206.

Luria, A. R. (1968). *The mind of mnemonist. A little book about a vast memory* (L. Solotaroff, Trans.). Chicago: Henry Regnery.

Lynch, G. (1986). *Synapses, circuits, and the beginnings of memory.* Cambridge, Mass.: MIT Press.

Lynch, G., & Baudry, M. (1984). The biochemistry of memory: A new and specific hypothesis. *Science, 224,* 1057–1063.

Margolis, R. K., & Margolis, R. U. (1983). Glycoproteins and proteoglycans. In A. Lajtha (Ed.), *Handbook of neurochemistry (2nd ed.): Vol. 5. Metabolic turnover in the nervous system* (pp. 177–204). New York: Plenum.

Menzel, R. (1983). Neurobiology of learning and memory: The honeybee as a model system. *Naturwissenschaften, 70,* 504–511.

Meyer, D. R. (1984). The cerebral cortex: Its role in memory storage and remembering. *Physiological Psychology, 12,* 81–88.

Mishkin, M. (1978). Memory in monkeys severely impaired by combined but not by separate removal of amygdala and hippocampus. *Nature, 273,* 297–298.

Mishkin, M., Malamut, B., & Bachevalier, J. (1984). Memories and habits: Two neural systems. In G. Lynch, J. L. McGaugh, & N. M. Weinberger (Eds.), *Neurobiology of learning and memory* (pp. 65–77). New York: Guilford.

Montarolo, P. G., Goelet, P., Castellucci, V. F., Morgan, J., Kandel, E. R., & Schacher, S. (1986). A critical period for macromolecular synthesis in long-term heterosynaptic facilitation in *Aplysia. Science, 234,* 1249–1254.

Morris, R. G. M. (1983). An attempt to dissociate "spatial-mapping" and "working-memory" theories of hippocampal function. In W. Seifert (Ed.), *Neurobiology of the hippocampus* (pp. 405–432). London: Academic Press.

Muller, R. U., Kubie, J. L., & Ranck, J. B. Jr. (1987). Spatial firing patterns of hippocampal complex-spike cells in a fixed environment. *Journal of Neuroscience, 7,* 1935–1950.

Murray, E. A. (1987). Normal learning set formation in monkeys with combined ablation of the amygdaloid complex and hippocampal formation. *Society for Neuroscience Abstracts, 13,* 206.

Murray, E. A., & Mishkin, M. (1983). Severe tactual memory deficits in monkeys after combined removal of the amygdala and hippocampus. *Brain Research, 270,* 340–344.

Nathan, P. W., & Smith, M. C. (1950). Normal mentality associated with a maldeveloped "rhinencephalon." *Journal of Neurology, Neurosurgery and Psychiatry, 13,* 191–197.

O'Keefe, J. (1983). Spatial memory within and without the hippocampal system. In W. Seifert (Ed.), *Neurobiology of the hippocampus* (pp. 375–403). London: Academic Press.

Olton, D. S. (1983). Memory functions and the hippocampus. In W. Seifert (Ed.), *Neurobiology of the hippocampus* (pp. 335–373). London: Academic Press.

Overman, W. H. Jr., & Doty, R. W. (1979). Disturbance of delayed match-to-sample in macaques by tetanization of anterior commissure versus limbic system or basal ganglia. *Experimental Brain Research, 37,* 511–524.

Patten, B. M. (1971). Transient global amnesia syndrome. *Journal of the American Medical Association, 217,* 690–691.

Pawlow, J. P. (1904). Psychische Erregung der Speicheldrüsen. *Ergebnisse der Physiologie, biologische Chemie und experimentelle Pharmakologie, 3,* 177–193.

Penfield, W., & Mathieson, G. (1974). Memory; autopsy findings and comments on the role of hippocampus in experiential recall. *Archives of Neurology, 31,* 145–154.

Ringo, J. L., & Doty, R. W. (1985). A macaque remembers pictures briefly viewed six months earlier. *Behavioural Brain Research, 18,* 289–294.

Ringo, J. L., Lewine, J. D., & Doty, R. W. (1986). Comparable performance by man and macaque on memory for pictures. *Neuropsychologia, 24,* 711–717.

Rosene, D. L., & Van Hoesen, G. W. (1987). The hippocampal formation of the primate brain: A review of some comparative aspects of cytoarchitecture and connections. In E. G. Jones & A. Peters (Eds.), *Cerebral cortex* (Vol. 6, pp. 345–456). New York: Plenum.

Russell, W. R. (1959). *Brain, memory and learning: A neurologist's view.* Oxford: Clarendon Press.

Sands, S. F., & Wright, A. A. (1982). Monkey and human pictorial memory scanning. *Science, 216,* 1333–1334.

Searle, J. (1984). *Minds, brains and science.* Cambridge, Mass.: Harvard University Press.

Squire, L. R., & Cohen, N. (1979). Memory and amnesia: Resistance to disruption develops for years after learning. *Behavioral and Neural Biology, 25,* 115–125.

Squire, L. R., & Cohen, N. J. (1984). Human memory and amnesia. In G. Lynch, J. L. McGaugh, & N. M. Weinberger (Eds.), *Neurobiology of learning and memory* (pp. 3–64). New York: Plenum.

Sternberg, S. (1966). High-speed scanning in human memory. *Science, 153,* 652–654.

Swadlow, H. A., Geschwind, N., & Waxman, S. G. (1979). Commissural transmission in humans. *Science, 204,* 530–531.

Thoenen, H., Otten, U., & Schwab, M. (1979). Orthograde and retrograde signals for the regulation of neuronal gene expression: The peripheral sympathetic nervous system as a model. In F. O. Schmitt & F. G. Worden (Eds.), *The neurosciences, fourth study program* (pp. 911–928). Cambridge, Mass.: MIT Press.

Thomas, G. J. (1984). Memory: Time binding in organisms. In L. R. Squire & N. Butters (Eds.), *Neuropsychology of memory* (pp. 374–384). New York: Guilford.

Vanderwolf, C. H., & Leung, L.-W. S. (1983). Hippocampal rhythmical slow activity: A brief history and the effects of entorhinal lesions and phencyclidine. In W. Seifert (Ed.), *Neurobiology of the hippocampus* (pp. 275–302). London: Academic Press.

Vertes, R. P. (1986). A new role for FTG neurons? *Behavioral and Brain Sciences, 9,* 425–426.

Wehner, R. (1981). Spatial vision in arthropods. In H. Autrum (Ed.), *Handbook of sensory physiology: Vol. VII/6C. comparative physiology and evolution of vision in invertebrates, C: Invertebrate visual centers and behavior II* (pp. 287–616). Berlin: Springer-Verlag.

Zaidel, D. W. (1987). Hemispheric asymmetry in memory for pictorial semantics in normal subjects. *Neurospsychologia, 25,* 487–495.

Zola-Morgan, S., Squire, L. R., & Amaral, D. G. (1986). Human amnesia and the medial temporal region: Enduring memory impairment following a bilateral lesion limited to field CA_1 of the hippocampus. *Journal of Neuroscience, 6,* 2950–2967.

8

Forms of Memory: Issues and Directions

ARTHUR P. SHIMAMURA

What constitutes evidence for different forms of memory? In behavioral neuroscience, memory forms are often distinguished by the kind of test paradigm that is used—from nonassociative learning paradigms such as habituation and sensitization to verbal learning paradigms such as word recall and recognition. A critical issue in understanding the neurobiological basis of memory is to identify and characterize the neural architecture that supports such behavioral expressions of memory. In this chapter I evaluate evidence that has been used to argue for different forms of memory, particularly in the domain of neuropsychological research.

TWO EXTREME VIEWS OF MEMORY REPRESENTATION

We can approach the idea of forms of memory from two extreme views. First, one could argue that there is only one, undifferentiated neural system for memory. This view is similar to that proposed by Lashley (1950). That is, the neural substrate of memory is so distributed and so interactive that one cannot locate any subcomponents or functional units within the system. Thus any damage within the system causes some level of memory impairment, and every part of this system is equally potent in producing impairment. An extreme version of this view predicts that performance on every test of memory should decrease to some extent as a result of damage to the brain.

It is easy to reject this extreme view on the basis of human neuropsychological data. Memory functions do not degrade in a nonspecific manner as a result of brain injury. That is, not all areas of the brain contribute equally to memory— there is some differentiation and specialization of memory function. In particular, damage to the medial temporal or diencephalic region produces a selective impairment of memory. Moreover, studies of memory in various animal models (see Chapters 2, 3, and 4, this volume) suggest that it is possible to dissociate the neural architecture underlying one form of memory from another.

The opposite extreme view is that all memory representations are unique, so that divisions of memory into two, three, or more forms are arbitrary and erroneous. In some sense, all memory representations should be differentiated from one another, otherwise they would produce exactly the same behavioral consequence. Yet some divisions in memory may be especially honored by the brain. That is, some memory forms may share similar yet not identical neural substrates, and others may be quite distinct. In this sense, it would be useful to develop classes or divisions of memory forms, just as it is useful to classify the multitude of animal species into a taxonomy. Even though all animal species are considered to be different to some extent, it has been useful to identify classes, orders, and families of species.

DIVISIONS OF MEMORY AND BEHAVIORAL DISSOCIATIONS

Many divisions of memory have been proposed, and some of them are listed in Table 8.1. These classifications are not mutually exclusive, and in fact there is much overlap between some of them. A common way to establish evidence for divisions of memory is to identify dissociations between two putatively different forms of memory. Figure 8.1 illustrates the ideal data set for establishing a single dissociation. Performance by a control group indicates normal performance on two tests (tests A and B). Group 1 could represent a group that has a damaged neural system. This group could be a group of experimentally lesioned animals, a group of neurologically impaired patients, or a group given a pharmacological agent. For example, Morris (Chapter 3, this volume) showed that rats are impaired on a spatial memory test (test A) but not on a visual discrimination test (test B) when they are injected with D-2-amino-5-phosphonovalerate (AP-5), a pharmacological agent that blocks N-methyl-D-aspartate (NMDA) receptor

TABLE 8.1   Divisions of Memory

Fact memory	Skill memory
Declarative	Procedural
Memory	Habit
Explicit	Implicit
Knowing that	Knowing how
Cognitive mediation	Semantic
Conscious recollection	Skills
Elaboration	Integration
Memory with record	Memory without record
Autobiographical memory	Perceptual memory
Representational memory	Dispositional memory
Vertical association	Horizontal association
Locale	Taxon
Episodic	Semantic
Working	Reference

Source: From Squire (1987).

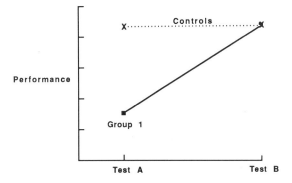

FIGURE 8.1. Idealized data for establishing a single dissociation. Group 1 exhibits impaired performance on test A but entirely normal performance on test B. Group 1 represents an impaired group, such as a group of experimentally lesioned animals, a group of neuropsychological patients, or a group given a pharmacological agent.

channels (see Foster & Fagg, 1984; Jahr & Stevens, 1987). This finding suggests that the behavioral impairment resulting from AP-5 is rather selective.

To demonstrate single dissociations, three important criteria must be satisfied. First, one must show *entirely normal* performance on a test—as shown by the performance on test B in Figure 8.1. If even a relatively small but significant impairment is observed in test B, a pure dissociation is not supported, because it must be allowed that at least some aspect of performance on test B depends on the neural system that is damaged in group 1. Second, tests A and B must be sensitive tests. In particular, equivalent performance should not be attributed to ceiling or floor effects. For example, an extremely easy or extremely hard test B could result in a spurious finding of no significant difference between groups. Third, it would be ideal to observe entirely normal performance in test B under a variety of manipulations, not just one condition, as is shown in Figure 8.1. For example, normal performance of group 1 might be observed on test B at various retention intervals along a forgetting curve or for different doses of a drug.

Studies of amnesia have shown that certain memory functions can be dissociated from other cognitive and memory functions. The central feature of organic amnesia is an impairment of new learning capacity (i.e., anterograde amnesia) that affects performance on a variety of standard memory tests, such as tests of free recall, cued recall, recognition, and paired-associate learning (for review, see Cermak, 1982; Shimamura, in press; Squire, 1987; Warrington & Weiskrantz, 1982). Severe anterograde amnesia can occur despite relatively intact intellectual and language functions. Importantly, recent findings suggest that certain memory forms are expressed in an entirely normal fashion in amnesic patients (see Cohen, 1984; Schacter, 1987a; Shimamura, 1986; Squire, 1987). Such dissociations follow the pattern shown in Figure 8.1 and satisfy all three criteria mentioned above.

One form of memory that is preserved in amnesia is priming: the unconscious facilitation or bias of recently presented information (for review, see Shimamura, 1986). Priming can be demonstrated in a word association priming task in which study words (e.g., *baby*) are cued with semantically related words (e.g., *child*). In one study (Shimamura & Squire, 1984), patients with Korsakoff's syndrome and alcoholic control subjects were presented a list of words but were not told to expect a memory test. Following list presentation, subjects were told, "Now I want to give you a different task. I will say a word and I want you to say the first word that comes to mind." Patients with Korsakoff's syndrome used previously presented words in the word association priming test as often as control subjects, despite severe impairment on a test of explicit recall memory (Fig. 8.2). In fact, both groups exhibited about a twofold increase in their use of study words, as compared to their baseline tendency to use these words when no prior presentation is given. When priming was tested after a 2-hr retention interval, word association performance in both groups was at baseline levels. Examples of entirely normal priming in amnesia can be found on a variety of other implicit tests (see Schacter, 1987a; Shimamura, 1986).

Skill learning is another form of memory that can be expressed by amnesic patients in an entirely normal manner. Pursuit rotor learning (Corkin, 1968) and mirror reading (Cohen & Squire, 1980) are two examples. What distinguishes tests of skills and priming from standard memory tests such as tests of recall and

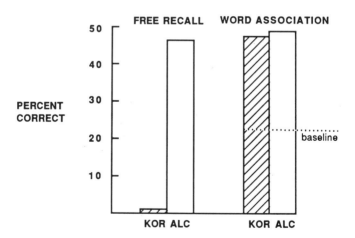

FIGURE 8.2. An example of a single dissociation in amnesia. Compared with alcoholic control subjects (ALC), patients with Korsakoff's syndrome (KOR) exhibited impaired performance on a free recall test but entirely normal performance on a word association priming test (data from Shimamura and Squire, 1984). In the word association test, subjects were presented words that were related to study words and simply asked to say the first word that came to mind.

recognition is that skills and priming can be tested without any explicit reference to the fact that memory is being tested. In tests of skills, patients can exhibit normal retention across days and even months, with no knowledge of ever having practiced the skill before. In priming tests, subjects are asked to say the first word that comes to mind and study words simply appear to pop to mind.

These findings have suggested that amnesic patients exhibit impairment whenever they are asked explicitly to declare or recollect previously presented information. Thus it has been suggested that amnesic patients exhibit a particular deficit in declarative, conscious, or explicit memory (see Baddeley, 1982; Schacter, 1987a; Squire, 1982b, 1987). Figure 8.3 illustrates this division of memory. Memory is divided into declarative and nondeclarative forms. Declarative memory includes episodic (i.e., autobiographical) memory and semantic (i.e., fact) memory (see Tulving, 1983). In addition, other divisions could be made within the declarative memory domain. For example, divisions could be made between recall and recognition memory in the sense that these two forms may require different kinds of processing, as Johnson (Chapter 5, this volume) suggested. Declarative memory deficits are found in any test where memory is explicitly requested. This deficit is found not only on standard tests such as word recall and recognition, but it also can be seen on tests of fact memory (Shimamura & Squire, 1987). In fact memory tests, subjects are presented obscure facts (e.g., Angel Falls is located in Venezuela) and then are asked explicitly to recollect the answer (e.g., Where is Angel Falls located?). A deficit occurs even when the question is presented as a test of general knowledge rather than making reference to an earlier learning session.

Nondeclarative memory comprises a heterogeneous group of memory functions, all of which can operate without the neural systems damaged in amnesia. It includes procedural memory or skill learning, simple classical conditioning, priming, and other forms of memory such as preceptual aftereffects. In the past,

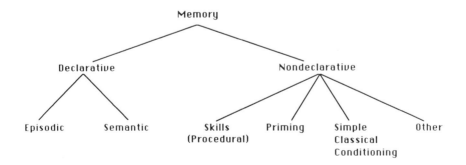

FIGURE 8.3. Forms of declarative and nondeclarative memory. Declarative memory depends on the medial temporal and diencephalic areas known to be damaged in amnesic patients. Nondeclarative memory comprises a heterogeneous group of memory forms; it can be expressed implicitly, that is, without awareness that memory is being tested.

the term "procedural memory" was used to classify all these spared functions. Yet because so little is known about the similarities and differences among these spared functions, it is not clear whether the phrase "procedural memory" can be appropriately applied to all these nondeclarative forms. Thus the more neutral classification of "nondeclarative memory" is used here.

Declarative memory functions are better understood. In particular, they depend critically on the diencephalic and medial temporal regions. Neuropathological studies of patients with Korsakoff's syndrome (Mair, Warrington, & Weiskrantz, 1979; Victor, Adams, & Collins, 1971) have implicated the diencephalic region as important for the establishment of declarative memory. Ever since the now-classic studies of patient H. M. (see Corkin, 1984; Scoville & Milner, 1957), we have known that damage to the medial temporal region—including the hippocampal gyrus, amygdala, and hippocampus proper—is important for new learning ability. Recently the importance of the hippocampus was demonstrated by amnesic case R.B., who in a postmortem study by Zola-Morgan, Squire, and Amaral (1986) was found to have bilateral lesions restricted to the CA1 subfield of the hippocampus.

Figure 8.4 illustrates why the medial temporal region may be so important for memory. It depicts the fact that unimodal and polymodal information from many areas of neocortex projects to entorhinal cortex either directly, as indicated by projections from neocortical areas such as orbitofrontal cortex, cingulate cortex, and superior temporal gyrus, or indirectly from other neocortical areas (e.g., Brodmann areas 9 and 23) that influence the entorhinal cortex through their projections to the parahippocampal gyrus or perirhinal cortex. The entorhinal cortex projects to the hippocampus via the perforant path. In addition, there are reciprocal projections back to cortical areas from the hippocampus via the subiculum and entorhinal cortex. Thus the medial temporal region—particularly the hippocampus—is privy to extensive cortical activity from a variety of areas. One possibility is that the hippocampus acts to integrate, associate, or index cortical events (for further discussion see Rolls, Chapter 9, this volume; Squire, Shimamura, & Amaral, 1989; Teyler & DiScenna, 1986).

It is presumed that the establishment of declarative memory depends critically on the medial temporal region. That is, when the medial temporal region is damaged, performance on memory tests that tap conscious or explicit memory should be impaired. Evidence suggests that within this domain, the severity of amnesia depends on the extent of damage. For example, compared with case R.B., H.M.'s medial temporal damage is more extensive and his amnesia is more severe. Similarly, damage to areas outside the medial temporal and diencephalic regions, such as the frontal cortex, may cause additional memory impairment. Additional damage could account for disproportionate deficits seen on two different declarative memory tests such as recall and recognition. That is, patients with more widespread damage may exhibit cognitive and memory impairment not seen in other amnesic patients with more circumscribed damage.

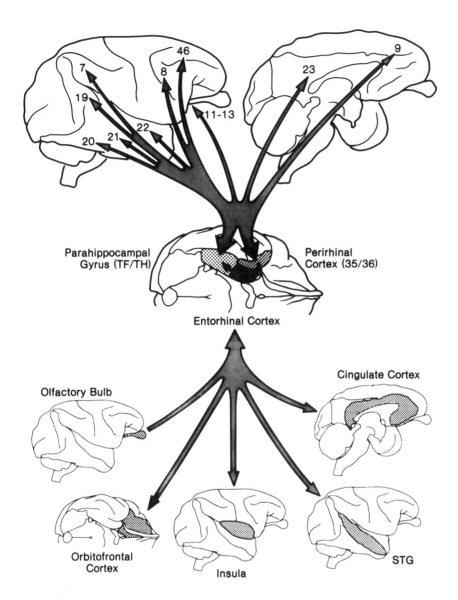

FIGURE 8.4. Many cortical areas project to entorhinal cortex either directly as shown by the projections at the bottom (e.g., orbitofrontal cortex, cingulate cortex) or indirectly by way of the parahippocampal gyrus or perirhinal cortex (e.g., Brodmann areas shown above). The entorhinal cortex projects to the hippocampus and also sends reciprocal projections back to cortical areas. (From Squire, Shimamura, and Amaral, 1989)

PARTIAL DISSOCIATIONS: TRUE OR SPURIOUS?

Disproportionate deficits on two declarative memory tests could resemble the data set illustrated in Figure 8.5. I will refer to such a pattern of results as a *partial dissociation*. In this example, group 1 exhibits impairment on tests A and B relative to control subjects. yet performance on test A is disproportionately low. This pattern of results is not uncommon (e.g., recall vs. recognition). In many comparisons between two tests of memory, amnesic patients appear to be more impaired on one test than another. A simple explanation is that one of the memory tests is a more sensitive measure than the other. Other scaling artifacts can also produce spurious dissociations (see Loftus, 1978). Yet another possibility is that amnesic patients in fact exhibit a qualitatively different (i.e., a disproportionate) deficit on one memory test compared to another. That is, they may indeed have more difficulty with the function measured by one test than with the function measured by the other.

To distinguish between these possibilities, one needs to know what would happen to control subjects if their memory were weakened so that performance on one of the memory tests was matched to the performance of amnesic patients. Memory could be weakened in control subjects by testing after a longer retention interval or by presenting information at faster exposure times (see Meudell & Mayes, 1982). Two possible outcomes that may occur with an additional group of "weakened" control subjects are shown in Figure 8.6. One possibility is that as memory weakens, performance on test A declines faster than performance on test B so that weakened control subjects actually perform like the amnesic patients on both tests. Figure 8.6B illustrates this outcome, which could occur as a result of differences in test sensitivity or differences in scaling effects between tests. For example, it was once thought that recognition memory performance was disproportionately impaired relative to cued recall performance (Warrington & Weiskrantz, 1974; see Mayes & Meudell, 1981). Yet when weakened control subjects were used, it was found that this apparent dissociation was spurious (Huppert & Piercy, 1978; Mayes & Meudell, 1981; Squire, Wetzel, & Slater, 1978). These findings suggest that some "disproportionate"

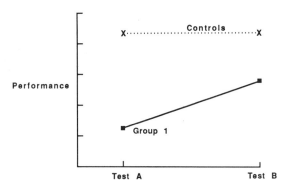

FIGURE 8.5. Partial dissociations occur when performance by an impaired group (group 1) is disproportionately impaired on one test (test A) relative to another (test B). Note, however, that a complete dissociation does not exist because entirely normal performance is not observed on test B.

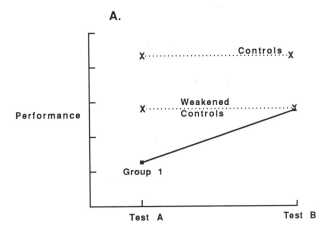

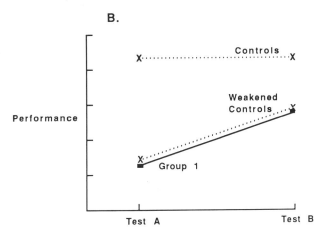

FIGURE 8.6. To determine if partial dissociations are true or spurious, an additional (weakened) control group is used to assess performance in control subjects who are matched to the impaired group on one test (test B). Performance can be weakened by using a longer retention interval. (A) A true dissociation occurs because even when performance is weakened in control subjects, group 1 still exhibits a disproportionate impairment on test A. (B) A spurious dissociation occurs when weakened control subjects exhibit a decline in performance on tests in the same manner as group 1.

effects may simply be a consequence of weak memory. That is, some differences between groups could be explained as a result of quantitative differences rather than qualitative differences between tests (for another example, see Shimamura & Squire, 1988).

Some phenomena in amnesia cannot be explained solely on the basis of weak memory. Figure 8.6A illustrates a situation in which the data suggest a true single dissociation. Amnesic patients (i.e., group 1) and weakened control subjects exhibited the same performance level on test B, yet amnesic patients exhibited a disproportionate deficit on test A. Such findings suggest a true (qualitative) dissociation between tests A and B. The deficit in free recall compared with recognition memory is one example (e.g., Hirst et al., 1986). Other examples include the disproportionate impairment in metamemory (the ability to know about one's own memory abilities) in some amnesic patients and the presence of source amnesia (a memory loss for where and when information was learned) in some patients (see Schacter, Harbluk, & McLachlan, 1984; Shimamura & Squire, 1986, 1987). Initially it was difficult to determine whether these phenomena were true or spurious dissociations. Upon further studies with weakened control subjects it was possible to conclude that a true dissociation had been observed.

The extent and severity of neurological damage in amnesic patients can vary greatly. One possibility is that partial dissociations reflect damage that occurs outside the medial temporal and diencephalic areas. One candidate structure that could contribute to memory impairment is the frontal lobes. Indeed, patients with Korsakoff's syndrome have cortical atrophy in frontal areas, as indicated by quantitative analyses of computed tomography (CT) scans (Shimamura, Jernigan, & Squire, 1988). Moreover, patients with Korsakoff's syndrome exhibit cognitive and memory deficits that are not seen in other amnesic patients (see Moscovitch, 1982; Oscar-Berman, 1980; Squire, 1982a; Talland, 1965). For example, Korsakoff patients exhibit particular deficits in the ability to remember the temporal order of events (Huppert & Piercy, 1978; Squire, 1982a) and in metamemory (Shimamura & Squire, 1986). Other amnesic patients do not exhibit these memory deficits. These deficits may be related to deficits in planning and in spatial/temporal memory which are characteristic of patients with frontal lobe damage (for review, see Milner & Petrides, 1984; Schacter, 1987b).

Perhaps the best neuropsychological method for addressing these issues would be to compare amnesic patients directly with patients with frontal lobe damage. By using two neurologically impaired groups, it may be possible to locate double dissociations as shown in Figure 8.7. For instance, group 1 could represent a group of patients with circumscribed medial temporal damage who show memory impairment on test A but not on test B. Conversely, group 2 could represent a group of patients with frontal damage who show the reverse pattern. Findings of double dissociations between groups would greatly strengthen our understanding of the role of various neural systems on memory processing. In fact, it may be that patients with Korsakoff's syndrome would constitute a third group in which performance is impaired on both tests A and B, because of their combined diencephalic and frontal damage.

Recent findings suggest that patients with frontal lobe damage exhibit impairment on some tests of memory (Janowsky, Shimamura, Kritchevsky, & Squire, 1989). A group of seven patients with relatively circumscribed frontal lobe lesions was studied. Two patients had left frontal damage, three had right frontal

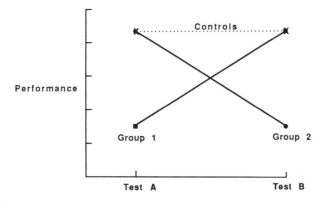

FIGURE 8.7.   Double dissociations provide strong behavioral evidence for the independence of performance on two tests. One impaired group exhibits normal performance on test B but impaired performance on test A, whereas another impaired group exhibits the reverse pattern.

damage, and two had bilateral damage. We found reliable memory dysfunction in these patients, though they do not come close to exhibiting the amnesic disorder seen in patients with diencephalic or medial temporal damage. For example, preliminary findings suggest that some aspects of metamemory are impaired in these frontal lobe patients (Janowsky, Shimamura, & Squire, 1989).

Patients with frontal damage also appear to have deficits on tests of free recall, despite relatively preserved performance on tests of recognition memory. Interestingly, relative to anoxic or ischemic patients, patients with Korsakoff's syndrome also appear to have a disproportionate deficit on free recall tests relative to performance on recognition memory tests. These findings provide evidence for the contribution of frontal lobes to performance on some memory tests. Free recall deficits may be linked to the planning and spatial/temporal memory deficits that are known to occur as a result of frontal lobe damage. Such deficits could affect retrieval processes or strategies which may be more important on tests of free recall.

FORMS OF MEMORY

Figure 8.8 summarizes in simple terms some of the points made here about different forms of memory. The figure shows what might be called three forms of memory. Each form depends on the interconnections of a number of brain structures or systems, which are identified by circles. Each is different, yet each shares some structures with others. Suppose structure B represents the hippocampus. Then by definition, memory forms 1 and 2 are two forms of declarative memory. For example, memory forms 1 and 2 could represent the processes that contribute to recall and recognition memory, respectively. Memory form 3 could

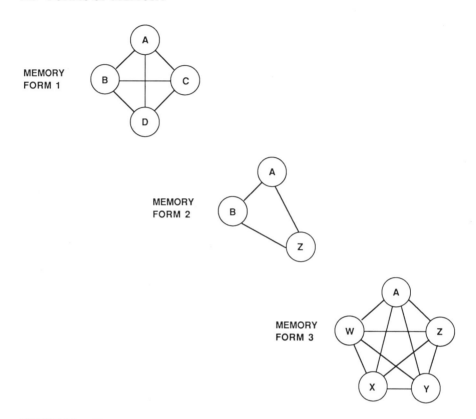

FIGURE 8.8.   Three forms of memory.

represent neural structures that contribute to priming. If structure B is damaged, then memory forms 1 and 2 should be affected (i.e., a declarative memory impairment). In contrast, performance on tests that tap memory form 3 should be entirely normal. In other words, single dissociations should be observed between memory form 3 and the other two memory forms (1 and 2).

Suppose further that structure C represents the frontal lobes such that memory form 1 depends critically on both the hippocampus and frontal lobes (structures B and C). Memory form 2 depends on the hippocampus but not on the frontal lobes. If structures B and C are damaged, then form 1 should be disproportionately affected on tests that involve both structures B and C. Yet both forms 1 and 2 should be affected on tests that involve structure B. Consequently, a partial dissociation would occur between memory forms 1 and 2, because both forms would be impaired on declarative tests, but on some tests form 1 would be more impaired than form 2. This scheme could help to explain dissociations between various forms of declarative memory, such as the dissociation between recall and recognition memory.

CONCLUSIONS

Evidence of different forms of memory as indicated by neuropsychological studies of amnesia can provide important clues about the organization of memory. Yet a complete understanding of memory cannot be achieved by such studies alone. It is extremely important to characterize the neural systems more explicitly using animal models—from invertebrate preparations to nonhuman primate models. Such models are important for providing information about basic principles of memory. Also, models in the nonhuman primate (see Mishkin, 1982; Squire & Zola-Morgan, 1983) may provide better information at the neural systems level because with such models one can gain more precise control of the structures that when damaged cause amnesia. Finally, the field seems ripe for computational models of memory. In particular, the advent of connectionistic or parallel distributed processing approaches (see Byrne & Berry, 1989; Rumelhart & McClelland, 1986) is a great boon for theories of memory because they can bring together information from neuroscience, neuropsychology, and cognitive science.

Acknowledgments
This work was supported by the Medical Research Service of the Veterans Administration, by National Institute of Mental Health Grant MH24600, and by the Office of Naval Research. I thank Larry Squire and Jeri Janowsky for helpful comments on earlier drafts.

REFERENCES

Baddeley, A. D. (1982). Domains of recollection. *Psychological Review, 89,* 708–729.
Byrne, J. H., & Berry, W. O. (Eds.). (1989). *Neural models of plasticity.* Orlando, Fla.: Academic Press.
Cermak, L. S. (1982). *Human memory and amnesia.* Hillsdale, N.J.: Erlbaum.
Cohen, N. J. (1984). Preserved learning capacity in amnesia: Evidence for multiple memory systems. In L. R. Squire & N. Butters (Eds.), *Neuropsychology of memory* (pp. 83–103). New York: Guilford.
Cohen, N. J., & Squire, L. R. (1980). Preserved learning and retention of pattern analyzing skill in amnesia: Association of knowing how and knowing that. *Science, 210,* 207–209.
Corkin, S. (1968). Acquisition of motor skill after bilateral medial temporal lobe excision. *Neuropsychologia, 6,* 225–265.
Corkin, S. (1984). Lasting consequences of bilateral medial temporal lobectomy: Clinical course and experimental findings in H.M. *Seminars in Neurology, 4,* 249–259.
Foster, A. C., & Fagg, G. E. (1984). Acidic amino acid binding sites in mammalian neuronal membranes: Their characteristics and relationship to synaptic receptors. *Brain Research Review, 7,* 103–164.
Hirst, W., Johnson, M. K., Kim, J. K., Phelps, E. A., Risse, G., & Volpe, B. T. (1986). Recognition and recall in amnesics. *Journal of Experimental Psychology: Learning, Memory, and Cognition, 12,* 445–451.

Huppert, F. A., & Piercy, M. (1978). The role of trace strength in recency and frequency judgements by amnesic and control subjects. *Quarterly Journal of Experimental Psychology, 30,* 346–354.

Jahr, C. E., & Stevens, C. F. (1987). Glutamate activates multiple single channel conductances in hippocampal neurons. *Nature, 325,* 522–525.

Janowsky, J. S., Shimamura, A. P., Kritchevsky, M., & Squire, L. R. (1989). Cognitive impairment following frontal lobe damage and its relevance to human amnesia. *Behavioral Neuroscience, 103,* 548–560.

Janowsky, J. S., Shimamura, A. P., & Squire, L. R. (1989). Memory and metamemory: Comparisons between patients with frontal lobe lesions and amnesic patients. *Psychobiology, 17,* 3–11.

Lashley, K. S. (1950). In search of the engram. *Symposia of the Society of Experimental Biology, 4,* 454–482.

Loftus, G. (1978). On the interpretations of interactions. *Memory and Cognition, 6,* 312–319.

Mair, W. G. P., Warrington, E. K., & Weiskrantz, L. (1979). Memory disorder in Korsakoff psychosis: A neuropathological and neuropsychological investigation of two cases. *Brain, 102,* 749–783.

Mayes, A. R., & Meudell, P. R. (1981). How similar is the effect of cueing in amnesics and normal subjects following forgetting? *Cortex, 171,* 113–124.

Meudell, P. R., & Mayes, A. R. (1982). Normal and abnormal forgetting: Some comments on the human amnesic syndrome. In L. A. Ellis (Ed.), *Normality and pathology in cognition function* (pp. 203–237). London: Academic Press.

Milner, B., & Petrides, M. (1984). Behavioural effects of frontal-lobe lesions in man. *Trends in Neuroscience, 7,* 403–407.

Mishkin, M. (1982). A memory system in the monkey. *Philosophical Transactions of the Royal Society (London), 298,* 85–95.

Moscovitch, M. (1982). Multiple dissociations of function in amnesia. In L. Cermak (Ed.), *Human memory and amnesia* (pp. 337–370). Hillsdale, N.J.: Erlbaum.

Oscar-Berman, M. (1980). The neuropsychological consequences of long-term chronic alcoholism. *American Scientist, 68,* 410–419.

Rumelhart, D. E., & McClelland, J. L. (1986). *Parallel distributed processing.* Cambridge, Mass.: MIT Press.

Schacter, D. L. (1987a). Implicit memory: History and current status. *Journal of Experimental Psychology: Learning, Memory and Cognition, 13,* 501–518.

Schacter, D. L. (1987b). Memory, amnesia, and frontal lobe dysfunction. *Psychobiology, 15,* 21–36.

Schacter, D. L., Harbluk, J. L., & McLachlan, D. R. (1984). Retrieval without recollection: An experimental analysis of source amnesia. Journal of Verbal Learning and Verbal Behavior, 23, 593–611.

Scoville, W. B., & Milner, B. (1957). Loss of recent memory after bilateral hippocampal lesions. *Journal of Neurology, Neurosurgery, and Psychiatry, 20,* 11–21.

Shimamura, A. P. (1986). Priming effects in amnesia: Evidence for a dissociable memory function. *Quarterly Journal of Experimental Psychology, 38A,* 619–644.

Shimamura, A. P. (in press). Disorders of memory: The cognitive science perspective. In F. Boller & J. Grafman (Eds.), *Handbook of clinical neuropsychology.* Amsterdam: Elsevier.

Shimamura, A. P., Jernigan, T. L., & Squire, L. R. (1988). Radiological (CT) findings in patients with Korsakoff's syndrome and their relationship to memory impairment. *Journal of Neuroscience, 8,* 4400–4410.

Shimamura, A. P., & Squire, L. R. (1984). Paired-associate learning and priming effects in amnesia: A neuropsychological study. *Journal of Experimental Psychology: General, 113,* 556–570.

Shimamura, A. P., & Squire, L. R. (1986). Memory and metamemory: A study of the feeling-of-knowing phenomenon in amnesic patients. *Journal of Experimental Psychology: Learning, Memory and Cognition, 12,* 452–460.

Shimamura, A. P., & Squire, L. R. (1987). A neuropsychological study of fact memory and source amnesia. *Journal of Experimental Psychology: Learning, Memory and Cognition, 13,* 464–473.

Shimamura, A. P., & Squire, L. R. (1988). Long-term memory in amnesia: Cued recall, recognition memory, and confidence ratings. *Journal of Experimental Psychology: Learning, Memory and Cognition, 14,* 763–770.

Squire, L. R. (1982a). Comparisions between forms of amnesia: Some deficits are unique to Korsakoff's syndrome. *Journal of Experimental Psychology: Learning, Memory, and Cognition, 8,* 560–571.

Squire, L. R. (1982b). The neuropsychology of human memory. *Annual Review of Neuroscience, 5,* 241–273.

Squire, L. R. (1987). *Memory and brain.* New York: Oxford University Press.

Squire, L. R., Shimamura, A. P., & Amaral, D. (1989). Memory and the hippocampus. In J. H. Byrne & W. O. Berry (Eds.), *Neural models of plasticity* (pp. 208–239). Orlando, Fla.: Academic Press.

Squire, L. R., Wetzel, C. D., & Slater, P.C. (1978). Anterograde amnesia following ECT: An analysis of the beneficial effect of partial information. *Neuropsychologia, 116,* 339–347.

Squire, L. R., & Zola-Morgan, S. (1983). The neurology of memory: The case for correspondence between the findings for human and nonhuman primates. In J. A. Deutsch (Ed.), *The physiological basis of memory* (2nd ed.). New York: Academic Press.

Talland, G. A. (1965). *Deranged memory.* New York: Academic Press.

Teyler, T. J., & DiScenna, P. (1986). The hippocampal memory indexing theory. *Behavioral Neuroscience, 100,* 147–154.

Tulving, E. (1983). *Elements of episodic memory.* Oxford: Clarendon Press.

Victor, M., Adams, R. D., & Collins, G. H. (1971). *The Wernicke-Korsakoff syndrome.* Philadelphia: Davis.

Warrington, E. K., & Weiskrantz, L. (1974). The effect of prior learning on subsequent retention in amnesic patients. *Neuropsychologia, 12,* 419–428.

Warrington, E. K., & Weiskrantz, L. (1982). Amnesia: A disconnection syndrome? *Neuropsychologia, 20,* 233–248.

Zola-Morgan, S., Squire, L. R., & Amaral, D. G. (1986). Human amnesia and the medial temporal region: Enduring memory impairment following a bilateral lesion limited to field CA1 of the hippocampus. *Journal of Neuroscience, 6,* 2950–2967.

II

Regulation of Cortical Function in Memory

Introduction

MARK R. ROSENZWEIG

A major theme that runs through this section is differential changes and differential activities in the nervous system in relation to learning and memory, and often in relation to specific kinds of learning and memory. These changes can occur during learning and formation of memory and during development and self-organization of the nervous system; morever, differential changes in the brain caused by diseases lead to predictable changes in specific abilities to learn and remember.

Let us look at a few examples of these differential effects from the following chapters. Rolls (Chapter 9) takes up specific kinds of learning known to involve the primate hippocampus. He reports that about one tenth of the neurons in the hippocampus come to respond differentially to the combination of a particular object with a particular location in space; about one seventh of the neurons in the hippocampus come to respond differentially to the rewarded combination of a particular object with a particular motor response. Moreover, it appears that although many hippocampal neurons originally respond to a new combination, the few that show sustained responses to it inhibit others that show only transient modification, so that relatively few neurons are allocated to a particular association. In turn, these hippocampal neurons may allocate memory storage to specific regions of cerebral cortex for efficient use of cortical capacity. Subsequent use of this stored material may produce progressively more specific representation. Thus all along the way, differential responsiveness is stressed.

Van Hoesen (Chapter 11) considers whether Alzheimer's disease (AD) dissects memory into distinct behavioral compartments and whether such compartments are related to damage in distinct locations in the brain. He points out that neither the course of the memory changes in AD nor the sequence of changes in the brain have been studied fully by rigorous methods; Van Hoesen nevertheless produces evidence for regularity in time courses and for relationships between the behavioral and the neuroanatomical changes. Here are a few examples. The earliest changes in AD may be deficiencies in anterograde episodic memories; this may be related to the fact that the most persistent and perhaps earliest neuroanatomical changes occur in the hippocampus, particularly in its subicular subdivision, and in the anterior parahippocampal gyrus including the entorhinal cortex. Impairments of retrograde episodic memories also occur relatively early in AD, and they often cause the victim or the family to seek medical advice. These losses appear to be related to pathology in posterior parahippocampal, lateral temporal, and anterior insular cortices. Still later, generic and semantic memory decline when the multimodal association cortices are involved. Even when a region of cortex is affected in AD, pathology is not uniformly distributed but is confined to specific cell types and to specific cortical layers. Specific subcortical formations and specific subregions within some of them are also involved in AD. In fact, although this section of the book deals with "Regulation of Cortical Function in Memory," the authors frequently treat the cortex in the context of its connections to other parts of the brain.

Singer (Chapter 10) considers some of the mechanisms of development of self-organization of the brain, especially the organization of binocularity in the visual system, and investigates the extent to which they may be precursors of mechansims that mediate learning in the adult. Singer points out that neural activity, including the results of information processing, becomes part of the environment relevant for self-organization, and the spiral of reciprocal interactions leads to ever more differentiated structures. At least early in life, both formation and withdrawal of synaptic connections are involved, and, especially in adult life, changes in the efficacy of synaptic connections are involved. Recording from individual cortical neurons, Singer and his colleagues studied changes during monocular visual deprivation and during reversed monocular occlusion. They conclude that two different processes are involved: rapid inactivation of deprived connections and slow increase in effectiveness of previously inactivated connections. (Chapter 15 by Cooper, Bear, Ebner, and Scofield suggests that the changes in visual dominance occur chiefly at excitatory synapses on excitatory cells, a type of synapse that is formed exclusively on dendritic spines, a feature that distinguishes it from other types of cortical synapse—again a highly specific site.) Singer reports that changes in ocular dominance occur only when the animal is alert and using its visual system, so postsynaptic modulatory inputs to the plastic cells are also important. Permissive gating signals may involve both cholingergic and noradrenergic modulatory systems and also Ca^{2+} fluxes governed by NMDA receptors, so a variety of neurochemical processes is involved.

A less overt theme in this section is the overcoming of certain older ideas about the nervous system, learning, and memory as new ideas are presented and demonstrated—as well as the revival of other old ideas. One dogma that had wide currency in the fifties was that the adult nervous system is quite stable and could not be altered in any measurable way by such benign activities as learning and formation of memory. In light of some of the reports and discussions in this section, it may be difficult for many readers to realize how fixed the adult nervous system seemed then. But I remember clearly how exciting it was for Edward Bennett, David Krech, and me when our data forced us to conclude that giving formal training or informal experience to experimental animals caused measurable changes in the biochemistry of their brains and that these changes were not caused by associated variables (Krech, Rosenzweig, & Bennett, 1960). Soon thereafter, along with Marian Diamond, we were startled to find that small but significant changes in gross anatomy of the cerebral cortex were induced by differential experience in enriched or impoverished environments (Rosenzweig, Krech, Bennett, & Diamond, 1962).

A further belief that gave way before empirical evidence was the idea that the brain, or at least the cerebral cortex, responded in a rather general, uniform way to training or differential experience. Our early experiments demonstrated that the cerebral cortex responded differently to experience than did noncortical tissue, and within the cerebral cortex different regions responded with reliably larger or smaller changes (Rosenzweig et al., 1962). Going to a finer level of resolution, we and others soon found that neurons show a variety of morphological responses to differential experience, using measures such as dendritic branching (e.g., Holloway, 1966; Volkmar & Greenough, 1972), numbers of synapses (e.g., Diamond, Lindner, Johnson, Bennett, & Rosenzweig, 1975; West & Greenough, 1972) and numbers of dendritic spines (Globus, Rosenzweig, Bennett, & Diamond, 1973). These morphological changes were accompanied by an increase in protein in the cortical regions involved (Bennett, Diamond, Krech, & Rosenzweig, 1964). Complementary experiments demonstrated that administering agents that inhibit protein synthesis in the brain shortly before either appetitive or aversive training prevents formation of long-term memory, although it does not prevent acquisition of short-term or intermediate-term storage (e.g., Barondes & Cohen, 1968; Flood, Bennett, Orme, & Rosenzweig, 1975; Flood, Bennett, Rosenzweig, & Orme, 1972, 1973). As pointed out at the First Irvine Conference, the synthesis of proteins required for formation of long-term memory usually occurs in the minutes following training, but "this synthesis can be deferred during a period of inhibition of protein synthesis . . . the stronger the training, the longer the synthesis can be deferred but still take place" (Rosenzweig & Bennett, 1984, p. 268).

Can differential experience cause changes in the numbers of cortical synapses? Morris (Chapter 3) raised this question earlier in this book, and it is also pertinent here. Although Singer doubts that the visual cortex can show changes in synaptic number in the adult, several laboratories have found changes in synaptic numbers in occipital cortex of the rat as a result of differential experience (e.g., Bhide & Bede, 1984; Diamond et al., 1975; Globus et al., 1973; Sirevaag & Greenough, 1986), and Colonnier and Beaulieu (1985) found similar results in the cat. Wenzel et al. (1977) also found increases in synaptic numbers in the hippocampus of the rat as a result of formal training. Stewart, Rose, Kind, Gabbott, and Bourne (1984) found that peck-avoidance training in chicks caused a significant increase in the number of synapses per unit volume of neuropil in the left cerebral hemisphere. These findings in vertebrates are now being repeated in invertebrates. Recently investigators studying the mechansims of long-term sensitization in *Aplysia* showed that the number of synapses on sensory neurons is significantly increased after training, and the number then declines over a few weeks in parallel with decreasing retention (Bailey & Chen, 1987). Nevertheless, opinion has fluctuated on this question ever since Tanzi (1893) proposed that the plastic changes in learning would be found at the junctions between neurons. I remember Eccles exclaiming at a conference, "Learning can produce only bigger and better synapses, not new ones." (He wrote much the same thing, but not quite so pithily [Eccles, 1973, p. 184].) On the contrary, Eccles's teacher Sherrington was an early proponent of the hypothesis that learning could result in formation of new synaptic connections. In the chapter in which he proposed the name "synapse," Sherrington offered this portrayal of educable neurons:

> Shut off from all opportunities of reproducing itself and adding to its number by mitosis or otherwise, the nerve cell directs its pent-up energy towards amplifying its connections with its fellows, in response to the events which stir up. Hence, it is capable of an education unknown to other tissues. (Foster & Sherrington, 1897, 1117)

I believe that Eccles was wrong on two counts when he asserted that learning involves only increasing the size of existing synapses. First, as noted, results from several laboratories show that training or enriched experience does cause the formation of new synapses. Second, it appears that enriched experience may cause some synapses to become smaller while others become larger, as we pointed out some time ago (Rosenzweig, Diamond, Bennett, & Mollgaard, 1972). The latter point is reminiscent of the findings on the inhibitory as well as excitatory changes during learning reported by Rolls and of the concept of pruning connections through experience as mentioned by Singer.

To claim that formation of new synapses (and elimination of existing synapses) is employed in some kinds of memory storage is not to hold that such changes occur in all memory storage. Some forms of memory (especially short-term) are very unlikely to require changes in synaptic number. Other kinds may very well employ this mechanism, as shown by the evidence cited earlier. Kety (1976) put the case for plurality of memory mechansims well:

> So profound and powerful an adaptation as learning or memory is not apt to rest upon a single modality. Rather, I suspect that advantage is taken of every opportunity provided by evolution. There were forms of memory before organisms developed nervous systems, and after that remarkable leap forward it is likely that every new pathway and neural complexity, every new neurotransmitter, hormone, or metabolic processes that played upon the nervous sytem and subserved a learning process was preserved and incorporated. (pp. 321–322)

Another old idea, now refuted, was that the two cerebral hemispheres of animals play essentially similar and equal roles in learning and memory formation. It is not so long ago that many investigators supposed that only the human being employs the two hemispheres in differential fashion, but now rodents and chicks show clear hemispheric differences in ways that we are still far from understanding (e.g., Horn, 1985; Patterson, Alvarado, Warner, Bennett, & Rosenzweig, 1986; Rose & Csillag, 1985; Stewart et al., 1984). In particular, Patterson et al. (1986) found that to form memories of peck-aversion learning in chicks, the left hemisphere is the one that counts in regard to one brain structure (the intermediate medial hyperstriatum ventrale) but the right hemisphere is the important one for another structure (the lateral neostriatum).

An old idea that keeps coming back is Tanzi's general concept that the same mechanisms may be involved in the development of the nervous system and in learning and memory storage. A strong statement of this hypothesis was made by Galambos (1961) at an international conference on brain mechanisms and learning in 1959:

> It could be argued . . . that no important gap separates the explanations for how the nervous sytem comes to be organized during embryological development in the first place; for how it operates to produce the innate responses characteristic of each species in the second place; and for how it comes to be reorganized, finally, as a result of experiences during life. If this idea should be correct, the solution of any one of these problems would mean that the answers to the others would drop like a ripe plum, so to speak, into our outstretched hands. (pp. 238–239)

Although this hypothesis has intrigued many investigators, it is only in recent years that substantial empirical support has been obtained for it, as exemplified by Singer's chapter in this book and many other current papers and symposia (e.g., Black & Greenough, 1986; Purves, Smith, Bailey, & Greenough, 1987).

It is worth noting that the kinds of learning and memory considered in this section, as well as in Part I, represent a considerable variety. This may seem quite natural these days, even though the discussions in this book show that we are far from agreeing about the categories of learning and memory or the definitions of various proposed categories. But in the 1940s, when behavioral "schools" of learning theory held sway, it was generally believed that all learning is basically similar and that one set of laws should be able to encompass all instances of learning. It was startling then for Edward Tolman to write an article entitled "There Is More Than One Kind of Learning" (1949), and he probably did not convince many readers. Considerably later, Neal Miller (1967) wrote about "Grade-A Certified Learning" (associative learning in mammals) as if that was *the* kind to be studied. Miller admitted that there are other phenomena such as habituation or even immune reactions "that may have some elements in common with learning and that may provide the key to an understanding of its physical basis. . . . In our present state of ignorance we cannot afford to discard any approaches" (p. 643). That almost exclusive focus on associative learning is certainly not the view of the authors in this volume. Carew, Marcus, Nolen, Ranking, and Stopfer (Chapter 2), for example, reported important results on the developmental emergence of habituation, dishabituation, and sensitization. The authors in Part II specify a number of different kinds of learning and memory, including certain types involving spatial location that require the hippocampus, anterograde and retrograde impairments in recall, episodic and semantic memories, working and long-term memories. In fact, when Singer draws up similarities between developmental self-organization and "adult learning," one wonders what kind or kinds of adult learning he has in mind.

So the following chapters consider various kinds of learning and memory and a variety of possible neurophysiological, neuroanatomical, and neurochemical correlates and mechansims. All this implies to me that much progress is being made in getting beyond oversimple generalities; investigators are beginning to reach the specifics of the processes involved in the many kinds of learning and memory that human beings and other animals demonstrate and experience. To celebrate these differential approaches and findings, let me conclude the introduction to the following chapters by expanding a famous aphorism: "Vivent *les* differences!"

REFERENCES

Bailey, C. H., & Chen M. (1987). The course of the structural changes at identified sensory neuron synapses during long-term sensitization in *Aplysia*. *Society for Neuroscience Abstracts, 13* (Part 1), 617.

Barondes, S. H., & Cohen, H. D. (1968). Memory impairment after subcutaneous injection of acetoxycycloheximide. *Science, 160,* 556–557.

Bennett, E. L., Diamond, M. C., Krech, D., & Rosenzweig, M. R. (1964). Chemical and anatomical plasticity of brain. *Science, 146,* 610–619.

Bhide, P. G., & Bede, K. S. (1984). The effects of a lengthy period of environmental diversity on well-fed and previously undernourished rats. II. Synapse-to-neuron ratios. *Journal of Comparative Neurology, 227,* 305–310.

Black, J. E., & Greenough, W. T. (1986). Developmental approaches to the memory process. In J. L. Martinez, Jr., 7 R. P. Kesner (Eds.), *Learning and memory: A biological view* (pp. 55–81). Orlando, Fla.: Academic Press.

Colonnier, M., & Beaulieu, C. (1985). The differential effect of impoverished and enriched environments on the number of "round asymmetrical" and "flat symmetrical" synapses in the visual cortex of cat. *Society for Neuroscience Abstracts, 11,* 226.

Diamond, M. C., Lindner, B., Johnson, R., Bennett, E. L., & Rosenzweig, M. R. (1975). Differences in occipital cortex synapses from environmentally enriched, impoverished, and standard colony rats. *Journal of Neuroscience Research, 1,* 109–119.

Eccles, J. C. (1973). *The understanding of the brain.* New York: McGraw-Hill.

Flood, J. F., Bennett, E. L., Orme, A. E., & Rosenzweig, M. R. (1975). Effects of protein synthesis inhibition on memory for active avoidance training. *Physiology and Behavior, 14,* 177–184.

Flood, J. F., Bennett, E. L., Rosenzweig, M. R., & Orme, A. E. (1972). Influence of training strength on amnesia induced by pretraining injections of cycloheximide. *Physiology and Behavior, 9,* 589–600.

Flood, J. F., Bennett, E. L., Rosenzweig, M. R., & Orme, A. E. (1973). The influence of duration of protein synthesis inhibition on memory, *Physiology and Behavior, 10,* 555–562.

Foster, M., & Sherrington, C. S. (1897). *A textbook of physiology: Part 3. The central nervous system.* New York: Macmillan.

Galambos, R. (1961). Changing concepts of the learning mechanism. In A. Fessard, R. W. Gerard, & J. Konorski (Eds.), *Brain mechanisms and learning* (pp. 231–241). Springfield, Ill.: Charles C. Thomas.

Globus, A., Rosenzweig, M. R., Bennett, E. L., & Diamond, M. C. (1973). Effects of differential experience on dendritic spine counts in rat cerebral cortex. *Journal of Comparative and Physiological Psychology, 82,* 175–181.

Holloway, R. L. (1966). Dendritic branching: Some preliminary results of training and testing in rat visual cortex. *Brain Research, 2,* 393–396.

Horn, G. (1985). *Memory, imprinting and the brain.* Oxford: Clarendon Press.

Kety, S. (1976). Biological concomitants of affective states and their possible role in memory processes. In M. R. Rosenzweig and E. L. Bennett (Eds.), *Neural mechanisms of learning and memory* (pp. 321–326). Cambridge, Mass.: MIT Press.

Krech, D., Rosenzweig, M. R., & Bennett, E. L. (1960). Effects of environmental complexity and training on brain chemistry. *Journal of Comparative and Physiological Psychology, 53,* 509–519.

Miller, N. E. (1967). Certain facts of learning relevant to the search for its physical basis. In G. C. Quarton, T. Melnechuk, & F. O. Schmitt (Eds.), *The neurosciences* (pp. 643–653). New York: Rockefeller University Press.

Patterson, T. A., Alvarado, M. C., Warner, I. T., Bennett, E. L., & Rosenzweig, M. R. (1986). Memory stages and brain asymmetry in chick learning. *Behavioral Neuroscience, 100,* 856–865.

Purves, D., Smith, S., Bailey, C. H., & Greenough, W. T. (1987). Symposium: Dynamic changes of synaptic structure under normal and experimental conditions. *Society for Neuroscience Abstracts, 13* (Part 2), 1001.

Rose, S. P. R., & Csillag, A. (1985). Passive avoidance training results in lasting changes in deoxyglucose metabolism in left hemisphere regions of chick brain. *Behavioral and Neural Biology, 44,* 315–324.

Rosenzweig, M. R. & Bennett, E. L. (1984). Basic processes and modulatory influences in the stages of memory formation. In G. Lynch, J. L. McGaugh, & N. M. Weinberger (Eds.), *Neurobiology of learning and memory* (pp. 263–288). New York: Guilford.

Rosenzweig, M. R., Diamond, M. C., Bennett, E. L. & Mollgaard, K. (1972). Negative as well as positive synaptic changes may store memory. *Psychological Review, 79,* 93–96.

Rosenzweig, M. R., Krech, D., Bennett, E. L., & Diamond, M. C. (1962). Effects of environmental complexity and training on brain chemistry and anatomy: A replication and extension. *Journal of Comparative and Physiological Psychology, 55,* 429–437.

Sirevaag, A. M., & Greenough, W. T. (1986). Multivariate analyses of morphological measurements can distinguish among rats reared in complex, social or individual environments. *Society for Neuroscience Abstracts, 12,* 1284.

Stewart, M. G., Rose, S. P. R., Kind, T. S., Gabbott, P. L. A., & Bourne, R. (1984). Hemispheric asymmetry of synapses in chick medial hyperstriatum ventrale following passive avoidance training: A stereological investigation. *Developmental Brain Research, 12,* 261–269.

Tanzi, E. (1893). I fatti e le induzioni nell'odierna istologia del sistema nervoso. *Revista Sperimentale di Freniatria e di Medicina Legale, 19,* 419–472.

Tolman, E. C. (1949). There is more than one kind of learning. *Psychological Review, 56,* 144–155.

Volkmar, F. R. & Greenough, W. T. (1972). Rearing complexity affects branching of dendrites in the visual cortex of the rat. *Science, 176,* 1447–1449.

Wenzel, J., Kammerer, E., Joschko, R., Joschko, M., Kaufmann, W., Kirsche, W., & Matthies, H. (1977). Der Einfluss eines Lernexperimentes auf die Synaptenzahl in Hippocampus der Ratte. Elekronenmikroskpische und morphometrische Untersuchungen. *Zeitschrift für mikroskopische-anatomische Forschung, 91,* 57–73.

West, R. W. & Greenough, W. T. (1972). Effects of environmental complexity on cortical synapses of rats: Preliminary results. *Behavioral Biology, 7,* 279–283.

9

Functions of Neuronal Networks in the Hippocampus and of Backprojections in the Cerebral Cortex in Memory

EDMUND T. ROLLS

FUNCTIONS OF THE PRIMATE HIPPOCAMPUS IN MEMORY

It is known that damage to certain regions of the temporal lobe in humans produces anterograde amnesia, manifested as a major deficit following the damage in learning to recognize new stimuli (Milner, 1972; Scoville & Milner, 1957; Squire, 1986, 1987). The anterograde amnesia has been attributed to damage to the hippocampus, which is within the temporal lobe, and to its associated pathways such as the fornix (Gaffan, 1974, 1977; Milner, 1972; Scoville & Milner, 1957; Zola-Morgan, Squire, & Amaral, 1986), but this has been questioned, and it has been suggested that damage to both the hippocampus and the amygdala is crucial in producing anterograde amnesia, in that combined but not separate damage to the hippocampus and amygdala produced severe difficulty with visual and tactual recognition tasks in the monkey (Mishkin, 1978, 1982; Murray & Mishkin, 1984). In investigations of the particular aspects of memory for which the hippocampus may be essential, it has been shown that monkeys with damage to the hippocampo-fornical system have a learning deficit on memory tasks that requires them to make associations between a stimulus, for example, a picture, and a spatial motor response such as touching one part of a screen (Gaffan, 1985; Rupniak & Gaffan, 1987); they are also impaired on memory tasks that require combinations of stimulus attributes with their locations in space to be processed together, such as memory not only for which object was shown but where it was shown (Gaffan & Saunders, 1985). Further, humans with right temporal lobe damage are also impaired in conditional spatial response and object–place memory tasks (Petrides, 1985; Smith & Milner, 1981).

To analyze the functions being performed by the hippocampus in memory, the activity of 1510 single hippocampal neurons was recorded in rhesus monkeys learning and performing these memory tasks known to be impaired by damage to the hippocampus or fornix (Cahusac, Miyashita, & Rolls, 1989; Miyashita, Rolls, Cahusac, & Niki, 1989; Rolls et al., 1989).

In an object–place memory task in which the monkey had to remember not only which object had been seen in the previous 7 to 15 trials, but also the position in which it had appeared on a video monitor, neurons were found which responded differentially depending on where on the monitor screen the objects were shown (Rolls et al., 1989). These neurons composed 9.3% of the population recorded. It is notable that these neurons responded to particular postions in space (whereas "place" cells in the rat respond when the rat is in a particular place; O'Keefe, 1984). In addition, 2.4% of neurons responded more to a stimulus the first time it was shown in a particular position than the second time. These neurons thus responded to a combination of information about the stimulus being shown and about position in space, for only by responding to a combination of this information could the neurons respond when a stimulus was shown for the first time in a certain position in space.

In tasks in which the monkeys had to acquire associations between visual stimuli and spatial responses, 14.2% of the neurons responded to particular combinations of stimuli and responses (Miyashita et al., 1989). For example, in a task in which the monkey had to perform one response (touching a screen three times) when one visual stimulus was shown, but had to perform a withholding response for 3 sec to obtain reward when a different stimulus was shown (Gaffan, 1985), 9.2% of the neurons responded to one of the stimuli if it was linked to one of the responses in this task. The same neurons typically did not respond if the same stimuli or the same responses were used in different tasks, or if other stimuli were associated with the same responses in this task. Thus these neurons responded to a combination of a particular stimulus with a particular spatial motor response (Miyashita et al., 1989).

It was possible to study the activity of 70 neurons in the hippocampus or parahippocampal gyrus while the monkeys learned new associations between visual stimuli and spatial responses. In some cases it was possible to show that the activity of these neurons became modified during this learning (Cahusac, Feigenbaum, Rolls, Miyashita, & Niki, 1986). Interestingly, 22% of the neurons acquired a sustained differential response during the learning, and 45% of the neurons differentiated between the stimuli only at or just before the monkey learned the task and stopped differentiating after 5 to 10 more trials. This is consistent with the possibility (discussed later) that the neurons which show large sustained differential responses inhibit the other neurons which show transient modification, so that as a result of competition not all neurons are allocated to one stimulus—spatial response association.

These results show that hippocampal neurons in the primate have responses related to certain types of memory. One type of memory involves complex conjunctions of environmental information, for example, when information about position in space (perhaps reflecting information from the parietal cortex) must

A

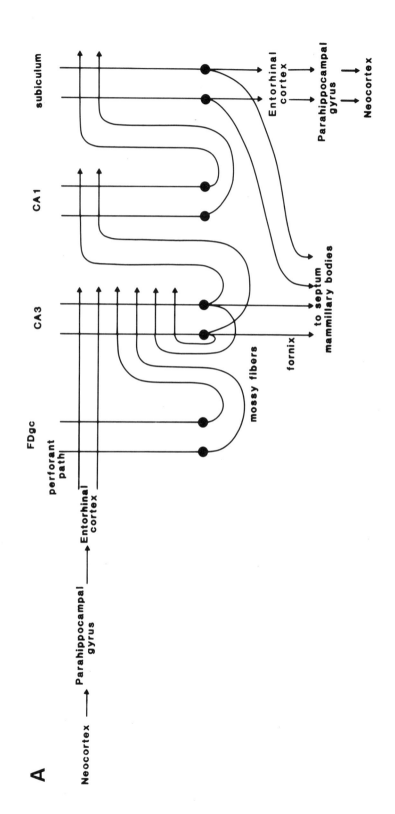

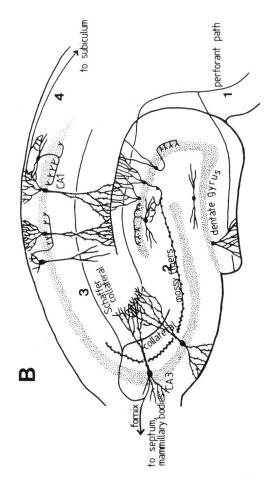

FIGURE 9.1. (A) Representation of connections within the hippocampus. Inputs reach the hippocampus through the perforant path, which makes synapses with the dendrites of the dentate granule cells and also with the apical dendrites of the CA3 pyramidal cells. The dentate granule cells project via the mossy fibers to the CA3 pyramidal cells. The well-developed recurrent collateral system of the CA3 cells is indicated. The CA3 pyramidal cells project via the Schaffer collaterals to the CA1 pyramidal cells, which in turn have connections to the subiculum. (B) Schematic representation of the connections of the hippocampus, showing also that the cerebral cortex (neocortex) is connected to the hippocampus via the parahippocampal gyrus and entorhinal cortex, and that the hippocampus projects back to the neocortex via the subiculum, entorhinal cortex, and parahippocampal gyrus.

be memorized in conjunction with what that object is (perhaps reflecting information from the temporal lobe visual areas) so that where a particular object was seen in space can be remembered. The hippocampus is ideally placed anatomically for detecting such conjuntions in that it receives highly processed information from association areas such as the parietal cortex (conveying information about position in space), the inferior temporal visual cortex (conveying a visual specification of an object), and the superior temporal cortex (conveying an auditory specification of a stimulus) (Van Hoesen, 1982; see Fig. 9.5). The positions of stimuli in space may be represented by the firing of hippocampal neurons as described above so that conjunctions of, for example, objects and their position can be formed. It is also suggested that one neurophysiological mechanism by which "place" cells in the rat (see O'Keefe, 1984) may be formed is by conjunction learning of sets of simultaneously occurring stimuli in different parts of space, each set of which defines a place.

COMPUTATIONAL THEORY OF THE HIPPOCAMPUS

A possible theoretical basis for these results, and in particular how the hippocampus may perform the conjunction or combination learning just described, is now considered. Figure 9.1A is schematic of the connections of the hippocampus. One feature is that there is a sequence of stages, in each of which there is a major set of input axons that connect by a form of matrix with the output neurons of that stage. The type of computation that could be performed by one of these stages is considered first.

The perforant path connections with the dentate granule cells may be taken as an example. A version of this is represented as a simplified matrix in Figure 9.2. Although the perforant path makes one set of synapses with the output neurons in the form of a matrix, the matrix is clearly very different from an association matrix memory in that in the hippocampal system there is no unconditioned stimulus that forces the output neurons to fire (see Rolls, 1987). Nor is there a climbing fiber for each output cell that acts as a teacher as in the cerebellum (see Ito, 1984). In the hippocampal circuit there is apparently no teacher; that is, this appears to be an example of an unsupervised learning system. One mode of operation for such a network is described next, and properties of the hippocampus which suggest that it may operate in this way are discussed later.

Consider a matrix memory of the form shown in Figure 9.2 in which the strengths of the synapses between horizontal axons and the vertical dendrites are initially random (postulate 1). Because of these random initial synaptic weights, different input patterns on the horizontal axons will tend to activate different output neurons (in this case, granule cells). The tendency for each pattern to select or activate different neurons can then be enhanced by providing mutual inhibition between the output neurons, to prevent too many neurons responding to that stimulus (postulate 2). This competitive interaction can be viewed as enhancing the differences in the firing rates of the output cells (cf. the

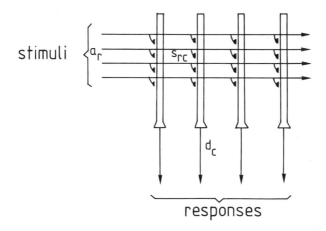

FIGURE 9.2.   A matrix for competitive learning in which the input stimuli are presented along the rows of the input axons (a_r), which make modifiable synapses (s_{rc}) with the dendrites of the output neurons, which form the columns (d_c) of the matrix.

contrast enhancement described by Grossberg, 1982). Synaptic modification then occurs according to the rules of long-term potentiation in the hippocampus; that is, synapses between active afferent axons and strongly activated postsynaptic neurons increase in strength (see Kelso, Ganong, & Brown, 1986; Levy, 1985; McNaughton, 1984; Wigstrom, Gustaffson, Huang, & Abraham, 1986) (postulate 3). The effect of this modification is that the next time the same stimulus is repeated, the neuron responds more (because of the strengthened synapses), more inhibition of other neurons occurs, and then further modification produces even greater selectivity. The response of the system as a classifier thus climbs over repeated iterations. One effect of this observed in simulations is that a few neurons then obtain such strong synaptic weights that almost any stimulus which has any input to that neuron will succeed in activating it. The solution to this is to limit the total synaptic weight that each output (postsynaptic) neuron can receive (postulate 4). In simulations this is performed by normalizing the sum of the synaptic weights on each neuron to a constant (e.g., 1.0) (see Rumelhart & Zipser, 1986; von der Malsburg, 1973). This has the effect of distributing the output neurons evenly between the different input patterns received by the network. In the brain this may be achieved by using a modified Hebb rule which produces some decrease in synaptic strength if there is high presynaptic but low postsynaptic activation (see Bear, Cooper, & Ebner, 1987).

   A simulation of the operation of such a competitive neuronal network is reproduced as Figure 9.3. It is shown that the network effectively selects different output neurons to respond to different combinations of active input horizontal lines. It thus performs a type of classification in which different complex input patterns are encoded economically onto a few output lines. It should be noted

INPUT: **|**   CYCLE: 202

COMPETITION MATRIX

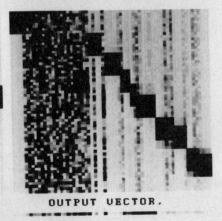

LEARNING STIMULUS :-
Overlap four A.

OUTPUT VECTOR.

AFTER FILTER.

INPUT: **J**   CYCLE: 202

COMPETITION MATRIX

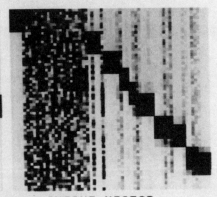

LEARNING STIMULUS :-
Overlap four B.

OUTPUT VECTOR.

AFTER FILTER.

that this classification finds natural clusters in the input events; orthogonalizes the classes so that overlap in input events can become coded onto output neurons with less overlap and in that many active input lines may be coded onto few active output lines; and does not allocate neurons to events that never occur (see Grossberg, 1982, 1987; Marr, 1970, 1971; Rumelhart & Zipser, 1986). It may be noted that there is no special correspondence between the input pattern and the output lines selected. Thus it is not useful for any associative mapping between an input and an output event and is thus different from associative matrix memories (Rolls, 1987). Instead, this type of matrix finds associations or correlations between input events (which are expressed as sets of simultaneously active horizontal input lines or axons), allocates output neurons to reflect the complex event, and stores the required association between the input lines onto the few output neurons activated by each complex input event.

There is evidence that in the hippocampus the synapses between inactive axons and active output neurons become weaker (see Bear et al., 1987; Levy, 1985; McNaughton, 1984). In the learning system described this would facilitate accurate and rapid classification, in that weakening synapses onto a postsynaptic neuron from axons that are not active when it is strongly activated would reduce the probability that it will respond to a stimulus which must be placed into a different class. It is also of interest that postulate 4 above (that the total synaptic strength onto a postsynaptic neuron is somewhat fixed) is not physiologically unreasonable (Levy & Desmond, 1985).

Another feature of hippocampal circuitry is the mossy fiber system, which connects the granule cells of the dentate gyrus to the CA3 pyramidal cells of the

←

FIGURE 9.3. Simulation of learning in a competitive matrix memory. The architecture is as shown in Figure 9.2, except that there are 64 horizontal axons and 64 vertical dendrites, which form the rows and columns respectively of the 64×64 matrix of synapses. The strength of each synapse, which was initially random, is indicated by the darkness of each pixel. The activity of each of the 64 input axons is represented in the 64-element vector at the left of the diagram by the darkness of each pixel. The output firing of the vertical neurons is represented in the same way by the output vectors at the bottom of the diagram. The upper output vector is the result of multiplying the input stimulus through the matrix of synaptic weights. The vector resulting from the application of competition between the output neurons (which produces contrast enhancement between the elements or neurons of the vector) is shown below by the vector labeled ''after filter.'' The state of the matrix is shown after 203 cycles in each of which stimuli with 8 of 64 active axons were presented, and the matrix was allowed to learn as described in the text. The stimuli, presented in random sequence, consisted of a set of vectors which overlapped in 0, 1, 2, 3, 4, 5, or 6 positions with the next vector in the set. The columns of the matrix were sorted after the learning to bring similar columns together, so that the types of neuron formed and the pattern of synapses formed on their dendrites can be seen easily. The dendrites with random patterns of synapses have not been allocated to any of the input stimuli. It is shown that application of one of the input stimuli (overlap four A) or vectors which overlapped in four of eight positions with another stimulus (overlap four B) produced one pattern of firing of the output neurons, and that application of input stimulus overlap four B produced a different pattern of firing of the output neurons. Thus the stimuli were correctly categorized by the matrix as being different.

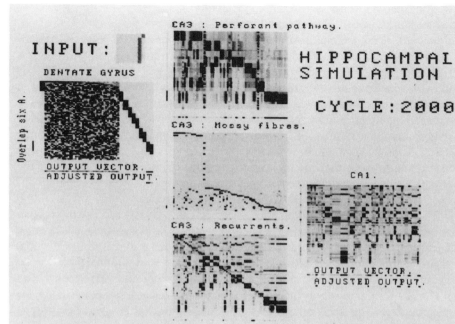

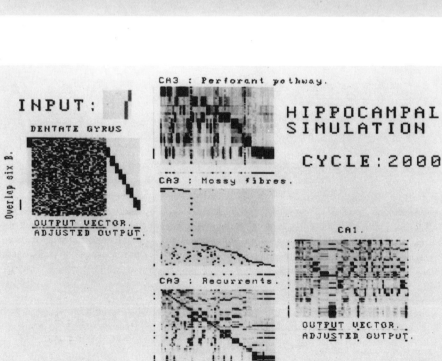

hippocampus. Each mossy fiber forms approximately 10 "mosses," in which there are dendrites of perhaps 5 different CA3 pyramidal cells. Thus each dentate granule cell may contact approximately 50 CA3 pyramidal cells (in the mouse; see Braitenberg & Schuz, 1984). In the rat, each mossy fiber forms approximately 14 mosses or contacts with CA3 cells, there are 1×10^6 dentate granule cells and thus 14×10^6 mosses onto 0.18×10^6 CA3 cells (D. G. Amaral, personal communication, 1988), and thus each dentate granule cell may contact approximately 78 CA3 pyramidal cells. This means that (in the rat) the probability that a CA3 cell is contacted by a given dentate granule cell is 78 synapses per 10^6 granule cells, or .000078. These mossy fiber synapses are very large, presumably because with such a relatively small number on each CA3 cell dendrite (and a much smaller number active at any one time), each synapse must be relatively strong. One effect that can be achieved by this low probability of contact of a particular dentate granule cell with a particular pyramidal cell is pattern separation. Consider a pattern of firing present over a set of dentate granule cells. The probability that any two CA3 pyramidal cells receive synapses from a similar subset of the dentate granule cells is very low (because of the low probability of contact of any one dentate granule cell with a pyramidal cell), so that each CA3 pyramidal cell is influenced by a very different subset of the active dentate granule cells. Thus each pyramidal cell effectively samples a very small subset of the active granule cells, and it is therefore likely that each CA3 pyramidal cell will respond differently to the others, so that in this way pattern separation is achieved. (The effect is similar to codon formation described in other contexts by Marr, 1970.) With modifiability of the mossy fiber synapses, CA3 neurons learn to respond to just those subsets of activity that do occur in dentate granule cells. Moreover, because of the low probability of contact, and because of the competition between the CA3 neurons, the patterns that occur are evenly distributed over different ensembles of CA3 neurons. This pattern separation effect can be seen in Figure 9.4. (It may be noted that even if competition does not

←————————————————————————————

FIGURE 9.4. Hippocampal stimulation. Conventions as in Figure 9.3. The dentate gyrus is shown as a competition matrix at the left, receiving input stimuli from the perforant path. The vertical dendrites of the CA3 pyramidal cells extend throughout the three submatrices shown in the middle. The middle submatrix, which operates as a competition matrix, receives the output of the dentate granule cells via the mossy fibers with potentially powerful synapses and a low contact probability. Pattern separation can be seen to operate in that input vectors are converted into output vectors with many elements activated by the inputs about which the submatrix has learned, and in that different output vectors are produced for even quite similar input vectors. The upper CA3 submatrix operates as a competition matrix with a direct perforant path input. The lower CA3 submatrix operates as an autoassociation matrix (formed by the recurrent collaterals). The output of the CA3 cells (summed vertically up and down the dendrite) is then used as the input (via the Schaffer collaterals) to the CA1 cells, which operate as a competition matrix. The states of the matrices after 2000 presentations of the same set of stimuli used for Figure 9.3. are shown. One point demonstrated is that two very similar stimuli, overlap six A and overlap six B, produce output vectors at CA1 which are relatively orthogonal to each other.

operate in this system to increase orthogonality, the low probability of connections just described would nevertheless mean that the hippocampus could operate to produce relatively orthogonal representations.)

It is notable that in addition to the mossy fiber inputs, the CA3 pyramidal cells receive inputs directly from perforant path fibers (see Figs. 9.1 and 9.2). This is not a sparse projection, in that each pyramidal cell may receive on the order of 2300 such synapses. (This is calculated using the evidence that of 15 mm of total dendritic length with 10,000 spines, approximately 3.5 mm [range 2.5–4.5 mm] is in the lacunosum moleculare and thus receives inputs from the perforant path; D. G. Amaral, personal communication, 1988). What would be the effect of this input together with the very sparse but strong synapses from the mossy fibers? One effect is that the mossy fiber input would cause the pattern of synapses (considered as a vector) on each pyramidal cell to point in a different direction in a multidimensional space. However, the precise direction in that multidimensional space could not be well specified by the relatively small number of mossy fiber synapses onto each CA3 pyramidal cell. But a particular cell, once pointed to that part of space by the mossy fibers, would show cooperative Hebbian learning between its activation by the mossy input and the direct perforant path input, allowing the direct input to come by learning to specify the exact direction of that cell in multidimensional space much more effectively than by the coarse mossy fiber input alone. This effect can be seen in Figure 9.4. The relative weighting in this simulation was that the mossy fiber input had an effect on each neuron which was five times greater than that of the direct perforant path input. Thus it is suggested that the combination of the sparse mossy fiber input and the direct perforant path input is to achieve pattern separation, and at the same time to allow the response of the neuron to be determined not just by the sparse mossy fiber input, but much more finely by making use of the direct perforant path input.

An additional feature of the hippocampus, developed in the CA3 pyramidal cells in particular, is the presence of strong recurrent collaterals, which return from the output of the matrix to cross over the neurons of the matrix, as shown in Figures 9.1 and 9.2. This anatomy immediately suggests that this is an autoassociation (or autocorrelation) matrix. The autoassociation arises because the output of the matrix, expressed as the firing rate of the CA3 pyramidal cells, is fed back along the horizontally running axons so that the pattern of activity in this part of the matrix (the CA3 pyramidal cells) is associated with itself (see, e.g., Kohonen, Oja, & Lehtio, 1981; Rolls, 1987). It can be noted here that for this suggestion to be the case, the synapses of the recurrent collaterals would have to be modifiable, and the modification rule would require alteration of synaptic strength when both the presynaptic fiber and the postsynaptic dendrite were strongly activated. Further, the probability of contact of the neurons in the autoassociation matrix must not be very low if it is to operate usefully (see Marr, 1971). Given that the region of the CA3 cell dendrites on which the recurrent collaterals synapse is long (approximately 11.5 mm), and that the total dendritic length is approximately 15 mm and has approximately 10,000 spines (D. G.

Amaral, personal communication, 1988), approximately 7700 synapses per CA3 pyramidal cell could be devoted to recurrent collaterals, which with 180,000 CA3 neurons in the rat makes the probability of contact between the CA3 neurons .043. This is high enough for the system to operate usefully as an autoassociation memory (see Marr, 1971). It is remarkable that the contact probability is so high, and also that the CA3 recurrent collateral axons travel so widely in all directions that they can potentially come close to almost all other CA3 neurons (D. G. Amaral, personal communication, 1988).

The importance of the autoassociation performed by this part of the matrix is that it forms a recognition memory, with all the advantageous emergent properties of a matrix memory, such as completion, generalization, and graceful degradation (see Kohonen, 1984; Kohonen et al., 1977, 1981; Rolls, 1987). One particularly relevant property here is completion: if part of a stimulus (or event) occurs, then the autoassociation part of the matrix completes that event. Completion may operate particularly effectively here, because it operates after the granule cell stage, which will reduce the proportion of neurons firing to represent an input event to a low number partly because of the low probability of contact of the granule cells with the CA3 pyramidal cells. Under these conditions the simple autocorrelation effect can reconstruct the whole of one pattern without interference, which would arise if too high a proportion of the input neurons was active. A scheme of this type, although not expressed this way in the autoassociation matrix formulation, was proposed by Marr in 1971. Another effect of the autoassociation matrix is that patterns of activity which are not similar to those already learned by this type of recogniton memory are lost, so that noisy patterns can be cleaned up by the autoassociation matrix. It is further notable that these completion and cleaning up processes may benefit from several iterations (repeated cycles) of the autoassociation feedback effect. It has been suggested by McNaughton (personal communication, 1987) that one function of hippocampal theta activity may be to allow this autoassociation effect produced by the recurrent collaterals to cycle for several iterations (in a period of approximately 50 msec) and then to stop, so that the system can operate again with maximal sensitivity to new inputs received on the mossy and perforant path systems by the CA3 cells.

The CA1 pyramidal cells that receive from the CA3 cells are considered to form a further stage of competitive learning, which has the effect of further classification of signals received, perhaps enabled by the pattern of connections within the hippocampus to form these classifications over inputs received from any part of the association neocortex. The firing of the CA1 cells would thus achieve a much more economical and orthogonal classification of signals than that present in the perforant path input to the hippocampus. These signals are then returned to the association neocortex through the subiculum, entorhinal cortex, and parahippocampal gyrus, as indicated in Figures 9.1 and 9.2. It is suggested below that one role which these economical (in terms of the number of activated fibers) and relatively orthogonal signals play in neocortical function is to guide information storage or consolidation in the neocortex.

Multilayer networks (such as the hippocampus) can potentially solve classes of problem that cannot be solved in principle by single-layer nets (Rumelhart & Zipser, 1986), because subcategories formed in an early stage of processing can enable a later stage to find solutions or categories that are not linearly separable in the input information space.

Having considered the computational theory of how the hippocampal circuitry may function, we can now turn to a systems level analysis, in which the inputs and outputs of the hippocampus are considered and the function performed by the hippocampus in relation to overall brain function can be formulated.

SYSTEMS LEVEL THEORY OF HIPPOCAMPAL FUNCTION

The anatomical connections of the primate hippocampus with the rest of the brain are considered first, to provide a basis for considering how the computational ability of the hippocampus could be used by the rest of the brain. The hippocampus receives inputs by two main routes, the entorhinal cortex and the fimbria/fornix. The entorhinal cortex (area 28) provides the hippocampus with extensive inputs from the neocortex (i.e., cerebral cortex; see Fig. 9.5). Thus all temporal neocortical areas project to area 35, the perirhinal cortex, or to area TF–TH, in the parahippocampal gyrus, in turn projecting to the entorhinal cortex (Amaral, 1987; Van Hoesen, 1982; Van Hoesen & Pandya, 1975a). The parietal cortex (area 7) projects to area TF–TH, and thus can potentially influence the hippocampus. The orbitofrontal cortex, areas 12 and 13, projects directly to the entorhinal cortex (Van Hoesen, Pandya, & Butters, 1975). In addition, the entorhinal cortex receives inputs from the amygdala. The entorhinal cortex itself projects via the perforant path to reach primarily the dentate granule cells of the hippocampus proper. By these routes the hippocampus receives information after it has been highly processed through the temporal, parietal, and frontal cortices. It must thus be of great importance for hippocampal function in the primate that by its main input, the perforant path, it receives information from the highest parts of the neocortex. There are also inputs to the hippocampus via the fimbria/fornix from the cholinergic cells of the medial septum and the adjoining limb of the diagonal band of Broca. The hippocampus also receives a noradrenergic input from the locus coeruleus and a 5-hydroxytryptamine (5-HT) input from the median raphe nucleus.

A major output of the hippocampus arises from the hippocampal pyramidal cells and projects back via the subiculum to the entorhinal cortex, which in turn has connections back to area TF–TH, which, in turn, projects back to the neocortical areas from which it receives inputs (Van Hoesen, 1982); see Figs. 9.1 and 9.5). Thus the hippocampus can potentially influence the neocortical regions from which it receives inputs. This is the pathway that seems to be involved in guiding memory storage in the neocortex. A second efferent projection of the hippocampal system reaches the subiculum from the CA1 pyramidal

AFFERENT CONNECTIONS   EFFERENT CONNECTIONS

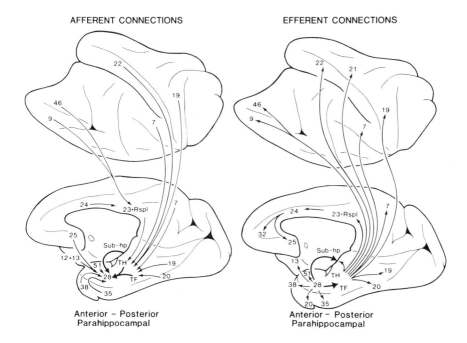

Anterior – Posterior
Parahippocampal   Anterior – Posterior
Parahippocampal

FIGURE 9.5. Connections of the primate hippocampus with the neocortex. A medial view of the macaque brain is shown below, and a lateral view is shown inverted above. The hippocampus receives its inputs via the parahippocampal gyrus, areas TF and TH, and the entorhinal cortex, area 28. The return projections to the neocortex (shown on the right) pass through the same areas. Cortical areas 19, 20, and 21 are visual association areas, 22 is auditory association cortex, 7 is parietal association cortex, and 9, 46, 12, and 13 are frontal cortical association areas. (From Van Hoesen, 1982)

cells and travels via the fimbria and (postcommissural) fornix to the anterior thalamus and to the mammillary bodies, which, in turn, project to the anterior thalamus. The anterior thalamus, in turn, projects into the cingulate cortex, which itself has connections to the supplementary motor cortex, providing a potential route for the hippocampus to influence motor output (Van Hoesen, 1982). Functions of the hippocampus in, for example, conditional spatial response learning apparently utilize this output path to the motor system.

The connections of the hippocampus with other parts of the brain and the internal connections and synaptic modifiability previously described, suggest that the hippocampus should be able to detect, and classify onto a few specifically responding neurons, specific conjunctions of complex (cortically processed) events, such as the information that a particular object (presumably reflecting temporal lobe visual processing) has appeared in a particular position in space (probably reflecting parietal input). Another example might be that a particular stimulus should be associated with a particular spatial motor response. It has been shown that this is the type of specific information which comes to activate different hippocampal neurons while monkeys are performing object–place memory and conditional spatial response learning tasks. Indeed, the neurophysiological findings discussed earlier provide evidence supporting the model of hippocampal function just described. The model is also supported by the evidence that during the learning of conditional spatial responses some hippocampal neurons start, but then stop showing differential responses to the different stimuli, consistent with competitive interactions between hippocampal neurons during learning, so that only some hippocampal neurons become allocated to any one learned event or contingency.

The foregoing analyses have shown that the hippocampus receives from high-order areas of association cortex; is able by virtue of the large number of synapses on its dendrites to detect conjunctions of events even when these are widely separated in information space, with their origin from different cortical areas; allocates neurons to code efficiently for these conjunctions probably using a competitive learning mechanism; and has connections back to the neocortical areas from which it receives, as well as to subcortical structures via the fimbria/ fornix system. What could be achieved by this system? It appears that the long-term storage of information is not in the hippocampus, at least in humans, where damage to the hippocampus does not necessarily result in major retrograde amnesia (Squire, 1986, 1987). On the other hand, the hippocampus does appear to be necessary for the storage of certain types of information (characterized by the description declarative, or knowing what, as contrasted with procedural, or knowing how). How could the hippocampus then be involved in the storage of information?

These and the other findings suggest that the hippocampus is specialized to detect the best way in which to store information and then, by the return paths to the neocortex, directs memory storage there. Clearly the hippocampus, with its large number of synapses on each neuron and its potentiation type of learning, is able to detect when there is coherence (i.e., conjunctive activation of arbitrary sets of its input fibers) and is able, as indicated both theoretically and by recordings made in the behaving monkey, to allocate neurons to economically (i.e., with relatively few neurons active) code for each complex input event. Such neurons could then represent an efficient way in which to store information, in that redundancy would effectively have been removed from the input signal. In a sense, the optimal way in which to build high-level feature analyzers could be determined by the hippocampus. It should be noted that this theory is not inconsistent with the possibility that the hippocampus provides a working memory, in that in the present theory the hippocampus sets up a representation using Hebbian learning, which is useful in determining how information can best be stored in the neocortex. (The representation found by the hippocampus could provide a useful working memory [see Olton, 1984]; indeed, in the object–place memory task described earlier, the object and place combinations formed onto single hippocampal neurons would provide a useful working memory. An understanding of the operations performed by the hippocampus at the neuronal network level may enable one to visualize how the hippocampus could contribute to several functions that are not necessarily inconsistent.)

Where the long-term storage occurs and how it may be directed by the hippocampus mut be considered next. The hippocampus is reciprocally connected via the subiculum and entorhinal cortex with the parahippocampal gyrus, which in turn is reciprocally connected with many high-order areas of association neocortex (see Fig. 9.5). It is therefore possible that the actual storage takes place in the parahippocampal gyrus and that this might be particularly appropriate for multimodal memories. However, having detected that, for example, a visual stimulus is regularly associated with an event in another modality such as a movement, it might be useful to direct the unimodal representation of that visual image, so that it is stored efficiently and can provide a useful input to the multimodal conjunction store. Thus return pathways (via, e.g., the parahippocampal gyrus) to unimodal cortex (e.g., inferior temporal visual cortex, area TE) might be used to direct unimodal storage by contributing to detection of the most economical way in which to store representations of stimuli.

The question of how the hippocampal output is used by the neocortex (i.e., cerebral cortex) will be considered next. Given that the hippocampal output returns to the neocortex, a theory of backprojections in the neocortex will be needed. By way of introduction, it may be noted that the particular hippocampal neurons that happen to represent a complex input event are not determined by any teacher or forcing (unconditioned) stimulus. The neocortex must be able to utilize the signal cleverly. One possibility is that any neocortical neuron with a number of afferents active at the same time that hippocampal return fibers in its vicinity are active modifies its responses so that it comes to respond better to those afferents the next time they occur. This learning by the cortex would involve a Hebb-like learning mechanism. One function served by what are thus in effect backprojections from the hippocampus is some guidance for or supervision of neocortical learning. It is a problem of unsupervised learning systems that they can efficiently detect local conjunctions, which are not necessarily those of most use to the whole system. It is exactly this problem that the hippocampus apparently helps to solve by detecting useful conjunctions globally (i.e., over the whole of information space) and then directing storage locally at earlier stages of processing so that filters are built locally which provide representations of input stimuli useful for later processing.

THEORETICAL SIGNIFICANCE OF BACKPROJECTIONS IN THE NEOCORTEX

The forward and backward projections that will be considered are shown in Figure 9.6 (for further anatomical information see Peters & Jones, 1984). In primary sensory cortical areas, the main extrinsic forward input is from the thala-

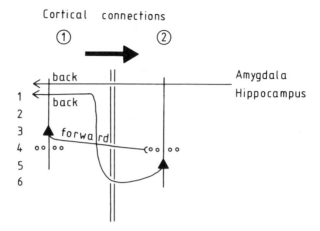

FIGURE 9.6.   Schematic diagram of forward and backward projections in the neocortex. The superficial pyramidal cells (triangles) in layers 2 and 3 project forward to terminate in layer 4 of the next cortical area. The deep pyramidal cells in the next area project back to layer 1 of the preceding cortical area, in which there are apical dendrites of pyramidal cells. The hippocampus and amygdala also are the source of backprojections which end in layer 1. Spiny stellate cells are represented by small circles in layer 4. See text for further details.

mus and ends in layer 4, where synapses are formed onto spiny stellate cells. These in turn project heavily onto pyramidal cells in layers 3 and 2, which in turn send projections forward to terminate strongly in layer 4 of the next cortical layer (on small pyramidal cells in layer 4 or on the basal dendrites of the layer 2 and 3 [superficial] pyramidal cells). Although the forward afferents end strongly in layer 4, the forward afferents have some synapses also onto the basal dendrites of the layer 2 pyramidal cells, as well as onto layer 6 pyramidal cells and inhibitory interneurons. Inputs reach the layer 5 (deep) pyramidal cells from the pyramidal cells in layers 2 and 3 (Martin, 1984), and the deep pyramidal cells send backprojections to end in layer 1 of the preceding cortical area (see Figure 9.6), where there are apical dendrites of pyramidal cells. There are few current theories about the functions subserved by the cortico-cortical backprojections, even though there are almost as many backprojecting as forward-projecting axons. It is important to note that in addition to the axons and their terminals in layer 1 from the succeeding cortical stage, there are also axons and terminals in layer 1 in many stages of the cortical hierarchy from the amygdala and (via the subiculum, entorhinal cortex, and papahippocampal cortex) from the hippocampal formation (see Fig. 9.6; Amaral, 1986, 1987; Amaral & Price, 1984; Turner, 1981; Van Hoesen, 1981). The amygdala and hippocampus are stages of information processing at which the different sensory modalities (such as vision, hearing, touch, and taste for the amygdala) are brought together, so that correlations between inputs in different modalities can be detected in these regions but not at prior cortical processing stages in each modality, since these cortical processing stages are unimodal. As a result of bringing together the two modalities, significant correspondences between the two modalities can be detected. For example, a particular visual stimulus may be associated with the taste of food; another visual stimulus may be associated with painful touch. Thus at these stages of processing, but not before, the significance of, say, visual and auditory stimuli can be detected and signaled, and sending this information back to the neocortex thus can provide a signal that indicates to the cortex that information should be stored, but—even more than this—it provides an orthogonal signal that could help the neocortex to store the information efficiently.

The way in which backprojections could assist learning in the cortex can be considered using the architecture shown in Figure 9.7. The (forward) input stimulus occurs as a vector applied to (layer 3) cortical pyramidal cells through modifiable synapses in the standard way for a competitive net. (If it is a primary cortical area, the input stimulus is at least partly relayed through spiny stellate cells, which may help to normalize and orthogonalize the input patterns in a preliminary way before the patterns are applied to the layer 3 pyramidal cells. If it is a nonprimary cortical area, the cortico-cortical forward axons may end more strongly on the basal dendrites of neurons in the superficial cortical layers.) The lower set of synapses on the pyramidal cells would then start by competitive learning to set up representations on the lower parts of these neurons, which would represent correlations in the input information space and could be said to correspond to features in the input information space, where a feature is defined simply as the representation of a correlation in the input information space.

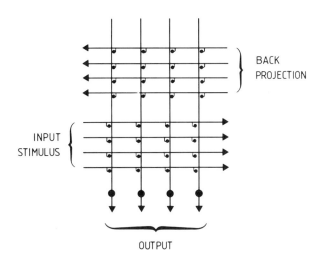

FIGURE 9.7. The architecture used to simulate the properties of backprojections. The forward (input stimulus) and backprojected axons make Hebb-modifiable synapses onto the same set of vertical dendrites, which represent cortical pyramidal cells.

Consider the application of one of the (forward) input stimulus vectors with the conjunctive application of a pattern vector via the backprojection axons with terminals in layer 1. Given that all the synapses in the matrix start with random weights, some of the pyramidal cells will by chance be strongly influenced both by the (forward) input stimulus and by the backprojecting vector. These strongly activated neurons will then compete with each other as in a standard competitive net, to produce contrast enhancement of their firing patterns. (The relatively short-range [50 μm] excitatory operations produced by bipolar and double bouquet cells, together with more widespread [300 to 500 μm] recurrent lateral inhibition produced by the smooth nonpyramidal cells and perhaps the basket cells, may be part of the mechanism of this competitive interaction.) Next, Hebbian learning takes place as in a competitive net, with the addition that not only are the synapses between forward-projecting axons and active postsynaptic neurons modified, but the synapses in layer 1 between the backward-projecting axons and the (same) active postsynaptic neurons are modified.

This functional architecture has the following properties. First, the backprojections, which are assumed to carry signals that are relatively information-rich (Rolls, 1987) and orthogonal to each other as a result of the conjunctions formed by the hippocampus, amygdala, or next cortical stage, help the neurons to learn to respond differently to (and thus separate) input stimuli (on the forward projection lines) even when the input stimuli are very similar. This is illustrated in the simulation seen in Figure 9.8, where input stimuli that overlap even in six positions out of eight can be easily learned as separate if presented conjunctively with different orthogonal backprojecting "tutors." (For a similar idea on the guidance of a competitive learning system see Rumelhart & Zipser, 1986.) Another way in which the learning of pyramidal cells can be influenced is that if two relatively different input stimuli are being received, but the same backprojecting signal occurs with these two somewhat different forward inputs, then the pyramidal cells, guided by the tutor, will build the representation of the forward input stimuli on the same pyramidal cells. If the representations of the forward inputs built by modification of the synapses on the pyramidal cells are considered as vectors in a multidimensional space, then the representations will be forced toward each other as a result of the operation of the common backprojecting tutor.

In the cerebral cortex, the backprojecting tutors can be of two types. One originates from the amygdala and hippocampus, and, by benefiting from cross-

→

FIGURE 9.8. Simulation of neocortical backprojection learning matrix. Conventions as in Figure 9.3. (A) During learning, both a forward input (chosen from the same set used in Figure 9.3) and a backprojected vector which was orthogonal to the other backprojected vectors are presented simultaneously. After 206 cycles with input stimulus–backprojected tutor pairs chosen in random sequence, the synapses had modified as shown. In (B,C) two similar input stimuli (overlap six A and six B) produce different outputs. The learning has been guided by the backprojected tutors presented during learning (D). If only the tutor originally paired with input stimulus overlap six A is presented, then recall of the output vector normally recognized by input stimulus overlap six A occurs.

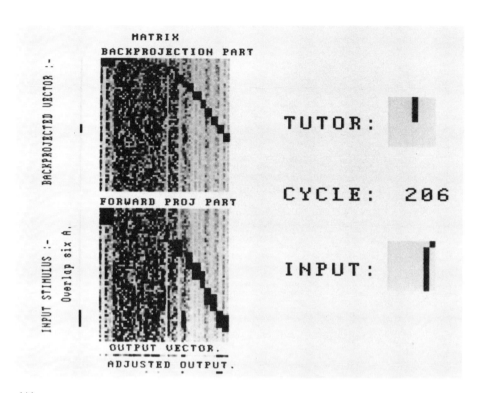

(A)

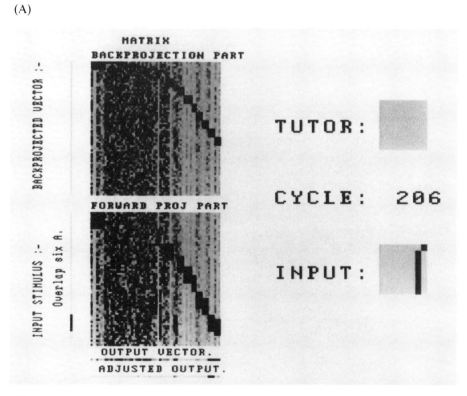

(B)

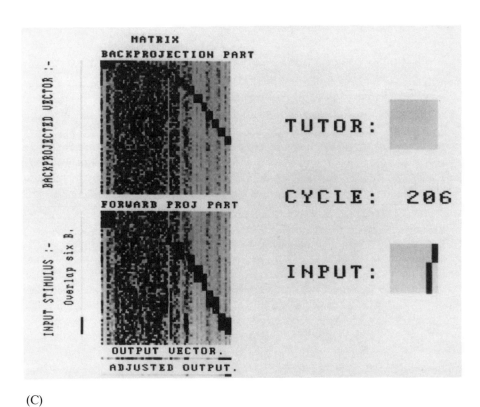

(C)

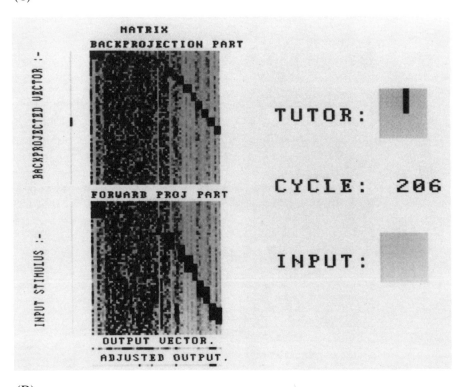

(D)

modal comparison, can provide an orthogonal backprojected vector. This backprojection, moreover, may be activated only if the multimodal areas detect that the visual stimulus is significant, for example, if it is associated with a pleasant taste. This provides one way in which a competitive learning system can be guided as to what it should learn, so that it does not attempt to lay down representations of all incoming sensory information, but only those shown to be significant as a result of comparison made with inputs originating in a different modality. Another way for this important function to be achieved is by activation of neurons that "strobe" the cortex when new or significant stimuli are shown. The cholinergic system originating in the basal forebrain (which itself receives information from the amygdala) and the noradrenergic input to layer 1 of the cortex from the locus coeruleus may also contribute to this function (see Bear & Singer, 1986; Rolls, 1987). However, in that there are relatively few neurons in these basal forebrain and noradrenergic systems, it is suggested that these projections provide only a simple strobe (see Rolls, 1987). In contrast, there are sufficient axons in the backprojecting systems from the hippocampus and amygdala to carry pattern-specific information, so that the hypothesis presented here is that these backprojections guide the consolidation of information by influencing how information is stored on pyramidal cells in the way described above. The situations in which the amygdala and hippocampal backprojections guide learning (as well as recall and attention, as discussed later) are probably different in the following way. The amygdala is particularly involved when associations are made between a neutral stimulus (such as a visual stimulus) and a reinforcing stimulus (e.g., from the taste or touch inputs it receives; see Rolls, 1985, 1987); in contrast, the hippocampus is particularly involved when conjunctions must be detected between spatial inputs (received by the major inputs of the hippocampus which originate from the parietal cortex) and its other inputs (e.g., the inferior temporal visual cortex), in, for example, conditional spatial response and object–place learning tasks.

The second type of backprojection is from the next cortical area in the hierarchy. The next cortical area operates in the same manner, and because it is a competitive system, it is able to further categorize or orthogonalize the stimuli it receives. This next cortical stage then projects back these more orthogonal representations as tutors to the preceding stage, to effectively build at the preceding stage better filters for the diagnosis of the categories being found at the next stage.

A second property of this architecture is that it provides for recall. Recall of a previously stored representation by another stimulus or event occurs in the following way. If only the tutor is presented, then the neurons originally activated by the forward-projecting input stimuli are activated. This occurs because the synapses from the backprojecting axons onto the pyramidal cells have been modified only where there was conjunctive forward-projected and backprojected activity during learning. Figure 9.8 is a simulation of this. Consider the situation when in the visual system the sight of food is forward projected onto pyramidal cells, and conjunctively there is a backprojected signal elicited by the taste of the food and originating from a multimodal area such as the amygdala. Neurons that have conjunctive inputs from these two stimuli set up representations of both, so that later if a backprojected signal produced by the taste occurs, then the visual neurons originally activated by the sight of that food will be activated, and thus recall of the visual representation is achieved. In this way many of the low-level details of the original visual stimulus can be recalled. Evidence that during recall relatively early cortical processing stages are activated comes from cortical blood flow studies in humans, in which it has been found, for example, that early visual cortical association areas are activated during recall of visual (but not auditory) information (Roland & Friberg, 1985; Roland, Vaernet, & Lassen, 1980). Recall could operate as a result of signals backprojected directly from the amygdala or parahippocampal gyrus or indirectly through series of back-connected cortical stages.

A third property of this architecture is that attention could operate from higher to lower levels to selectively facilitate only certain pyramidal cells by using the backprojections. Indeed, the backprojections described could produce many of the "top-down" influences common in perception. A fourth property is that semantic priming could operate by using the backprojecting neurons to provide a small activation of just those neurons in earlier stages which are appropriate for responding to that semantic category of input stimulus.

A fifth property of such a return mechanism, which, on detecting a conjunction (perhaps across modalities), improves unimodal representations of the input stimuli, would be a form of positive feedback that would gradually improve storage through the reciprocal interactions, as the feedback effect produced a better representation at the preceding level to be fed forward, with this occurring repeatedly. This might provide a neurophysiological and computational basis for any gradient of retrograde amnesia that occurs for the period just before disruption of temporal lobe function (Squire, 1986, 1987). A sixth property of the backprojections is that they would assist the stability of the preceding competitive networks by providing a relatively constant guiding signal as a result of associations made at a higher stage, for example, to an unconditioned taste or somatosensory input.

This theory of the functions of backprojections in the cerebral cortex requires a large number of backprojecting axons, as pattern-specific information (used to guide learning by providing a set of mutually orthogonal guidance signals, or to produce recall) must be provided by the backprojections. It also solves the dead-dressing problem, for the hippocampus does not need to know exactly where in the cortex information should be stored. Instead, the backprojection signal spreads widely in layer 1, and the storage site is simply on those neurons that happen to receive strong (and precise) forward activity as well as backprojected activity, so that Hebbian learning by conjunction occurs there. This scheme is consistent with neocortical anatomy, in that it requires the same pyramidal cell to receive both forward-projected and (more diffuse) backprojected activity, which the arrangement of pyramidal cells with apical dendrites extending all the way up into layer 1 achieves (see Peters & Jones, 1984). Indeed, in contrast to the relatively localized terminal distributions of forward cortico-cortical and thalamo-cortical afferents, the cortico-cortical backward projections that end in layer 1 have a much wider horizontal distribution, of up to several millimeters (Amaral, 1986). The suggestion is thus that this enables the backward-projecting neurons to search over a large number of pyramidal cells in the preceding cortical area for activity conjunctive with their own. Note that the theory utilizes a Hebbian learning scheme, which provides for learning to occur when conjointly there is forward and backprojected input to a pyramidal cell resulting in sufficient postsynaptic activation to provide for modification of synapses that happen to be active. This provides the opportunity to make it clear that the theoretical ideas introduced here make clear predictions that can be empirically tested. For example, the theory of backprojections just proposed predicts that the backprojections in the cerebral cortex have modifiable synapses on pyramidal cells in the previous cortical area. If this were found not to be the case in empirical tests, then the theory would be rejected.

The ideas introduced here also have many theoretical implications. One is that if the backprojections are used for recall, as seems likely (as discussed above; see also Roland & Friberg, 1985), then this would place severe constraints on their use for functions such as error backpropagation. Error backpropagation is an interesting and powerful algorithm in parallel distributed processing networks for setting the weights in hidden units (i.e., nodes in layers which are not input and output layers) to allow networks to learn useful mappings between input and output layers (Rumelhart, Hinton, & Williams, 1986). However, the backprojections in the architecture in which this algorithm is implemented have precise functions in conveying error from the output layer back to the earlier, hidden layers. It would be difficult to use the weights (synaptic strengths) from the backprojecting neurons to neurons in earlier layers both to convey the error correctly and to have the appropriate strengths for recall.

CONCLUSIONS

In this chapter, experimental evidence on and theoretical approaches to the function of the hippocampus and of backprojections in the cerebral cortex were considered. Theories of how the hippocampus functions and of the functions of backprojections in the neocortex were proposed. The theories are at the level of neuronal networks, and are based on evidence on the fine architecture of the networks, on the rules of synaptic modifiability incorporated, and on the systems level connections. It is suggested that this approach will be useful in linking anatomical evidence on structure to physiological evidence on modifiability, understanding the global properties of the networks, and thus understanding the role of the networks in brain function and behavior.

Acknowledgments
The author has worked on some of the experiments and neuronal network modeling described here with P. Cahusac, D. Cohen, J. Feigenbaum, R. Kesner, Y.

Miyashita, and H. Niki, and their collaboration is sincerely acknowledged. Discussions with David G. Amaral of the Salk Institute, La Jolla, were also much appreciated. This research was supported by the Medical Research Council.

REFERENCES

Amaral, D. G. (1986). Amygdalohippocampal and amygdalocortical projections in the primate brain. In R. Schwarz and Y. Ben-Ari, (Eds.), *Excitatory amino acids and epilepsy* (pp. 3–17) New York: Plenum.

Amaral, D. G. (1987). Memory: Anatomical organization of candidate brain regions. In F. Plum (Ed.), *Handbook of physiology: Sec. 1. The nervous system* (pp. 211–294). Bethesda, Md.: American Physiological Society.

Amaral, D., & Price, J. L. (1984). Amygdalo-cortical projections in the monkey *(Macaca fascicularis). Journal of Comparative Neurology, 230,* 465–496.

Bear, M. F., Cooper, L. N., & Ebner, F. B. (1987). A physiological basis for a theory of synapse modification. *Science, 237,* 42–48.

Bear, M. F., & Singer, W. (1986). Modulation of visual cortical plasticity by acetylcholine and noradrenaline. *Nature, 320,* 172–176.

Braitenberg, V., & Schuz, A. (1982). Some anatomical comments on the hippocampus. In W. Seifert (Ed.), *Neurobiology of the Hippocampus* (pp. 21–37), London: Academic Press.

Cahusac, P. M. B., Feigenbaum, J., Rolls, E. T., Miyashita, Y., & Niki, H. (1986). Modifications of neuronal activity during learning in the primate hippocampus. *Neuroscience Letters, S24,* S29.

Cahusac, P. M. B., Miyashita, Y., & Rolls, E. T. (1989). Responses of hippocampal neurons in the monkey related to delayed spatial response and object-place memory tasks. *Behavioural Brain Research 33,* 229–240.

Corkin, S. (1984). Lasting consequences of bilateral medial temporal lobectomy: Clinical course and experimental findings in H. M. *Seminars in Neurology, 4,* 249–259.

Gaffan, D. (1974). Recognition impaired and association intact in the memory of monkeys after transection of the fornix. *Journal of Comparative and Physiological Psychology, 86,* 1100–1109.

Gaffan, D. (1977). Monkeys' recognition memory for complex pictures and the effects of fornix transection. *Quarterly Journal of Experimental Psychology, 29,* 505–514.

Gaffan, D. (1985). Hippocampus: Memory, habit and voluntary movement. *Philosophical Transactions of the Royal Society B, 308,* 87–99.

Gaffan, D., & Saunders, R. C. (1985). Running recognition of configural stimuli by fornix transected monkeys. *Quarterly Journal of Experimental Psychology, 37B,* 61–71.

Grossberg, S. (1982). *Studies of mind and brain.* New York: Reidel.

Grossberg, S. (1987). Competitive learning: From interactive activation to adaptive resonance. *Cognitive Science, 11,* 23–63.

Hinton, G. E., & Anderson, J. A. (1981). *Parallel models of associative memory.* Hillsdale, N.J.: Erlbaum.

Ito, M. (1984). *The cerebellum and neural control.* New York: Raven.

Jones, E. G., & Peters, A. (Eds.). (1984). *The cerebral cortex: Vol. 2. Functional properties of cortical cells.* New York: Plenum.

Kelso, S. R., Ganong, A. H., & Brown, T. H. (1986). Hebbian synapses in the hippocampus. *Proceedings of the National Academy of Sciences, 83,* 5326–5330.

Kohonen, T. (1984). *Self-organization and associative memory.* Berlin: Springer-Verlag.

Kohonen, T., Lehtio, P., Rovamo, J., Hyvarinen, J., Bry, K., & Vainio, L. (1977). A principle of neural associative memory. *Neuroscience, 2,* 1065–1076.

Kohonen, T., Oja, E., & Lehtio, P. (1981). Storage and processing of information in distributed associative memory systems. In G. E. Hinton & J. A. Anderson (Eds.), *Parallel models of associative memory* (pp. 105–143). Hillsdale, N.J.: Erlbaum.
Levy, W. B. (1985). Associative changes in the synapse: LTP in the hippocampus. In W. B. Levy, J. A. Anderson, & S. Lehmkuhle (Eds.), *Synaptic modification, neuron selectivity, and nervous system organization* (pp. 5–33). Hillsdale, N.J.: Erlbaum.
Levy, W. B., & Desmond, N. L. (1985). The rules of elemental synaptic plasticity. In W. B. Levy, J. A. Anderson, & S. Lehmkuhle (Eds.), *Synaptic modification, neuron selectivity, and nervous system organization* (pp. 105–121). Hillsdale, N.J.: Erlbaum.
Marr, D. (1970). A theory for cerebral cortex. *Proceedings of the Royal Society B, 176,* 161–234.
Marr, D. (1971). Simple memory: A theory for archicortex. *Philosophical Transactions of the Royal Society B, 262,* 23–81.
McNaughton, B. L. (1984). Activity dependent modulation of hippocampal synaptic efficacy: Some implications for memory processes. In W. Seifert (Ed.), *Neurobiology of the hippocampus* (pp. 233–252). London: Academic Press.
Martin, K. A. C. (1984). Neuronal circuits in cat striate cortex. In E. G. Jones & A. Peters (Eds.), *The cerebral cortex: Vol 2. Functional properties of cortical cells* (pp. 241–285). New York: Plenum.
Milner, B. (1982). Disorders of learning and memory after temporal lobe lesions in man. *Clinical Neurosurgery, 19,* 421–446.
Mishkin, M. (1978). Memory severely impaired by combined but not separate removal of amygdala and hippocampus. *Nature, 273,* 297–298.
Mishkin, M. (1982). A memory system in the monkey. *Philosophical Transactions of the Royal Society B, 298,* 85–95.
Miyashita, Y., Rolls, E. T., Cahusac, P. M. B., & Niki, H. (1989). Activity of hippocampal formation neurons in the monkey related to a stimulus-response association task. *Journal of Neurophysiology, 61,* 669–678.
Murray, E. A., & Mishkin, M. (1984). Severe tactual as well as visual memory deficits follow combined removal of the amygdala and hippocampus in monkeys. *Journal of Neuroscience, 4,* 2565–2580.
Murray, E. A., & Mishkin, M. (1985). Amygdalectomy impairs crossmodal association in monkeys. *Science, 228,* 604–606.
O'Keefe, J. (1984). Spatial memory within and without the hippocampal system. In W. Seifert (Ed.), *Neurobiology of the Hippocampus* (pp. 375–403). London: Academic Press.
Olton, D. S. (1984). Memory functions and the hippocampus. In W. Seifert (Ed.), *Neurobiology of the hippocampus,* (pp. 335–373). London: Academic Press.
Palm, G. (1982). *Neural assemblies.* Berlin: Springer-Verlag.
Peters, A., & Jones, E. G. (1984). *The cerebral cortex: Vol. 1. Cellular components of the cerebral cortex.* New York: Plenum.
Petrides, M. (1985). Deficits on conditional associative-learning tasks after frontal- and temporal-lobe lesions in man. *Neuropsychologia, 23,* 601–614.
Roland, P. E., & Friberg, L. (1985). Localization of cortical areas activated by thinking. *Journal of Neurophysiology, 53,* 1219–1243.
Roland, P. E., Vaernet, K., & Lassen, N. A. (1980). Cortical activations in man during verbal report from visual memory. *Neuroscience Letters* (Suppl. 5), S478.
Rolls, E. T. (1985). Connections, functions and dysfunctions of limbic structures, the prefrontal cortex, and hypothalamus. In M. Swash & C. Kennard (Eds.), *The scientific basis of clinical neurology* (pp. 201–213). London: Churchill Livingstone.
Rolls, E. T. (1987). Information representation, processing and storage in the brain: Analysis at the single neuron level. In J.-P. Changeux & M. Konishi (Eds.), *The neural and molecular bases of learning* (pp. 503–540). Chichester: Wiley.
Rolls, E. T. (1988). Visual information processing in the primate temporal lobe. In M. Imbert (Ed.), *Models of visual perception: From natural to artificial.* Oxford: Oxford University Press.

Rolls, E. T., Miyashita, Y., Cahusac, P. M. B., Kesner, R. P., Niki, H., Feigenbaum, J., & Bach, L. (1989). Hippocampal neurons in the monkey with activity related to the place in which a stimulus is shown. *Journal of Neuroscience, 9,* 1835–1845.

Rumelhart, D. E., Hinton, G. E., & Williams, R. J. (1986). Learning internal representations by error propagation. In D. E. Rumelhart & J. L. McClelland (Eds.), *Parallel distributed processing: Vol. 1. Foundations* (pp. 318–362). Cambridge, Mass.: MIT Press.

Rumelhart, D. E., & Zipser, D. (1986). Feature discovery by competitive learning. In D. E. Rumelhart & J. L. McClelland (Eds.), *Parallel distributed processing: Vol. 1. Foundations* (pp. 151–193). Cambridge, Mass.: MIT Press.

Rupniak, N. M. J., & Gaffan, D. (1987). Monkey hippocampus and learning about spatially directed movements. *Journal of Neuroscience, 7,* 2331–2337.

Scoville, W. B., & Milner, B. (1957). Loss of recent memory after bilateral hippocampal lesions. *Journal of Neurology Neurosurgery & Psychiatry, 20,* 11–21.

Smith, M. L., & Milner, B. (1981). The role of the right hippocampus in the recall of spatial location. *Neuropsychologia, 19,* 781–793.

Squire, L. (1986). Mechanisms of memory. *Science, 232,* 1612–1619.

Squire, L. (1987). Complex connections involved in memory functions. In J. Byrne & W. O. Berry (Eds.), *Neural models of plasticity: Theoretical and empirical approaches.* Orlando, Fla.: Academic Press.

Turner, B. H. (1981). The cortical sequence and terminal distribution of sensory related afferents to the amygdaloid complex of the rat and monkey. In Y. Ben-Ari (Ed.), *The amygdaloid complex.* Amsterdam: Elsevier.

Turner, B. H., Mishkin, M., & Knapp, M. (1980). Organization of the amygdalopetal modality-specific cortical association areas in the monkey. *Journal of Comparative Neurology, 191,* 515–543.

Van Hoesen, G. W. (1981). The differential distribution, diversity and sprouting of cortical projections to the amygdala in the rhesus monkey. In Y. Ben-Ari (Ed.), *The amygdaloid complex* (pp. 79–90). Amsterdam: Elsevier.

Van Hoesen, G. W. (1982). The parahippocampal gyrus. New observations regarding its cortical connections in the monkey. *Trends in Neurosciences, 5,* 345–350.

Van Hoesen, G. W., & Pandya, D. N. (1975a). Some connections of the entorhinal (area 28) and perirhinal (area 35) cortices in the monkey. I. Temporal lobe afferents. *Brain Research, 95,* 1–24.

Van Hoesen, G. W., & Pandya, D. N. (1975b). Some connections of the entorhinal (area 28) and perirhinal (area 35) cortices in the monkey. III. Efferent connections. *Brain Research, 95,* 39–59.

Van Hoesen, G. W., Pandya, D. M., & Butters, N. (1975). Some connections of the entorhinal (area 28) and perirhinal (area 35) cortices in the monkey. II. Frontal lobe afferents. *Brain Research, 95,* 25–38.

Von der Malsburg, C. (1973). Self-organization of orientation-sensitive columns in the striate cortex. *Kybernetik, 14,* 85–100.

Wigstrom, H., Gustaffson, B., Huang, Y.-Y., & Abraham, W. C. (1986). Hippocampal long-term potentiation is induced by pairing single afferent volleys with intracellularly injected depolarizing currents. *Acta Physiologica Scandinavica, 126,* 317–319.

Zola-Morgan, S., Squire, L. R., & Amaral, D. G. (1986). Human amnesia and the medial temporal region: Enduring memory impairment following a bilateral lesion limited to field CA_1 of the hippocampus. *Journal of Neuroscience, 6,* 2950–2957.

10

Ontogenetic Self-Organization and Learning

WOLF SINGER

From a reductionist point of view, learning consists of a stimulus- and hence activity-dependent neuronal process that leads to a lasting change of stimulus–response relations. The formation of a memory trace may thus be considered a modification of the neuronal program that specifies input–output functions. This program is contained in the architecture of interneuronal connectivity and in the differential weighing of the transfer functions of these connections. Thus any activity-dependent process that modifies, in a sufficiently stable and long-lasting way, the excitatory or inhibitory interactions between pairs of neurons could serve as a mechanism of learning, and any long-lasting alteration of inter-cellular communication can be considered an engram.

Activity-dependent long-term changes of neuronal interactions have been observed in a number of brain structures of adult animals. They are a ubiquitous phenomenon during early ontogeny, where they play a crucial role in the self-organization of the brain. It is the goal of this short review to illustrate some of the mechanisms of developmental self-organization and to investigate the extent to which they can be considered precursors of mechanisms that mediate learning in the adult.

PRINCIPLES OF SELF-ORGANIZATION

It has often been emphasized that genes cannot contain, in any naive sense, the full information necessary to describe the brain. Cerebral cortex alone contains on the order of 10^{14} synapses. Forgetting considerations of genome size, one can hardly imagine how ontogeny could select the correct wiring diagram out of all alternatives if these were of equal likelihood. Besides, judging from the variability of the vertebrate brain structure, the precision of the ontogenetic process is not sufficient to specify individual connections. This implies that ontogeny has to make use of self-organization: of general rules for pattern generation and of simple principles of error correction.

The development of organs and organisms is based on a permanent interactive exchange between the information stored in the genome and the information available in the cellular "environment" of the genome.

The cellular environment determines which of the genetic commands should be expressed at particular developmental stages. As the developmental process proceeds and organs differentiate, the microenvironment of the genome changes and hence modifies continuously the further expression of the genes. During early phases of brain development gene expression and posttranslational modifications of gene products are controlled as in any other organ by the biochemical signals produced in the cellular microenvironment. Later, however, brain development starts to differ radically from the development of other organs because electrical activity is added to the biochemical messengers as a further signaling system in the self-organizing dialogue between the genes and their respective environment. It has to be assumed that these electrical signals are capable of influencing gene expression and posttranslational modifications.

This has a number of extremely important implications. Electrical signals are transported by neuronal processes over great distances and with high topological selectivity. This enlarges dramatically the range and the complexity of the environment that is available to the self-organization process. From a certain developmental stage on the brain possesses functioning sense organs that convert signals from within the organism and even from extracorporal space into electrical messages. Thus the environment relevant for brain self-organization ultimately includes all domains with which the evolving brain is capable of interacting and from which it can receive messages. Another important aspect is that the very same electrical signals which convey sensory messages are used by the brain as information carriers for computational processes. Hence the powerful capacities of nerve nets to perform complex logic operations on large-parameter sets become available to the self-organization process. As the complexity of the brain increases, the computational power and the complexity of its interactions with its environment increase as well. As a consequence, the set of parameters determining further brain development becomes more complex and capable of supporting self-organization toward even more differentiated structures. Because of this spiral of reciprocal interactions between the genome and its increasingly complex environment, a rather small set of genetic rules suffices to promote the development of such highly differentiated structures as the human brain. As will become clear later, these very processes that support experience-dependent self-organization during development are closely related to the more general processes that serve to adapt the mature brain to its environment and are commonly known as learning.

THE VISUAL SYSTEM AS A MODEL

Most of our knowledge of activity-dependent specification of neuronal connections comes from the visual system. "Seeing" has to be learned during a critical period of early postnatal development. The most dramatic evidence for this comes from patients who suffered from congenital opacities of the eyes during early childhood and therefore were unable to perceive contours. With the development of lens transplants the optical media of these patients' eyes could be restored, but unexpectedly these patients were unable to recover visual functions when operated on as juveniles or adults. Experiments in visually deprived animals revealed that these functional deficits are primarily due to abnormalities in visual centers of the cerebral cortex. The reason is that certain cortical functions can be developed only if visual experience is available.

The following example illustrates this. Higher mammals and humans who have frontally positioned eyes with overlapping visual fields can compute the distance of objects in space from the differences between the images in the two eyes. This ability has two obvious advantages. First, the distance of an object in space can be assessed with great precision even if object and observer are stationary and do not produce any motion parallaxes. Second, the separation of figures from ground, a primordial prerequisite for pattern recognition, is greatly facilitated by evaluating spatial distance. The basis for this function are neurons in the visual cortex which possess two receptive fields, one in each eye, that have the same features and are precisely superimposed in visual space. Thus during development the 1 million afferents arriving from each eye have to be arranged so that only those pairs of afferents converge onto cortical cells which originate from precisely corresponding retinal loci. The problem is that there is no way to predict with any great precision which retinal loci will actually be corresponding in the mature visual system. Retinal correspondence depends on parameters such as the size of the eyeballs, the position of the eyeballs in the orbit, and the interocular distance. Clearly, these parameters are strongly influenced by epigenetic factors. It follows that genetic instructions alone, even if they are quantitatively sufficient, cannot in principle suffice to determine with the required precision the pattern of interocular connections. An elegant possibility exists, however, to identify fibers as coming from corresponding retinal loci by evaluating their electrical activity. When a target is fixated with both eyes, corresponding retinal loci are stimulated by the same contours. Therefore, neuronal responses in afferents from corresponding retinal loci are more correlated than those in afferents from noncorresponding loci. What is required then is a developmental mechanism capable of consolidating selectively those retinal afferents which convey correlated activation patterns.

ACTIVITY-DEPENDENT CONSOLIDATION AND DISRUPTION OF FUNCTIONAL BINOCULARITY

In the following paragraphs I shall briefly review evidence suggesting that such mechanisms do indeed exist in the mammalian brain. I shall further demonstrate that these processes are not solely dependent on local interactions but are in addition controlled by more globally organized modulatory systems, which are implicated in the control of central states such as arousal, attention, and motivation.

Before visual experience becomes effective in influencing the ocularity of cortical neurons, most cells in the visual cortex of cats and monkeys respond to stimulation of both eyes. This condition is maintained with normal experience but also with dark rearing. With monocular deprivation, however, the large majority of cortical cells loses the ability to respond to the deprived eye (Blakemore, Garey, & Vital-Durand, 1978; Wiesel & Hubel, 1965a). The cells that continue to respond to the deprived eye are located preferentially within layer IV in the center of the shrunken termination fields of the deprived eye (Shatz & Stryker, 1978). This suggests that only those cells which have been monocularly driven by this eye right from the beginning continue to respond to the deprived eye. With reverse suture, if it occurs early enough, the previously closed eye may recover control over most cortical neurons while the previously open eye in turn becomes ineffective (Blakemore et al., 1978; Wiesel & Hubel, 1965b).

When induced early in development, at times when axonal segregation is not yet completed, these functional changes go in parallel with the retraction and expansion of thalamic afferents within layer IV and reflect to some extent the formation and withdrawal of synaptic connections between thalamic afferents and cortical target cells. However, these modifications of ocular dominance most certainly also include changes in the efficacy of intracortical synaptic connections, this latter mechanism becoming relatively more prominent at later stages of development when axonal segregation is already in an advanced stage. This has to be inferred from the evidence that marked changes in the ocularity of cortical neurons can occur without or with only minor modifications of the termination patterns of thalamic afferents in layer IV (for review see Tieman, 1985). One example is the late change of ocular dominance in dark-reared kittens. In normally reared kittens monocular deprivation is effective only during a critical period that lasts about 3 months (Olson & Freeman, 1980). In dark-reared kittens monocular deprivation induces changes of ocular dominance even after the end of this period (Cynader, 1983). These late changes of ocularity are, however, not associated with changes of columnar patterns in layer IV (Mower, Caplan, Christen, & Duffy, 1985; Mower & Christen, 1985). Another example for such a dissociation is the modification occurring with strabismus. Here the morphological pattern of ocular dominance columns in layer IV is nearly unchanged (LeVay, Stryker, & Shatz, 1978), while the functional ocularity of cortical neurons is drastically altered. Most cells are monocular and driven either by the right or the left eye (Hubel & Wiesel, 1965). Finally, there is evidence from single-cell recording and deoxyglucose mapping in monocularly deprived cats that activity is still present within the deprived eye's columns but is confined to layer IV, indicating transmission failure at the level of intracortical connections (Bonds, Silverman, Sclar, & Tootell, 1980; Shatz & Stryker, 1978). It is these latter changes in excitatory transmission rather than the macroscopic rearrangements of columnar patterns that will be dealt with in the following section.

THE EFFECTS OF MONOCULAR OCCLUSION ON INDIVIDUAL CORTICAL NEURONS

Thus far the changes resulting from monocular deprivation have never been followed in individual neurons. All interpretations and conclusions are based on the comparison of independently analyzed samples of neurons which in most cases have been recorded from different animals that were raised under different conditions. We have therefore developed a method for chronic recording which allows us to determine repeatedly the receptive field properties of cortical neurons in alert and only lightly restrained kittens. This made it possible to study the effects of monocular deprivation and reverse occlusion in individual cortical cells (Mioche & Singer, 1989).

The first effect of monocular deprivation was the disappearance of binocular summation, that is, the superiority of binocular over monocular responses. Overt changes of ocular dominance have been observed as soon as 6 hr after the beginning of monocular deprivation and a complete loss of excitatory responses to deprived eye stimulation was seen as early as 12 hr after occlusion. These changes in ocularity resulted mainly from a gradual decrease of the excitatory response to deprived eye stimulation and were only occasionally associated with a moderate increase of responses to the normal eye. During this shift neurons preserved their orientation and direction selectivity. Interestingly, stimulation of the deprived eye continued to evoke inhibitory responses even after excitatory responses had vanished completely. The interval required for the manifestation of these alterations appeared to be independent of the duration of preceding visual exposure, suggesting that the duration of visual stimulation required for the induction of a change is shorter than the time needed for subsequent expression of the change. Neurons that had already been monocular before deprivation were found resistant to monocular deprivation and showed changes neither in responsiveness nor in ocularity.

The recovery of responses to the previously deprived eye in the case of reverse occlusion had a considerably slower time course: at least 24 hr of reverse occlusion was required before the responses to the deprived eye reappeared and growth of these responses continued for up to 74 hr, the longest period investigated. The first change after reversal was a reduction of the response to the newly deprived eye. In numerous neurons responses to the newly open eye reappeared only after the cell had ceased to be excitable from the previously open eye. Thus these neurons passed through a phase during which they were entirely unresponsive to visual stimulation. In the remaining cells responses to the newly open eye reappeared before responses to the now deprived eye had disappeared. During this reversal of ocular dominance all cells preserved their original orientation preference, but there were indications for a reduction of orientation tuning.

The results of the monocular deprivation experiments suggest several conclusions. First, the downregulation of the deprived afferents cannot be considered the result of a homeostatic response to the upregulation of inputs from the viewing eye. Our results rather favor a mechanism that leads to primary inactivation of deprived inputs. This may either be due to weakening of excitatory or to strengthening of inhibitory inputs. The observation that inhibitory responses persisted once the excitatory response had disappeared is compatible with the latter interpretation. Also compatible is the finding that blockade of GABAergic inhibition reverses the early effects of monocular deprivation (Sillito, Kemp, & Blakemore, 1983). However, the alternative—inhibitory connections remain unmodified while excitatory transmission is weakened—has to be considered as equally likely.

The second conclusion is that the time required for the manifestation of changes in ocular dominance does not depend solely on the amount of visual stimulation but seems to be determined by the time constants of a process that is independent of experience. This has a bearing on the controversial discussion about the existence of a consolidation period for the expression of ocular dominance changes. Our data favor the notion of the involvement of two different processes: an early, vision-dependent induction phase and a subsequent vision-independent manifestation period. The recent finding of Rauschecker and Hahn (1987) that anesthesia, if induced within 1 hr after monocular exposure, prevents the manifestation of ocular dominance changes also points in this direction.

Finally, the results of the study of monocularly deprived kittens showed that the breakdown of binocular summation precedes the first signs of an ocular dominance shift. This suggests that binocular cooperativity is a particularly vulnerable network property. The earlier reports that short periods of monocular deprivation led to a reduction of binocular neurons rather than to a shift of ocular dominance toward the open eye may be relevant in this context (Freeman & Olson, 1982).

The results of the reversal experiments support the conclusion that the reduction of transmission in deprived afferents is not a direct consequence of increased efficiency of afferents from the open eye since the former process seemed to precede the latter. Differential gain changes in deprived and nondeprived afferents do not appear to result from a normalizing process aimed at keeping the overall excitatory input to a neuron constant. Rather it appears as if there are two processes which have different time constants and interact with each other through some still unidentified links: one leads to a rapid inactivation of deprived afferents while the other promotes a slow increase in the efficacy of the previously inactivated connections. The latter process appears to take over only after competing excitatory inputs are weakened.

THE ROLE OF POSTSYNAPTIC ACTIVATION

It has become clear that changes in ocular dominance do not depend solely on the level of activity in the afferent connections (Cynader & Mitchell, 1977;

Modification Rules

Input selection by coherency matching

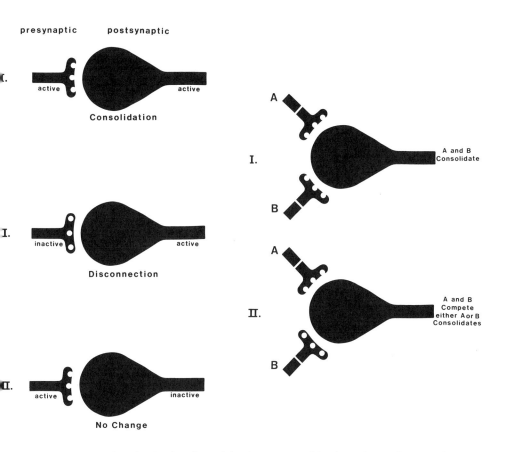

FIGURE 10.1.   The rules that describe activity-dependent modifications of synaptic connections in the developing visual cortex. As the rules in the left column indicate, connections consolidate if the probability is high that presynaptic and postsynaptic elements are active in temporal contiguity (rule I), while connections destabilize if the probability is high that the presynaptic terminal is inactive at the same time as the postsynaptic target is activated (rule II). In the absence of post-synaptic responses there appears to be no selective change in input connection irrespective of the state of the activation of the presynaptic input (rule III). When applied to conditions where two inputs converge on the same target (right column) these local rules lead to selective stabilization of converging inputs that convey correlated activity (condition I) while they lead to competition between converging inputs if these convey noncorrelated activity (condition II). In this case one input will consolidate at the expense of the other.

Greuel, Luhmann, & Singer, 1988; Singer, Rauschecker, & Werth, 1977). It rather appears that the critical variable is the state of activation of the postsynaptic neuron and in particular the degree of temporal correlation between presynaptic and postsynaptic activation (Rauschecker & Singer, 1979, 1981). The use-dependent modifications of excitatory transmission actually seem to follow rules that closely resemble those postulated by Hebb (1949) for adaptive neuronal connections (Rauschecker & Singer, 1981). As summarized in Figure 10.1, the basic assumption is that the direction of the change—increase or decrease of efficacy—depends on the correlation between presynaptic and postsynaptic activation. The efficacy of excitatory transmission appears to increase when presynaptic afferents and the postsynaptic cell are active in temporal contiguity and to decrease when the postsynaptic target is active while the presynaptic terminal is silent. These rules, when applied to circuits where two (or more) afferent pathways converge onto a common postsynaptic target cell, have the effect of selectively stabilizing and hence associating pathways that convey correlated activity. Similarly, these selection criteria lead to competition between converging pathways if these convey uncorrelated activity. In that case one subset of afferents is always inactive while the other is driving the postsynaptic cell. Hence one subset will increase its gain at the expense of the other. Eventually those afferents that have the highest probability of being active in temporal contiguity with the postsynaptic target cell will win.

THE DURATION OF THE INTEGRATION INTERVAL
FOR HEBBIAN MATCHING

The modification rules predict that pathways consolidate only when they are active in contingency with the postsynaptic cell. For converging pathways, such as those arriving from the two eyes, this implies that they have to be active simultaneously if they are to remain connected to a common target cell. As soon as they get out of phase they will compete with each other and one pathway will become repressed. We recently attempted to determine the cutoff point beyond which asynchrony between the activity patterns from the two eyes leads to disruption of binocularity. For that purpose high-speed solid-state shutters were mounted in goggles that were fitted to the head of freely moving kittens and allowed for rapidly alternating monocular occlusion (Altmann, Luhmann, Greuel, & Singer, 1987). The maximal interval of asynchrony still compatible with the maintenance of binocular connections was found to be on the order of 200 to 400 msec. This agrees with the psychophysical evidence that the neuronal representation of a stimulus persists for 300 to 400 msec (Altmann, Eckhorn, & Singer, 1986); signals can be integrated over such long time spans. The implication is that the signal which is generated by one eye persists, presumably in the cortical cells, for a few hundred milliseconds. This excludes individual action potentials as a basis for contingency matching. The neuronal processes subserving persistence have not yet been identified. Long-lasting postsynaptic conductance changes, persistence of second messenger signals, and reverberation in reciprocally coupled neuron ensembles are likely candidates.

THE ROLE OF CENTRAL GATING MECHANISMS

It is obvious that such activity-dependent selection can solve our specification problem and stabilize selectively those afferents from the two eyes which originate from corresponding retinal loci. It is further clear that such experience-dependent pruning of neuronal circuits is a very powerful and versatile mechanism to establish associations and hence has all the potential to serve as a basis for learning. Before discussing this fascinating aspect, however, further constraints on the experience-dependent developmental process have to be considered. In our special case selection of afferent connections from the two eyes can be successful only if it occurs while the animal is actually fixating a nonambiguous target with both eyes. Pruning must not take place when the two eyes are moving in an uncoordinated way. In this latter case, the images processed by the two eyes are different and hence all retinal signals, even those originating from corresponding retinal loci, are uncorrelated. All afferents from the two eyes would therefore compete with one another and the consequence would be complete disruption of binocular connections. The same would be the case if the spontaneously produced bursts of activity that occur, for example, in the geniculate afferents during certain sleep stages, were capable of inducing changes in circuitry. Moreover, to assure a sufficient degree of overlap of the images in the two eyes, some evaluation of the best match between the coarsely prespecified retinotopic representations ought to be made prior to selection. This requires preprocessing and control of eye movements and hence an aroused and attentive brain. The selection process must therefore be gated by nonretinal control systems capable of determining the instances at which retinal activity may induce changes in circuitry. In agreement with these postulates it has been found that nonretinal afferents to striate cortex play a crucial role in gating ocular dominance plasticity.

Even when contour vision is unrestricted and retinal signals readily elicit responses in the neurons of the visual cortex, vision-dependent modifications of excitatory transmission fail to occur in a variety of conditions. Thus neurons of the kitten's striate cortex may remain binocular despite monocular deprivation when the proprioceptive input from extraocular muscles is disrupted (Buisseret & Singer, 1983), when the open eye is surgically rotated within the orbit (Singer, Tretter, & Yinon, 1982), when large-angle squint is induced in both eyes (Singer, von Grünau, & Rauschecker, 1979), or when strabismus is induced by bilateral cyclotorsion (Crewther, Crewther, Peck, & Pettigrew, 1980). In these cases contour vision per se is unimpaired but the abnormal eye position and motility lead to massive disturbances of the kittens' visuomotor coordination. Initially the inappropriate retinal signals cause abnormal visuomotor reactions and during this period are effective in influencing cortical ocular dominance. Subsequently, however, the kittens rely less and less on visual cues and develop a near complete neglect of the visual modality. In this phase, retinal signals no longer modify ocular dominance, and they also fail to support the development of orientation-selective receptive fields.

These results suggest that retinal signals influence the development of cortical functions only when the animal uses them for the control of behavior. Indeed, retinal signals do not lead to changes of cortical functions when the kittens are paralyzed and/or anesthetized while exposed to visual patterns (Buisseret, Gary-Bobo, & Imbert, 1978; Freeman & Bonds, 1979; Singer, 1979; Singer & Rauschecker, 1982). Vision-dependent modifications also failed to occur in kittens in which a sensory hemineglect was induced by unilateral surgical lesions of the intralaminar nuclear complex of the thalamus (Singer, 1982). Following monocular deprivation, neurons in the visual cortex of the normal hemisphere had become monocular, as is usual with monocular deprivation. However, neurons in the visual cortex of the hemisphere with the lesion had remained binocular. Thus although both hemispheres had received identical signals from the open eye, these signals induced the expected modifications in the normal hemisphere only, remaining rather ineffective in the hemisphere which—because of the diencephalic lesion—"attended" less to retinal stimulation. Recent experiments revealed that these effects of the thalamic lesion cannot be attributed to the projections originating from the intralaminar nuclei alone (Bear, Kleinschmidt, & Singer, 1988). Cortical plasticity was found unimpaired when the intralaminar lesions were made by injections of the cytotoxin NMDA, which selectively destroys neurons but leaves fibers of passage intact. This suggests that the surgical lesions were effective because they comprised both thalamic neurons and fiber systems traversing the intralaminar nuclei.

THE CHEMICAL NATURE OF PERMISSIVE GATING SIGNALS

Kasamatsu and Pettigrew (1979) showed that neurons of the kitten striate cortex remain binocular despite monocular deprivation when cortical norepinephrine (NE) is depleted by local infusion of the neurotoxin 6-hydroxydopamine (6-OHDA). Since they could demonstrate that microperfusion of the depleted cortical tissue with NE reinstalls ocular dominance plasticity (Kasamatsu, Pettigrew, & Ary, 1979), these authors proposed that normal NE levels are a necessary prerequisite for ocular dominance plasticity.

Subsequent independent investigations indicated that ocular dominance changes can be induced despite NE depletion. In these investigations 6-OHDA was either injected prior to monocular deprivation or the noradrenergic input to cortex was blocked by means other than local 6-OHDA application (Adrien et al., 1985; Bear & Daniels, 1983; Bear et al., 1983; Daw, Robertson, Rader, Videen, & Cosica, 1984; Daw, Videen, Parkinson, & Rader, 1985). Apparent controversy may have been resolved by the demonstration that ocular dominance plasticity is influenced both by noradrenergic and cholinergic mechanisms (Bear & Singer, 1986). Ocular dominance plasticity is abolished only if both the noradrenergic pathway from locus coeruleus and the cholinergic projection from the basal forebrain are lesioned. Disruption of either system alone is not sufficient to arrest plasticity. These results suggest that both neuromodulators acetylcholine and norepinephrine have a permissive function in cortical plasticity, either system being capable of replacing the other.

INVOLVEMENT OF NMDA RECEPTOR ACTIVATION AND Ca^{2+} FLUXES IN USE-DEPENDENT PLASTICITY

The lesion experiments reported above indicated that use-dependent modifications of synaptic transmission require a certain amount of cooperativity between retinal input and additional internally generated signals. This suggested that the process mediating cortical plasticity has a threshold which is reached only when retinal signals are coincident with additional facilitatory input. As a possible substrate for such a threshold process the high-threshold voltage-dependent Ca^{2+} channels were considered. Their voltage threshold is higher than that of the Na^+ channels which mediate the regenerative action potential, and they appear to be located in dendritic rather than in somatic membranes (Llinas, 1979). Moreover, there is evidence from developing Purkinje cells and from binding studies in the kitten visual cortex (Bode-Greuel & Singer, 1988) that these channels are particularly numerous in the membranes of developing neurons (Llinas & Sugimori, 1979). An attempt was made, therefore, to determine with ion-selective electrodes whether stimuli known to modify cortical response properties also led to an activation of Ca^{2+} channels. The results revealed that stimulation conditions leading to changes in neuronal response properties also caused activation of Ca^{2+} fluxes from extracellular to intracellular compartments. Measurable Ca^{2+} fluxes occurred only when patterned retinal activity was coincident with electrical activation of the brain stem reticular core or of the intralaminar nuclei (Geiger & Singer, 1986). These Ca^{2+} fluxes were much more pronounced in 4- to 5-week-old kittens than in adult cats. This is compatible with the hypothesis that the respective Ca^{2+} conductances are related to mechanisms involved in developmental plasticity (see also below).

The hypothesis that Ca^{2+} currents are involved in activity-dependent long-term changes of neuronal excitability receives further support from the recent finding that the activation of the NMDA receptor, a subtype of the receptors for excitatory amino acids, is also crucial for the induction of ocular dominance changes (Kleinschmidt, Bear, & Singer, 1987). Infusion of 2-amino-5-phosphonovaleric acid (APV), a selective antagonist of the NMDA receptor, completely blocks any experience-dependent modifications of striate cortex functions without abolishing neuronal responses to light. The NMDA receptor is activated by excitatory amino acids and has a selective affinity for NMDA. It is coupled to an ionophore that is permeable for Ca^{2+} ions. A special property of this NMDA-

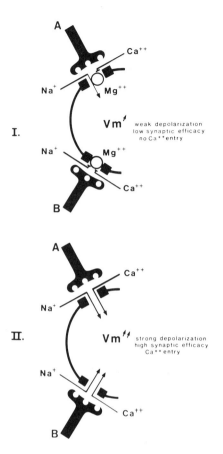

FIGURE 10.2. Functional properties of the NMDA receptor. The ionophore associated with the NMDA receptor becomes permeable for calcium ions only if the receptor is occupied by its endogenous ligand *and* if the membrane potential of the postsynaptic neuron is sufficiently depolarized to remove the magnesium block of the NMDA channel. In condition I, only input A is active and the membrane potential is not sufficiently positive to remove the magnesium block. In condition II, inputs A and B are active simultaneously; membrane depolarization is now sufficient for the removal of the magnesium block, and the NMDA ionophores become permeable for calcium-ions. The result is a strong depolarization of the membrane and influx of calcium. By virtue of its voltage dependence the NMDA mechanism is capable of evaluating the temporal contiguity of activity in converging pathways and promoting calcium entry if there is sufficient cooperativity.

sensitive channel is its voltage dependence (Fig. 10.2). It is activated only when the receptor is occupied by its endogenous ligand and when the membrane is sufficiently depolarized. Thus this mechanism is ideally suited to "evaluate" the contingency of presynaptic and postsynaptic activation. It contributes to the cells' depolarization only if there is sufficient cooperativity between converging afferents. Hence the NMDA mechanism could be the substrate for the threshold that needs to be reached in order to obtain long-term modifications of neuronal excitability.

Experiments in slices of the visual cortex seem to confirm this interpretation. They show that the conventional single spike responses to orthodromic stimulation of the optic radiation do not depend on the activation of the NMDA mechanism. However, NMDA channels seem to be involved in triggering the high-frequency bursts that may also be evoked by orthodromic stimulation, especially when stimuli are applied at higher frequency or when postsynaptic inhibition is reduced by application of bicuculline. These burst discharges are likely to depend on the activation of Ca^{2+} conductances and are blocked by application of the NMDA receptor blocker APV. In a substantial fraction of cortical cells prolonged application of burst-generating stimuli induces a long-term enhancement of excitatory transmission that is similar to long-term potentiation in the hippocampus. When the NMDA receptors are blocked by APV these same stimuli no longer generate burst discharges and also no longer induce changes in synaptic transmission (Artola & Singer, 1987). Thus the activation of the NMDA-dependent excitatory postsynaptic potential (EPSP) and the resulting burst discharge appear to be necessary conditions for the induction of long-term modifications. Since both phenomena are most likely associated with postsynaptic Ca^{2+} fluxes through NMDA-dependent ionophores and/or high-threshold Ca^{2+} channels, these results support the hypothesis that activity-dependent modifications require a surge of intracellular Ca^{2+} ions. Since APV also blocked experience-dependent modifications of cortical response properties in vivo, it is likely that these adaptive processes are based on mechanisms similar to those observed in vitro.

Supporting evidence for this possibility comes from experiments in which attempts were made to induce lasting changes of neuronal response properties by combining retinal stimulation with direct pharmacological modulation of the excitability of cortical neurons (Greuel et al., 1988). In anesthetized, paralyzed kittens cortical cells were activated from the retina with light while at the same time they were exposed to ionophoretically applied pulses of the excitatory amino acids NMDA and glutamate and the neuromodulators acetylcholine (ACh) and NE. In more than half of the neurons 30 min of conditioning with combined light and pharmacological stimulation were sufficient to induce a selective enhancement of the responses to the light stimulus used for conditioning and to produce a concomitant depression of responses to nonconditioned stimuli. Thus with appropriate light stimulation, drastic changes in ocular dominance and/or orientation and direction preference could be obtained that outlasted the end of the conditioning sequence by more than 30 min. These results support the notion that induction of use-dependent long-term modifications of response properties requires cooperativity between retinal input and further, internally generated, facilitatory influences. The permissive effects of NMDA, particularly, are suggestive of an involvement of Ca^{2+} currents in these processes.

CONSTRAINTS FOR THE INDUCTION
OF EXPERIENCE-DEPENDENT MODIFICATIONS

The data reviewed thus far could be used to define some of the constraints of use-dependent modifications of neuronal connectivity. These are summarized schematically in Figure 10.3. Local correlations between the activity patterns in modifiable afferents and their target cells determine the sign of the modification. Connections increase their gain and/or stabilize if their activity is correlated with that of their target cell. If presynaptic and postsynaptic activities are not

Factors influencing Neuronal Plasticity

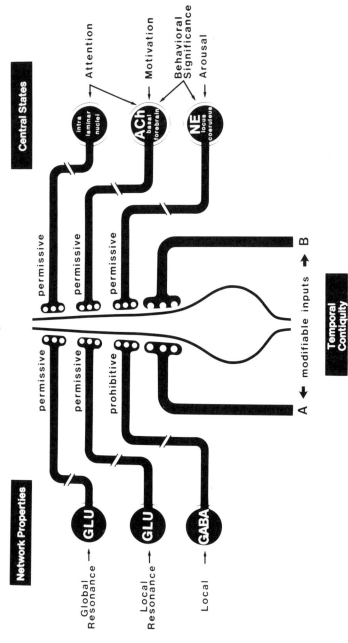

sufficiently contiguous, the respective connection weakens and if this weakening occurs during a critical period of development, it leads to physical removal of the synaptic connection. The integration interval during which presynaptic and postsynaptic activation must coincide in order to lead to stabilization of a pathway has a duration of maximally 200 to 300 msec. However, the decision as to whether such local patterns of activity lead to modifications depends on additional hierarchically organized gating systems. Thus it can be inferred from the requirement to reach the activation threshold of the NMDA mechanism that a critical level of postsynaptic depolarization has to be reached. This probability increases to the extent that excitatory and inhibitory inputs to the same dendrite are activated and silenced, respectively. Since all inhibitory inputs to cortical neurons and a large number of nonretinal excitatory afferents originate within the same and nearby cortical columns, this implies that those stimuli will be most effective in inducing modifications which match best the resonance properties of local arrays of excitatory cortical neurons. Since some of the excitatory input to individual cortical neurons is recruited also from remote cortical and subcortical centers, it can further be expected that the efficiency of stimuli to induce modifications of cortical circuitry will increase to the extent that the stimuli not only match the response properties of local neuron clusters in the striate cortex, but also conform with the resonance properties of more distributed neuronal assemblies.

Even if these local and global requirements for cooperativity are fulfilled, modifications may not occur unless the permissive modulatory systems—the noradrenergic, the cholinergic, and probably also the intralaminar projections—are in the appropriate state of activation. These systems in turn receive input from most centers in the brain and hence can be expected to influence local adaptive changes as a function of a very global evaluation of the adequacy of just processed and potentially change-inducing activity. The probability that a sensory pattern will induce a long-lasting modification of cortical circuitry thus depends both on the nature of this pattern and the central state of the brain that is maintained during sensory activation. The change will occur only if there is sufficient cooperativity among the inputs converging onto the cell whose modifiable inputs are to change; this in turn will be the case only if the pattern of sensory activation matches sufficiently well with the resonance properties of both local circuits in striate cortex and more distributed but interconnected neuronal assemblies. The gating of local adaptive changes is thus a distributed func-

←

FIGURE 10.3.   Factors influencing use-dependent modifications of neuronal circuits in the developing visual cortex. The sign of the change in modifiable connections A and B depends on the temporal correlation of activity conveyed by the modifiable inputs. Whether a change occurs in response to this activity depends on the state of activation of additional synaptic inputs to the same neuron. These comprise feedback loops originating within the same cortical column, the same cortical area, and probably also remote cortical and subcortical structures. Additional gating inputs are derived from the more globally organized modulatory systems which originate in central core structures of the brain.

tion in which numerous centers of the brain participate. This distributed nature of the gating process accounts well for the evidence that so many different interventions disrupt adaptive changes in response to sensory stimulation. From a teleological point of view such a multilevel control of plasticity appears indispensable in order to assure that local changes remain adapted to the global requirements of the developing brain.

FACTORS LIMITING DEVELOPMENTAL PLASTICITY

A characteristic feature of developmental plasticity is its rapid decline with age. The notion that cortical plasticity is influenced substantially by cholinergic mechanisms suggested the possibility that the age-dependent decline of malleability is the result of selective changes in the cholinergic projection to striate cortex. In this case, one expects a withdrawal of cholinergic afferents from particular subsets of neurons and/or a removal of muscarinic receptors. These changes ought to be particularly pronounced in layer IV because the circuit modifications that lead to ocularity changes occur mainly within this layer. Experimental data support this hypothesis. The density and laminar distribution of high-affinity binding sites for muscarinic agonists change during development in a way that suggests a relation to the time course of the critical period (Shaw, Needler, & Cynader, 1984). However, this redistribution of receptors is not paralleled by the laminar pattern of cholinergic afferents. The density of fibers with CHAT-like immunoreactivity increases with age, and there are no indications for a selective reduction of cholinergic fibers or terminal boutons from layer IV (Stichel & Singer, 1987). One reason for this could be that in layer IV, ACh acts mainly on the nicotinic receptors, which are prominant in this layer and most probably located on the thalamic afferents (Prusky, Shaw, & Cynader, 1987; Parkinson, Kratz, & Daw, 1988). However, a problem with this interpretation is that so far no axo-axonic synapses have been identified in the neocortex, which implies that the cholinergic influence on thalamic afferents would have to be mediated through nonconventional ways. The morphological data thus suggest that developmental changes of the cholinergic input to striate cortex are not responsible for the temporal limitation of ocular dominance plasticity. The interpretation that developmental changes in modulatory systems are not a limiting factor of plasticity is supported by electrophysiological evidence. Combining ionophoretic application of NE and ACh with patterned light stimuli has been found rather ineffective in producing substantial modifications of response properties in neurons of the visual cortex of adult cats, although this procedure has been effective in kittens (Greuel et al., 1988). Since ACh and NE were as effective in adult cats as in kittens in facilitating responses to light, it appears unlikely that the age-dependent decline in plasticity is a result of reduced availability of permissive modulatory signals. Recent evidence indicates, however, that a redistribution of calcium-dependent mechanisms might account for reduced plasticity in the adult. A first and indirect hint for this possibility came from the observation that it is much more difficult to induce calcium fluxes from extracellular to intracellular compartments in the visual cortex of adult cats than kittens.

More direct support for an age-dependent redistribution of calcium-dependent mechanisms comes from investigations of calcium-binding proteins and of calcium channels. An analysis of developmental changes in the distribution of the calcium binding proteins parvalbumin and vitamin D-dependent calcium-binding protein revealed that these calcium-buffering systems are particularly rich in developing neurons (Stichel, Singer, Heizmann, & Norman, 1987).

We recently obtained evidence that binding sites for organic calcium channel blockers of the dihydropyridin class are much more frequent in the visual cortex of kittens than of adults. The highest concentrations of these binding sites have been observed in layer IV at the peak of the critical period for ocular dominance plasticity. In good correlation with the age-dependent decline in ocular dominance plasticity, these binding sites disappeared from layer IV and eventually became restricted essentially to supragranular layers. If one accepts the interpretation that binding sites for organic calcium channel blockers reflect the location of postsynaptic voltage-dependent high-threshold calcium channels, this observation suggests that voltage-dependent calcium conductances redistribute during development and may even disappear from certain neuronal profiles altogether.

A similar pattern of developmental redistribution has been found for binding sites with a high affinity for APV, a potent antagonist of the NMDA receptor (Bode-Greuel & Singer, 1988). These binding sites were also much more frequent in kittens than in adults and more evenly distributed throughout the cortical depth in the former than in the latter. In the adult they were again restricted essentially to supragranular layers. If one assumes that high-affinity binding sites for APV reflect NMDA receptors, this would indicate that transmitter-activated calcium conductances also redistribute during development and become reduced with age. Both the presumptive reduction of voltage-sensitive calcium channels and that of transmitter-dependent calcium channels would be compatible with the reduced calcium fluxes in the adult. Taken together, these results suggest that certain neuronal profiles lose their calcium conductances and hence are no longer exposed to activity-dependent calcium influx. Since the latter is likely to serve as a messenger in activity-dependent long-term modifications of neuronal response properties, removal of calcium conductances could be one cause for the decline of plasticity with age.

SELF-ORGANIZATION AND LEARNING:
THE BRAIN AS AN EVER-CHANGING ORGAN

One interesting aspect of experience-dependent self-organization processes is their formal similarity with learning. At a descriptive and perhaps even mechanistic level the activity-dependent refinement of connectivity patterns shares certain characteristic features of associative learning. Two sets of variables, in our special case the afferents from the two eyes, become permanently associated with a common effector, the cortical target cell. The criterion for this association is coherency of activation, just as in classical or operant conditioning.

Another similarity between "developmental" self-organization and "adult" learning is that the activity patterns have to match some predispositions of the learning organism in order to establish associations. In our case the minimal requirement was that the retinal signals conform with the response properties of cortical neurons; that is, the visual stimuli had to contain spatial contrast gradients. The same is true in adult learning. Stimulus configurations have to fulfill some minimal criteria for saliency and unambiguity in order to be effective. Finally, there is the parallel that selective associations occur only when the stimulus patterns are contingent with internally generated gating signals that are available only when the brain is awake and attentive. As has been established in numerous behavioral experiments, a similar dependence on central states holds true for adult learning. As elaborated later, comparison with other model systems of neuronal plasticity suggests that even the molecular mechanisms involved in developmental self-organization and adult plasticity may be the same.

THE INVOLVEMENT OF Ca^{2+} IONS

In all cases where long-term changes of excitability and/or synaptic efficacy can be induced by neuronal activity, Ca^{2+} ions appear to serve as messengers translating membrane depolarization into biochemical signals. Both in *Aplysia* and *Hermissenda* the surge of free Ca^{2+} in the cytosol appears to function as the molecular equivalent of the conditional stimulus (Alkon, 1983; Carew, Hawkins, Abrams, & Kandel, 1984). The same is likely to be the case in the cerebellum since the complex spike of Purkinje cells which follows climbing fiber activation is associated with the activation of high-threshold Ca^{2+} channels (Ito, Sakurai, & Tongroach, 1982). Long-term potentiation (LTP) in the hippocampus also appears to require free Ca^{2+} ions in the cytosol of postsynaptic dendrites (Lynch & Baudry, 1984; Lynch, Larson, Kelso, Barrioneuvo, & Schottler, 1983). Finally, a Ca^{2+}-dependent process has also been implicated in activity-dependent long-term modifications of excitability of motor cortex neurons (Woody, 1984). The evidence suggesting an involvement of Ca^{2+} ions in ocular dominance plasticity was reviewed above. Recent evidence suggests that hippocampal LTP is also reduced when NMDA receptors are blocked with APV, thus adding a rather specific item to the list of similarities between developmental learning and plasticity (Collingridge, Kehl, & McLennan, 1983).

THE INVOLVEMENT OF NEUROMODULATORS
AND RECEPTOR-DEPENDENT SECOND MESSENGER SYSTEMS

In *Aplysia,* serotonin has been suggested as the molecular signal mediating the response to the conditional stimulus. It activates a membrane-bound cyclase and causes a surge of intracellular cAMP (for review see Carew et al., 1984). An increase of cAMP also appears as a necessary step in hippocampal LTP (Lynch & Baudry, 1984). In this case it is unclear whether the rise of cAMP is due to activation of a receptor-coupled cyclase or whether it is secondary to activation of a Ca^{2+}-dependent cyclase. Since NE facilitates LTP, the former possibility deserves consideration (Bliss, Goddard, & Riives, 1983; Hopkins & Johnston, 1984). Finally, NE has also been shown to facilitate the experience-dependent reorganization of templates in the rabbit olfactory bulb (Gray, Freeman, & Skinner, 1984). The evidence for a permissive role of NE and ACh in ocular dominance plasticity was reviewed above.

THRESHOLD PHENOMENA, TEMPORAL CONTIGUITY, AND COOPERATIVITY

There are indications from all vertebrate model systems that adaptive modifications have a threshold which is reached only if a sufficiently strong activation is achieved. Available evidence suggests that this threshold process is located at the posysynaptic side. In neurons of the motor cortex, changes in response to synaptic activation are facilitated when the postsynaptic neuron is depolarized by intracellular current injections, by antidromic stimulation, or by activation of additional excitatory inputs (Baranyi & Feher, 1981; Woody, 1984; Woody, Alkon, & Hay, 1984). In the cerebellum, changes in the efficiency of parallel fiber synapses required concomitant activation of Purkinje cells by climbing fibers (Ito et al., 1982). In the hippocampus, LTP is facilitated if converging excitatory inputs are coactivated simultaneously (Lee, 1983; Levy & Steward, 1983; McNaughton, Douglas, & Goddard, 1978), if glutamate is applied directly, or if postsynaptic inhibition is reduced while the afferents that are to be potentiated are stimulated (for references on cooperativity in LTP see Wigström & Gustafsson, 1985). All these manipulations are likely to enhance local dendritic depolarization. The evidence for threshold processes in ocular dominance plasticity was reviewed above.

These numerous similarities between developmental and adult plasticity prompt the hypothesis that learning in the adult might be considered as the continuation of the self-organizing processes that serve at first to adopt the building blocks of our nervous system to each other and that subsequently serve to adapt the whole system to its environment. This viewpoint predicts that there should be a continuity between early self-organization and adult learning not only at the level of formal description but also at the level of molecular mechanisms.

REFERENCES

Adrien, J., Blanc, G., Buisseret, P., Frégnac, Y., Gary-Bobo, E., Imbert, M., Tassin, J. P., & Trotter, Y. (1985). Noradrenaline and functional plasticity in kitten visual cortex: A reexamination. *Journal of Physiology, 367*, 73–98.

Alkon, D. L. (1983). Learning in a marine snail. *Scientific American, 249,* 70.

Altmann, L., Eckhorn, R., & Singer, W. (1986). Temporal integration in the visual system: Influence of temporal dispersion on figure-ground discrimination. *Vision Research, 26,* 1949–1957.

Altmann, L., Luhmann, H. J., Greuel, J. M., & Singer, W. (1987). Binocularity in kittens with rapidly and alternating monocular occlusion. *Journal of Neurophysiology, 16,* 965–980.

Artola, A., & Singer, W. (1987). Long-term potentiation and NMDA receptors in rat visual cortex. *Nature, 330,* 649–652.

Baranyi, A., & Feher, O. (1981). Long-term facilitation of excitatory synaptic transmission in single cortical neurones of the cat produced by repetitive pairing of synaptic potentials following intracellular stimulation. *Neuroscience Letters, 23,* 303–308.

Bear, M. F., & Daniels, I. D. (1983). The plastic response to monocular deprivation persists in kitten visual cortex after chronic depletion of norepinephrine. *Journal of Neuroscience, 3,* 407–416.

Bear, M. F., Kleinschmidt, A., & Singer, W. (1988). Experience-dependent modifications of kitten striate cortex are not prevented by thalamic lesions that include the intralaminar nuclei. *Experimental Brain Research, 70,* 627–631.

Bear, M. F., Paradiso, M. A., Schwartz, M., Nelson, S. B., Carnes, K. M., & Daniels, J. D. (1983). Two methods of catecholamine depletion in kitten visual cortex yield different effects on plasticity. *Nature, 302,* 245–247.

Bear, M. F., & Singer, W. (1986). Modulation of visual cortical plasticity by acetylcholine and noradrenaline. *Nature, 320,* 172–176.

Blakemore, C., Garey, L. J., & Vital-Durand, F. (1978). The physiological effects of monocular deprivation and their reversal in the monkey's visual cortex. *Journal of Physiology, 282,* 223–262.

Bliss, T. V. P., Goddard, G. V., & Riives, M. (1983). Reduction of long-term potentiation in the dentate gyrus of the rat following selective depletion of monoamines. *Journal of Physiology, 334,* 475–491.

Bode-Greuel, K. M., & Singer, W. (1988). Developmental changes of the distribution of binding sites for organic Ca^{2+}-channel blockers in cat visual cortex. *Experimental Brain Research, 70,* 266–275.

Bonds, A. B., Silverman, M. S., Sclar, G., & Tootell, R. B. (1980). Visually evoked potentials and deoxyglucose studies of monocularly deprived cats. Proceedings of the Association for Research in Vision and Ophthalmology, 225.

Buisseret, P., Gary-Bobo, E., & Imbert, M. (1978). Ocular motility and recovery of orientational properties of visual cortical neurones in dark-reared kittens. *Nature, 272,* 816–817.

Buisseret, P., & Singer, W. (1983). Proprioceptive signals from extraocular muscles gate experience-dependent modifications of receptive fields in the kitten visual cortex. *Experimental Brain Research, 51,* 443–450.

Carew, T. J., Hawkins, R. D., Abrams, T. W., & Kandel, E. R. (1984). A test of Hebb's postulate at identified synapses which mediate classical conditioning in *Aplysia. Journal of Neuroscience, 4,* 1217–1224.

Collingridge, G. L., Kehl, S. J., & McLennan, H. (1983). Excitatory amino acids in synaptic transmission in the Schaffer collateral–commissural pathway of the rat hippocampus. *Journal of Physiology* (London), *334,* 33–46.

Crewther, S. G., Crewther, D. P., Peck, C. K., & Pettigrew, J. D. (1980). Visual cortical effects of rearing cats with monocular or binocular cyclotorsion. *Journal of Neurophysiology, 44,* 97–118.

Cynader, M. (1983). Prolonged sensitivity to monocular deprivation in dark-reared cats: Effects of age and visual exposure. *Developmental Brain Research, 8,* 155–164.

Cynader, M., & Mitchell, D. E. (1977). Monocular astigmatism effects on kitten visual cortex development. *Nature, 270,* 177–178.

Daw, N. W., Robertson, T. W., Rader, R. K., Videen, T. O., & Cosica, C. J. (1984). Substantial reduction of noradrenaline by lesions of adrenergic pathway does not prevent effects of monocular deprivation. *Journal of Neuroscience, 4,* 1354–1360.

Daw, N. W., Videen, T. O., Parkinson, D., & Rader, R. K. (1985). DSP-4 depletes noradrenaline in kitten visual cortex without altering the effects of monocular deprivation. *Journal of Neuroscience, 5,* 1925–1933.

Freeman, R. D., & Bonds, A. B. (1979). Cortical plasticity in monocularly deprived immobilized kittens depends on eye movement. *Science, 206,* 1093–1095.

Freeman, R. D., & Olson, C. (1982). Brief periods of monocular deprivation in kittens: Effects of delay prior to physiological study. *Journal of Neurophysiology, 47,* 139–150.

Geiger, H., & Singer, W. (1986). A possible role of Ca^{++}-currents in developmental plasticity. *Experimental Brain Research,* Ser. 14, 256–270.

Gray, C. M., Freeman, W. J., & Skinner, E. (1984). Associative changes in the spatial amplitude patterns of rabbit olfactory EEG are norepinephrine dependent. *Society for Neuroscience Abstracts, 10,* 121.

Greuel, J. M., Luhmann, H. J., & Singer, W. (1987). Evidence for a threshold in experience-dependent long-term changes of kitten visual cortex. *Developmental Brain Research, 34,* 141–149.

Greuel, J. M., Luhmann, H. J., & Singer, W. (1988). Persistent changes of single-cell responses in kitten striate cortex produced by pairing sensory stimulation with ionophoretic application of neurotransmitters and neuromodulators. In C. D. Woody, D. L. Alkon, & J. L. McGaugh (Eds.), *Cellular mechanisms of conditioning and behavioral plasticity* (pp. 425–436). New York: Plenum.

Hebb, D. O. (1949). *The organization of behavior.* New York: Wiley.

Hopkins, W. F., & Johnston, D. (1984). Frequency dependent noradrenergic modulation of long-term potentiation in the hippocampus. *Science, 226,* 350–351.

Hubel, D. H., & Wiesel, T. N. (1965). Binocular interaction in striate cortex of kittens reared with artificial squint. *Journal of Neurophysiology, 28,* 1041–1059.

Ito, M., Sakurai, M., & Tongroach, P. (1982). Climbing fibre induced depression of both mossy fibre responsiveness and glutamate sensitivity of cerebellar Purkinje cells. *Journal of Physiology, 324,* 113–134.

Kasamatsu, T., & Pettigrew, J. D. (1979). Preservation of binocularity after monocular deprivation in the striate cortex of kittens treated with 6-hydroxydopamine. *Journal of Comparative Neurology, 185,* 139–161.

Kasamatsu, T., Pettigrew, J. D., & Ary, M.-L. (1979). Restoration of visual cortical plasticity by local microperfusion of norepinephrine. *Journal of Comparative Neurology, 185,* 163–182.

Kleinschmidt, A., Bear, M. F., & Singer, W. (1987). Blockade of "NMDA" receptors disrupts experience-dependent plasticity in kitten striate cortex. *Science, 238,* 355–358.

Lee, K. S. (1983). Cooperativity among afferents for the induction of long-term potentiation in the CA_1 region of the hippocampus. *Journal of Neuroscience, 3,* 1369–1372.

LeVay, S., Stryker, M. P., & Shatz, C. J. (1978). Ocular dominance columns and their development in layer IV of the cat's visual cortex: A quantitative study. *Journal of Comparative Neurology, 179,* 223–244.

Levy, W. B., & Steward, O. (1983). Temporal contiguity requirements for long-term associative potentiation/depression in the hippocampus. *Neuroscience, 8,* 791–797.

Llinas, R. (1979). The role of calcium in neuronal function. In F. O. Schmitt & F. G. Worden (Eds.), *The Neurosciences fourth study program* (pp. 555–571). Cambridge, Mass.: MIT Press.

Llinas, R., & Sugimori, M. (1979). Calcium conductances in Purkinje cell dendrites: Their role in development and integration. *Progress in Brain Research, 51,* 323–334.

Lynch, G., & Baudry, M. (1984). The biochemistry of memory: A new and specific hypothesis. *Science, 224,* 1057–1063.

Lynch, G., Larson, J., Kelso, S., Barrionuevo, G., & Schottler, F. (1983). Intracellular injections of EGTA block induction of hippocampal long-term potentiation. *Nature, 305,* 719–721.

McNaughton, B. L., Douglas, R. M., & Goddard, G. V. (1978). Synaptic enhancement in fascia dentata: Cooperativity among coactive afferents. *Brain Research, 157,* 277–293.

Mioche, L., & Singer, W. (1989). Chronic recordings from single sites of kitten striate cortex during experience-dependent modification of receptive field properties. *Journal of Neurophysiology, 62.*

Mower, G. D., Caplan, C. J., Christen, W. G., & Duffy, F. H. (1985). Dark rearing prolongs physiological but not anatomical plasticity of the cat visual cortex. *Journal of Comparative Neurology, 235,* 448–466.

Mower, G. D., & Christen, W. G. (1985). Role of visual experience in activating critical period in cat visual cortex. *Journal of Neurophysiology, 53,* 572–589.

Olson, C., & Freeman, R. D. (1980). Profile of the sensitive period for monocular deprivation in kitten. *Experimental Brain Research, 39,* 17–21.

Parkinson, D., Kratz, K. E., & Daw, N. W. (1988). Evidence for a nicotinic component to the actions of acetylcholine in cat visual cortex. *Experimental Brain Research, 73,* 553–568.

Prusky, G. T., Shaw, C., & Cynader, M. S. (1987). Nicotinic receptors are located on lateral geniculate nucleus terminals in cat visual cortex. *Brain Research, 412,* 131–138.

Rauschecker, J. P., & Hahn, S. (1987). Ketamine-xylazine anesthesia blocks consolidation of ocular dominance changes in kitten visual cortex. *Nature, 326,* 183–185.

Rauschecker, J. P., & Singer, W. (1979). Changes in the circuitry of the kitten's visual cortex are gated by postsynaptic activity. *Nature, 280,* 58–60.

Rauschecker, J. P., & Singer, W. (1981). The effects of early visual experience on the cat's visual cortex and their possible explanation by Hebb synapses. *Journal of Physiology, 310,* 215–239.

Shatz, C. J., & Stryker, M. P. (1978). Ocular dominance in layer IV of the cat's visual cortex and the effects of monocular deprivation. *Journal of Physiology, 281,* 267–283.

Shaw, C., Needler, M. C., & Cynader, M. (1984). Ontogenesis of muscarinic acetylcholine binding sites in cat visual cortex: Reversal of specific laminar distribution during critical period. *Developmental Brain Research, 14,* 295–299.

Shaw, C., Wilkinson, M., Cynader, M., Needler, M. C., Aoki, C., & Hall, S. E. (1986). The laminar distributions and postnatal development of neurotransmitter and neuromodulator receptors in cat visual cortex. *Brain Research Bulletin, 16,* 661–672.

Sillito, A. M., Kemp, J. A., & Blakemore, C. (1983). The role of GABAergic inhibition in the cortical effects of monocular deprivation. *Nature, 291,* 318–322.

Singer, W. (1979). Central core control of visual cortex functions. In F. O. Schmitt & F. G. Worden (Eds.), *The Neurosciences Fourth Study Program* (pp. 1093–1109). Cambridge, Mass.: MIT Press.

Singer, W. (1982). Central core control of developmental plasticity in the kitten visual cortex: I. Diencephalic lesions. *Experimental Brain Research, 47,* 209–222.

Singer, W., & Rauschecker, J. P. (1982). Central core control of developmental plasticity in the kitten visual cortex. II. Electrical activation of mesencephalic and diencephalic projections. *Experimental Brain Research, 47,* 223–233.

Singer, W., Rauschecker, J., & Werth, R. (1977). The effect of monocular exposure to temporal contrasts on ocular dominance in kittens. *Brain Research, 134,* 568–572.

Singer, W., Tretter, F., & Yinon, U. (1982). Central gating of developmental plasticity in kitten visual cortex. *Journal of Physiology, 324,* 221–237.

Singer, W., von Grünau, M., & Rauschecker, J. (1979). Requirements for the disruption of binocularity in the visual cortex of strabismic kittens. *Brain Research, 171,* 536–540.

Stichel, C. C., & Singer, W. (1987). Quantitative analysis of the choline acetyltransferase-immunoreactive axonal network in the cat primary visual cortex. II. Pre- and postnatal development. *Journal of Comparative Neurology, 258,* 99–111.

Stichel, C. C., Singer, W., Heizmann, C. W., & Norman, A. W. (1987). Immunohistochemical localization of calcium-binding proteins, parvalbumin and calbindin-D 28 K, in the adult and developing visual cortex of cats: A light and electron microscopic study. *Journal of Comparative Neurology, 262,* 563–577.

Tiemann, S. B. (1985). The anatomy of geniculocortical connections in monocularly deprived cats. *Cellular and Molecular Neurobiology, 5,* 35–45.

Wiesel, T. N., & Hubel, D. H. (1965a). Comparison of the effects of unilateral and bilateral eye closure on cortical unit responses in kittens. *Journal of Neurophysiology, 28,* 1029–1040.

Wiesel, T. N., & Hubel, D. H. (1965b). Extent of recovery from the effects of visual deprivation in kittens. *Journal of Neurophysiology, 28,* 1060–1072.

Wigström, H., & Gustafsson B. (1985). On long-lasting potentiation in the hippocampus: A proposed mechanism for its dependence on coincident pre- and postsynaptic activity. *Acta Physiologica Scandinavica, 123,* 519–522.

Woody, C. D. (1984). The electrical excitability of nerve cells as an index of learned behavior. In D. L. Alkon & J. Farley (Eds.), *Primary neural substrates of learning and behavioral change* (pp. 101–127). New York: Cambridge University Press.

Woody, C. D., Alkon, D. L., & Hay, B. (1984). Depolarization-induced effects of Ca^{2+}-calmodulin-dependent protein kinase injection, in vivo, in single neurons of cat motor cortex. *Brain Research, 321,* 192–197.

11

The Dissection by Alzheimer's Disease of Cortical and Limbic Neural Systems Relevant to Memory

GARY W. VAN HOESEN

Since the mid-1970s, Alzheimer's disease (AD) has been recognized as the most common form of dementia (Katzman, 1976). The clinical manifestations of AD are characterized by an unremitting decline in higher mental function, dominated typically by a memory impairment. However, the tempo of the changes vary and early onset AD is associated with a rapid decline (Corsellis, 1976; Tomlinson & Corsellis, 1984). Historically, this contributed to the confusion surrounding the term presenile dementia. Both this and senile dementia are now considered behaviorally and pathologically as AD, which recognizes that dementia can occur abnormally early, but that neither dementia nor extensive brain pathology is a necessary concomitant of senility. This is not to say that behavioral changes and structural changes to the brain do not occur in aging; of course they do, but an aberrant pace in terms of cognitive decline and an aberrant quantity of structural changes are abnormal, and together they form much of the essence of AD (Katzman, 1986).

Behaviorally, the cardinal change in AD is an impairment in memory, and it characterizes the disorder throughout its course. Aside from a relatively well preserved capacity for skill memory (Eslinger & Damasio, 1986; Knopman & Nissen, 1987) until late in the illness, few details are available regarding the course and character of the memory disorder. Episodic or contextual memory is clearly impaired and some believe that changes in their anterograde compartment are among AD's first manifestations (Van Hoesen & Damasio, 1987). Forgetting appointments, new names, new obligations, and news events are all examples. Episodic or contextual memory loss in the retrograde compartment is also common and in many instances seems to be the trigger that sufficiently alarms the victim to seek a medical opinion. An inability to remember a well-known route or the face of a relative or good friend is an example of such a change.

Disorders of generic or semantic memory are seen frequently in AD, especially in its later stages. The conceptual class to which a stimulus belongs—including the simple identity and function of common natural and man-made objects—might be lost. For practical purposes, this disability is an agnosia (Damasio, 1984).

Although this may strike a familiar chord with clinicians who examine patients with AD, or families and health care professionals who attend to their needs, the exact nature and sequence of the changes have not been studied fully. Similarly, the course of the memory changes has not been documented fully. For example, it is tempting to believe that the initial memory changes occur in the anterograde compartments of memory and entail episodic or contextual events and excessive forgetfulness. Later one might expect an involvement of the retrograde compartments of memory in the episodic or contextual realms, so that previously familiar stimuli, their relationships, and even previously overlearned spatial aspects of memory are impaired. As incapacitation approaches, generic and semantic memory are affected typically so that the identity and function of common environmental objects are lost, as is the patient's self-identity.

If this is the sequence of behavioral changes that characterize AD, it has important implications that would lead to predictions about the loci of pathological changes that occur as the illness progresses. Theoretically, these would be verifiable in longitudinal studies of AD where all data points, both behavioral and pathological, throughout the course of the disease were represented. For example, in the early stages where the memory impairment is for episodic or contextual events in the anterograde compartment, one might predict a focus of pathology in temporal lobe structures such as the hippocampus, amygdala, and parahippocampal gyrus (Scoville & Milner, 1957). Such changes would also be compatible with diencephalic pathology (Squire, 1986, 1987). Some of these changes—particularly those involving excessive forgetfulness—might also be related to pathological changes in basal forebrain structures (Damasio, Graff-Radford, Eslinger, Damasio, & Kassell, 1985).

The neural correlates for episodic and contextual memory impairments in the retrograde compartment and impairments for generic and semantic memory are not entirely understood. Clearly, neither depends exclusively on medial temporal or medial diencephalic structures. Damage to these areas can produce a partial retrograde change for events prior to the injury or surgery, but it is either incipient or lasts for only a few years (Damasio, 1984; Scoville & Milner, 1957; Squire, 1986). Recent evidence from survivors of herpes simplex encephalitis suggests that the posterior parahippocampal, lateral temporal, temporal polar, and anterior insular cortices may play a role in the preservation of retrograde memories (Damasio, Eslinger, Damasio, Van Hoesen, & Cornell, 1985).

Finally, generic memory is seldom affected with medial temporal injury even if it is bilateral. One would expect that the additive features in AD, which lead to a total breakdown in memory mechanisms, including all aspects of episodic and contextual memory plus generic and semantic memory, would be a consequence of additional pathological changes in the various association cortices, and particularly the multimodal areas of the frontal, parietal, and temporal lobes (see Damasio, 1984; Goldman-Rakic, 1987; Squire, 1986; Tulving, 1987).

Given our knowledge of the neural correlates of memory, derived from animal experimentation and the study of human patients with surgical, accidental, or infectious damage to selective parts of the brain, predictions can be made about the anatomical changes expected in AD. Although this would necessarily be skewed in the direction of end-stage AD where all forms of episodic and generic memory are impaired, the neural correlates of separate forms of memory might be highlighted in patients who die before end-stage AD of other illnesses. Thus a careful analysis of the specific cortical and subcortical changes in AD is warranted along with an analysis of the known neural connectivity of affected areas. However, before doing this it is essential to highlight certain aspects of the neural connectivity of the primate brain and, even more, the brain of a nonhuman primate like the rhesus monkey, since this species provides our best approximation to humans in terms of experimental knowledge.

SOME BASICS OF CORTICAL CONNECTIVITY IN PRIMATES

Experimental studies in nonhuman primates since the late 1960s have revealed an orderly sequence of intrahemispheric corticocortical neural systems that link the primary sensory cortices with both the association cortices and limbic system structures. These form an intricate series of multisynaptic neural pathways that provide both unimodal and multimodal sensory processing and that provide limbic structures with a refined digest of cortical activity (Van Hoesen, 1982).

The primary sensory areas all give rise to powerful, short intrahemispheric corticocortical connections to the adjacent primary sensory association cortex (Jones & Powell, 1970; Pandya & Kuypers, 1969). This connection begins a feedforward system (Maunsell & Van Essen, 1983; Van Essen & Maunsell, 1983) that characterizes the visual (Rockland & Pandya, 1981; Van Essen & Maunsell, 1983), auditory (Galaburda & Pandya, 1983), and somatosensory cortices (Pandya & Seltzer, 1982b). It is the first step in the dissemination of sensory information to other parts of the cortex. After successive relays in other sensory association areas, these projections end in the nonprimary association cortex of the forntal, temporal, and parietal lobes. Many also have as a target multimodal association areas, in that their input is characterized by projections from multiple primary sensory association cortices each committed functionally to a single modality (Chavis & Pandya, 1976; Jones & Powell, 1970; Pandya & Seltzer, 1982a; Seltzer & Pandya, 1976). Another target of the association cortices, including those of a multimodal variety, is the limbic system (Goldman-Rakic, Selemon, & Schwartz, 1984; Jones & Powell, 1970; Van Hoesen, Pandya, & Butters, 1972). For example, nearly the entire limbic lobe (posterior orbital and medial frontal cortex, cingulate cortex, parahippocampal cortex, temporal polar cortex, and anterior insular cortex) receives as a major input projections from the association cortices. Additional direct limbic projections from the association cortices converge on several nuclei of the amygdala (Aggleton, Burton, & Passingham, 1980; Herzog & Van Hoesen, 1976; Turner, Mishkin & Knapp, 1980; Whitlock & Nauta, 1956). Together with powerful projections from the cortex of the limbic lobe (Van Hoesen, 1982), these provide the amygdala with a sizable cortical input. One of the final limbic system linkages of the neural systems of the association cortices is with the allocortex that forms the hippocampal formation. These are mediated via projections from the limbic lobe and association cortex to the entorhinal cortex, as illustrated in Figure 11.1 (Amaral, 1987; Amaral, Insausti, & Cowan, 1983; Goldman-Rakic et al., 1984; Van Hoesen, 1982; Van Hoesen & Pandya, 1975a, 1975b; Van Hoesen et al., 1972; Van Hoesen, Pandya, & Butters, 1975). This area (Brodmann's area 28) gives rise to the perforant pathway that terminates along the distal dendrites of the dentate gyrus granule cells and hippocampal pyramidal cells (Van Hoesen, 1985; Van Hoesen & Pandya, 1975a, 1975b; Van Hoesen et al., 1975).

Although less information is available, it is clear that many of these connections are reciprocated by a feedback series of neural systems (Galaburda & Pan-

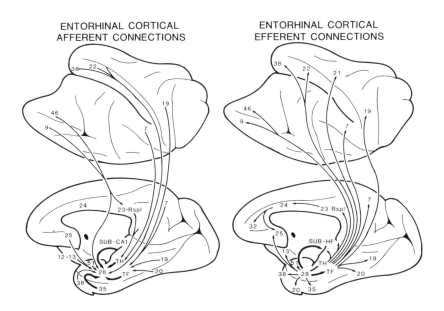

FIGURE 11.1.   Major cortical afferent and efferent neural systems of the entorhinal cortex in the rhesus monkey on medial and lateral views of the cerebral hemisphere. Identification of cortical areas corresponds to those of Brodmann and Bonin and Bailey. Note that cortical neural systems from the frontal, parietal, occipital, temporal, and limbic lobes converge on Brodmann's area 28, the entorhinal cortex. Layer IV of the entorhinal cortex receives a powerful output from the subiculum (Sub) and CA1 parts of the hippocampal formation (HF) and gives rise to neural systems that feed back to widespread limbic and association cortical areas.

dya, 1983; Maunsell & Van Essen, 1983; Pandya & Yeterian, 1985; Rockland & Pandya, 1981; Van Essen & Maunsell, 1983). To conceptualize this, recall that the major output of the hippocampal formation arises from its subicular subdivision. This cortex has several projections to subcortical structures (Swanson & Cowan, 1975, 1977) and to other parts of the limbic lobe, including a strong one to the deeper cell layers (layer IV) of the entorhinal cortex (Rosene & Van Hoesen, 1977; Shipley & Sorensen, 1975). The cortical areas of the limbic lobe all project to various parts of the association cortices, which in turn project back to the various primary sensory cortices (Mesulam, Van Hoesen, Pandya, & Geschwind, 1977; Pandya, Van Hoesen, & Mesulam, 1981; Vogt & Miller, 1983).

In short, corticocortical intrahemispheric pathways clearly form neural systems that serve to transmit sensory information that ultimately reaches the oldest of cortices, the allocortex of the hippocampal formation. On the other hand, output from the allocortex begins a reciprocation of these projections that eventually can be traced back to the primary sensory area (Van Hoesen, 1982). Some of these relationships are illustrated in Figures 11.1 and 11.2. In this context it

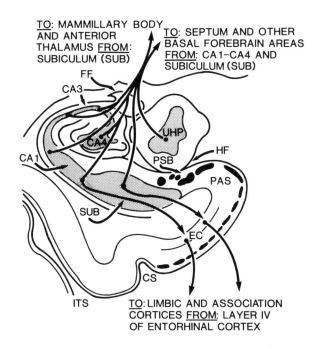

FIGURE 11.2.   Major efferent neural systems of the hippocampal formation. The major cortical target is the entorhinal cortex (EC). Both the subiculum and entorhinal cortex are major targets for neurofibrillary tangles in AD. CS = collateral sulcus; FF = fimbria fornix; HF = hippocampal fissure; ITS = inferior temporal sulcus; PAS = parasubiculum; PSB = presubiculum; UHP = uncal hippocampus.

is also important that recent investigations have shown that the amygdala also gives rise to widespread projections to the association cortices as well (Amaral & Price, 1984; Porrino, Crane, & Goldman-Rakic, 1981).

The cells of origin that give rise to intrahemispheric neural systems are not entirely known. However, available evidence (*see* Andersen, Asanuma, & Cowan, 1985; Bugbee & Goldman-Rakic, 1983; Goldman-Rakic & Schwartz, 1982; Jones, 1981, 1984; Maunsell & Van Essen, 1983; Rockland & Pandya, 1979; Schwartz & Goldman-Rakic, 1982) indicates that the feedforward system, involved in the outflow of sensory information and other intrahemispheric projections, arises from both supragranular and infragranular cortical layers, whereas the feedback system arises largely from infragranular layers. More specifically, the small pyramids that form layer II, many of the medium-sized pyramids of layer III, and a subset of the larger pyramids of layer V give rise to the feedforward system of corticocortical connections. In contrast, the feedback system arises largely from layers V and VI (Fig. 11.3).

TOPOGRAPHICAL DISTRIBUTION OF PATHOLOGICAL CHANGES IN ALZHEIMER'S DISEASE IN RELATION TO CORTICAL TYPES

The observation of severe pathological changes in the cerebral cortex in Bielchowsky-stained tissue was the major pathologic feature that motivated Alzheimer (1907) to publish his now classic report on "a singular disease of the cerebral cortex." His findings have never been disputed seriously. Cortical changes quantitatively overshadow those in subcortical areas, although it is clear that the cortex is not affected uniformly. All types of cortex are affected in AD, but the changes within a given type of cortex are selective. A review of the major types of cortex and their involvement in AD follows.

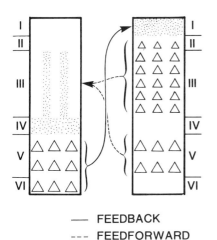

— FEEDBACK
--- FEEDFORWARD

FIGURE 11.3. Cortical laminar origin (triangles) for feedback and feedforward corticocortical neural systems and laminar distribution of their terminals within the cortex (dots). Neurofibrillary tangles in AD are found in great abundance in layers III and V and neuritic plaques are seen often in layers I and III. There is a strong suggestion that corticocortical association neural systems are compromised in AD.

Allocortical Changes

The allocortices are a conspicuous component of the cerebral cortex. They are composed of two to three layers, of which one or two are cellular. Pyramidal neurons are the dominant cell type. Characteristically, polarized apical dendrites extend toward the pia mater and form a wide molecular layer. The dentate gyrus, hippocampus, subiculum, olfactory, and periamygdaloid cortices are examples. In AD these fields are heavily but selectively compromised (Ball, 1976, 1977, 1978; Hyman, Damasio, Van Hoesen, & Barnes, 1984; Kemper, 1978; Wilcock, 1983). For example, within the hippocampal formation, the pryamids that form the subiculum and CA1 sector of the hippocampus are usually invested heavily with neurofibrillary tangles. Neuritic plaques are found among them and in their molecular layer (Burger, 1983; Gibson, 1983). In contrast, the adjoining CA3 sector of the hippocampus and the dentate gyrus may contain only an occasional neuron with neurofibrillary tangles (Hyman et al., 1984). There is also evidence that the olfactory allocortices are damaged heavily in AD (Esiri & Wilcok, 1984).

Periallocortical Changes

The periallocortical parts of the cerebral cortex are characterized by atypical laminar arrangements and cell types. The deep layers are related closely to the adjacent allocortex, whereas the superficial layers are reminiscent of the isocortex. The entorhinal, parasubicular, presubicular, and retrosplenial cortices are the best examples of periallocortex. As with allocortices, the involvement of the periallocortices in AD is not uniform. For example, the entorhinal cortex is involved heavily with many neurofibrillary tangles and neuritic plaques (Hirano & Zimmerman, 1962; Hyman et al., 1984; Van Hoesen, Hyman, & Damasio, 1986). Typically the changes are so extensive that the normal and unique cytoarchitecture of this cortex is unrecognizable. The same may be said for the adjacent and closely related parasubicular cortex. In contrast, the adjacent presubicular cortex is largely spared in AD (Hyman, Van Hoesen, Kromer, & Damasio, 1985). It may contain an occasional neuritic plaque and neurofibrillary tangle, but these are in random locations without a predilection for a specific layer or cell type.

Proisocortical Changes

The proisocortices, a sizable component of the cerebral cortex, along with the periallocortices and allocortices form the limbic lobe. The posterior parts of the orbitofrontal cortex, the cingulate cortex, the retrocalcarine, posterior parahippocampal, perirhinal, temporal polar, and anterior insular cortices constitute major examples. These areas resemble the isocortex in that there are multiple cellular layers. However, some of these may be atypical, because they are accentuated or incipient, and generally layers V and VI contain large and poorly differentiated neurons. These areas are the most uniformly affected cortices in AD. For example, the posterior part of the parahippocampal cortex (Brodmann's area 36) is a common site of pathological change and contains an abundance of neurofibrillary tangles and neuritic plaques. These are continuous into the more anteriorly located perirhinal cortex (Brodmann's area 35) and the temporal polar cortex (Brodmann's area 38) (Braak & Braak, 1985; Kemper, 1978).

The dysgranular part of the insular cortex and the posterior orbital cortex are likewise involved to a major degree, as is the subcallosal part of the cingulate gyrus (Brodmann's area 25). Some investigators report that the posterior part of the cingulate gyrus (Brodmann's area 23) is one of the more heavily affected cortical areas in AD (Brun & Englund, 1981). However, there is a major exception regarding the anterior parts of this gyrus (Brodmann's area 24). This cortex does not appear affected until later in the disorder and may be spared entirely (Brun & Englund, 1981; Brun & Gustafson, 1976). Interestingly, this part of the proisocortices is related closely to the motor cortices (supplementary, premotor, and primary motor cortices), which typically are spared in AD.

Isocortical Changes

The nonuniform involvement of the isocortex in AD often can be detected by visual inspection of the gross brain (Tomlinson & Corsellis, 1984). In brief, pathological changes in the form of neurofibrillary tangles, neuritic plaques, and cell loss are abundant in the association areas of the temporal and parietal lobes in many Alzheimer's brains, and additional changes in the frontal and occipital lobes are common. In contrast, the primary sensory areas (Fig. 11.4) and the

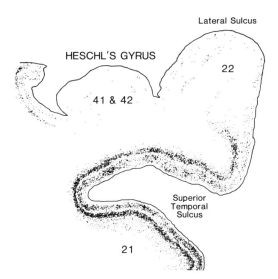

FIGURE 11.4. Cross section of the pattern and laminar distribution of neurofibrillary tangles in the auditory cortex from a case of AD charted with an X–Y recorder coupled to the axes of the microscopic stage. Each dot represents a tangle. Note that the primary auditory cortex (Brodmann's areas 41 and 42) that forms Heschl's gyrus is largely spared. The dorsal and lateral parts of area 22, the primary sensory association cortex, are also relatively spared. More distal auditory association areas in the upper bank of the superior temporal sulcus contain extensive pathology.

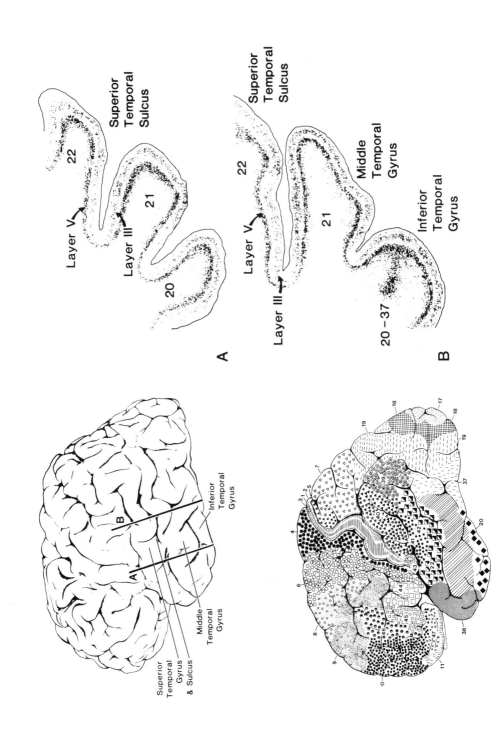

primary motor cortices are not affected greatly. The relative sparing of these sensory and motor areas is consistent with the paucity of motor and sensory impairment in AD. Nonetheless, the heavy and possibly early involvement of the olfactory cortex in AD (Esiri & Wilcock, 1984) suggests that odor detection is an exception (Corwin, Serby, Conrad, & Rotrosen, 1985; Doty, Reyes, & Gregor, 1987; Warner, Peabody, Flattery, & Tinklenberg, 1986).

The association cortices affected in AD are of the so-called homotypical variety (Pearson, Esiri, Hiorns, Wilcock, & Powell, 1985; Rogers & Morrison, 1985). In the frontal lobe the homotypical cortical areas form Brodmann's areas 9, 10, 11, 12, 13, 14, and 46. In the parietal lobe, they form Brodmann's areas 7, 39, and 40. In the occipitotemporal region, Brodmann's area 37 contains the major expanse of homotypical isocortex. Areas 20, 21, and 22 represent the major examples of this type of cortex in the temporal lobe (Fig. 11.5). These regions are characterized by a similarity of architectural plan and form the largest part of the cerebral cortex in the human brain. They represent the classic six-layered pattern of isocortex. Layer II is well developed and has small neurons, mostly of the pyramidal variety. Layer III is generally wide and only slightly differentiated, with the major cell type being medium-sized pyramids. Layer IV is composed of small neurons of pyramidal or stellate variety. Layer V is composed largely of pyramidal neurons of varying sizes with prominent apical dendrites and is distinguishable from layer VI, which is formed by multiform elements of varying size and shape. These areas give rise to a majority of the long cortico-cortical association projections that mediate interconnectivity between the various lobes and with the limbic cortical areas (Jones & Powell, 1970; Pandya & Kuypers, 1969). They participate prominently in both feedforward and feedback cortical connections (see Fig. 11.3).

The degree of pathological involvement of the association cortices in AD can vary greatly, ranging from extensive involvement to only selective involvement in one or two lobes. However, the involvement of the proisocortex of the limbic lobe, the periallocortex of the anterior parahippocampal gyrus, and the allocortex of the hippocampal formation is more consistent. Whether this represents early involvement of these types of cortex or a differential degree of intensity once the disease process starts is not yet apparent. Among isocortical association areas the parietotemporal and occipitotemporal regions seem affected heavily in AD (Brun & Englund, 1981).

FIGURE 11.5.   Two X–Y chartings of neurofibrillary tangle distribution through the anterior (A) and middle (B) parts of the temporal lobe in AD. Brodmann's numbers denote auditory (22) and visual (20, 21, and 37) association areas. In each case these are so-called distal association areas and are known to be involved in complex sensory processing. The cortex that lines the banks of the superior temporal sulcus is multimodal and is also associated with higher order functions. Note the layer III and V laminar pattern of tangles and their dense distribution in the distal and multimodal association cortices.

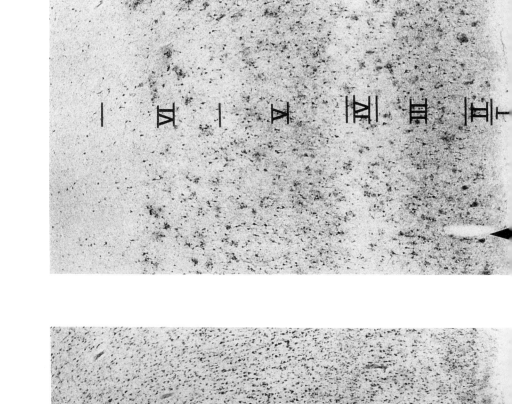

LAMINAR SPECIFICITY AND PATTERNS OF CORTICAL PATHOLOGY IN ALZHEIMER'S DISEASE

The topographical specificity of Alzheimer's pathology in terms of cortical types is paralleled by a cellular and laminar specificity within affected areas (Figs. 11.5 and 11.6). This is clearly the case for neurofibrillary tangles. For example, neurons that form predominantly one or two cortical layers contain this cytoskeletal alteration, whereas their immediate neighbors in adjacent layers may be unaltered (Braak & Braak, 1985; Hyman et al., 1984; Lewis, Campbell, Terry, & Morrison, 1987; Pearson et al., 1985; Van Hoesen et al., 1986). The same applies to some extent for neuritic plaque distribution (Rogers & Morrison, 1985). Although this pathological marker may have a broader distribution in terms of laminar location (Pearson et al., 1985), there are many examples in the cerebral cortex where plaques are found largely in selective cortical layers. It is less clear whether cell loss, in addition to that attributable to neurofibrillary tangles, follows a laminar-specific pattern (Mann, Yates, & Marcyniuk, 1985; Terry, 1983; Terry, Peck, DeTeresa, Schechter, & Horoupian, 1981), but it appears that larger cortical neurons are lost to a greater degree than small neurons in both AD and normal aging. Because large neurons are located primarily in layers III, V, and VI, it would follow that at least some laminar specificity occurs in age-related cell loss whether AD is present or not.

It is apparent that pathological changes in AD are decidedly skewed toward the association and limbic cortices. As summarized in Figure 11.1, homotypical cortical areas that form the association cortices are a major source of input to the limbic system (Van Hoesen, 1982) and represent a major recipient of limbic system output (Amaral & Price, 1984; Kosel, Van Hoesen, & Rosene, 1982; Porrino et al., 1981; Van Hoesen, 1982). Moreover, they provide a major source of long cortical projections that link together the various parts of the cerebral cortex. Their destruction of the magnitude noted in AD would suggest that devastating cognitive change should ensue. Morever, the laminar distribution of cortical pathology in AD correlates closely with the laminar origin of cortical projections and the laminar distribution of cortical association efferents.

The critical nature of these changes can be appreciated if one considers the connectional relationship between the hippocampal formation and the cerebral cortex. The hippocampus receives few direct inputs from cortical association areas. Instead, its major cortical input arises from the entorhinal cortex (Brodmann's area 28), which forms the anterior parahippocampal gyrus. The entorhinal cortex gives rise to the perforant pathway, a major neural system of the temporal lobe, which terminates on the outer parts of the dendritic trees of den-

←——————————————————————————————————

FIGURE 11.6. (left) Nissl-stained cross section through the cortex of the inferior temporal gyrus in AD. (right) The same microscopic field (note the vessel track in the lower left corner of each photo at arrowhead) with the tissue processed for Alz-50 immunoreactivity. This monoclonal antibody recognizes a tissue antigen found in high concentrations in certain somas and their processes in AD but not in age-compatible normals. Note the high density of Alz-50 immunoreactive somas in layers III, V, and VI.

tate gyrus granule cells and hippocampal pyramidal cells. It has been stressed since the time of Ramón y Cajal's original description of the perforant pathway in Golgi-stained material that it carries the strongest source of input to the hippocampal formation and forms its exclusive link to the remainder of the cortex. The input to the entorhinal cortex thus becomes a critical issue and many of its sources have been described recently (see Amaral, 1987; Van Hoesen, 1982). Most afferents arise from neighboring cortical areas such as the presubiculum, parasubiculum, periamygdaloid, and prepiriform cortex and proisocortical areas of the temporal lobe. The latter includes area 35, the perirhinal cortex; area 36, the posterior parahippocampal cortex; area 37, the occipitotemporal cortex; and area 38, the temporal polar cortex. All of these areas are the recipients of powerful corticocortical association input from sensory association and multimodal cortical association areas and in turn project powerfully to the superficial layers of the entorhinal cortex. The critical relay neurons in areas 35, 36, 37, and 38 are the pyramids in layers III and V. Briefly, it is probably accurate to state that a sizable component of the feedforward system of cortical sensory connections converges onto the entorhinal cortex, where it is relayed to the hippocampal formation by the perforant pathway.

Nearly all of the key components of these neural systems are affected in AD. For example, in areas 35, 36, 37, and 38, the most common distribution of neurofibrillary tangles is in cortical layers III and V. Neuritic plaques are abundant in their terminal zone in the entorhinal cortex layers I to III, and particularly layer III. Moreover, the cells of origin for the perforant pathway, the large layer II stellate neurons and the more superficial layer III pyramids, are laden with neurofibrillary tangles (Figs. 11.7 and 11.8) and often are destroyed totally in AD (Hyman, Van Hoesen, Kromer, & Damasio, 1986). There is a strong likelihood that the specific cortical neurons that form neural systems conveying cortical association input to the hippocampal formation are destroyed in AD. The reciprocal of this relationship also seems compromised greatly (Hyman et al., 1984). This feedback system arises primarily from the subicular and CA1 part of the hippocampal formation and from layer IV of the entorhinal cortex, which itself receives a large subicular projection (see Figs. 11.1 and 11.2). Both the subiculum and layer IV of the entorhinal cortex typically contain neurofibrillary tangles in AD. Such observations led researchers to state previously that the pathological distribution of neurofibrillary tangles and neuritic plaques in AD dissects neural systems of the temporal lobe with a cellular precision that effectively isolates the hippocampal formation from the remainder of the cerebral cortex (Hyman et al., 1984; Van Hoesen & Damasio, 1987; Van Hoesen et al., 1986).

In conclusion, there seems to be little doubt that the cerebral cortex is damaged heavily in AD, but in a very selective manner. In the allocortex, it takes the form of selective manner. In the allocortex, it takes the form of selective destruction of the subicular and CA1 zones of the hippocampal formation but with preservation of the neighboring CA3 zone. In the periallocortex it can be seen by conspicuous alterations of the entorhinal (see Fig. 11.7) and parasu-

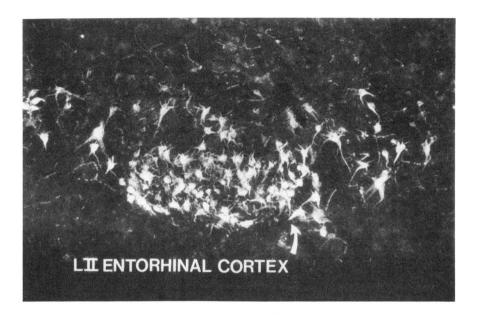

FIGURE 11.7.   Thioflavin S–stained neurofibrillary tangles in layer II of the entorhinal cortex in AD. These neurons give rise to major component of the perforant pathway that links the cortex with the dentate gyrus of the hippocampal formation.

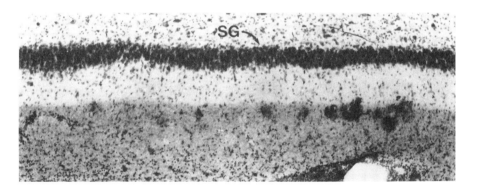

FIGURE 11.8.   Alz-50 terminal immunoreactivity in the outer two thirds of the molecular layer of the dentate gyrus in an area that would correspond to the terminal zone of the perforant pathway. This pattern of immunoreactivity suggests that the AD antigen recognized by Alz-50 is located in the terminals of layer II entorhinal neurons. Note the presence of Alz-50 immunoreactive neuritic plaques in the immunoreactive zone. The vessel profile marks the location of the hippocampal fissure. The granule cells of the dentate gyrus, or stratum granulosum (SG), have been stained with thionin.

bicular cortex but preservation of the adjacent presubicular periallocortex. In the proisocortex, Brodmann's cingulate areas 25 and 23 may be heavily damaged. In the isocortex, the homotypical association cortices of all four lobes may contain cell loss, neurofibrillary tangles, and neuritic plaques, whereas adjacent primary sensory and motor cortices remain well preserved.

Imposed on these selective changes is a remarkable degree of laminar specificity within affected areas, such that often only certain layers contain neurofibrillary tangles or an unusually large number of neuritic plaques. This is best demonstrated in the entorhinal cortex, where layers II and IV are damaged heavily, whereas neighboring layers are less heavily damaged. It is also manifested in the homotypical isocortical association areas, where neurofibrillary tangles occur primarily in cell layers III and V (see Figs. 11.4 to 11.6).

On the basis of studies of cortical connectivity in nonhuman primates such as the monkey, it is plausible to argue that the pathological targets of AD especially affect the long association systems that are responsible for linking the various association areas of the hemisphere among themselves and with the cortex of the limbic lobe. Both the feedforward systems of connections that disseminate cortical information throughout the cortex and the feedback systems that reciprocate them are implicated (see Fig. 11.3). Indeed, the laminar origins and some of the terminal fields of these systems correspond remarkably with the patterns of pathology observed in the cortex in AD (Hyman et al., 1984; Lewis et al., 1987; Pearson et al., 1985; Rogers & Morrison, 1985).

Many questions can be asked about the patterns of cortical pathology in AD. The most obvious is whether the changes occur as invariant features of the disorder, and they seem to, provided that the illness lasts long enough. In such cases, or end-stage AD, one might expect a major lesion of the cortical association and related limbic connections combined with an overall devastating impairment of cognition. Variations in both pathology and cognitive impairment occur for victims who die of other causes at earlier stages after onset of the illness (Wilcock & Esiri, 1982). The rate and amount of accrual of pathological change also vary. Certain neural systems are more involved than others. Naturally, different patterns of cognitive impairment should be expected in relation to such differential pathological involvement. The question of whether there is a single focus for the initiation of the process, or whether it starts in different parts of the nervous structure simultaneously, should be asked. Observations suggest that there is a single early focus that resides in the temporal lobe, particularly in the parahippocampal gyrus and hippocampal formation. The isolated, early changes in episodic and contextual memory, which represent the hallmark of the disease, are the cognitive counterpart to this pathological change.

ANATOMICAL ALTERATIONS IN SUBCORTICAL STRUCTURES IN ALZHEIMER'S DISEASE

Although more lesions in AD involve the cortex than other regions, subcortical changes should not be overlooked. Well-studied cognitive abnormalities have been reported with purely subcortical lesions, and they can affect processes such as memory (Damasio, 1984; von Cramon, Hebel, & Schuri, 1985). In addition, many of the subcortical structures implicated in AD provide sources of input for the cortex. Other affected subcortical structures include critical relays in neural systems that convey limbic and hypothalamic influences directly to the cortex.

Telencephalic Structures

Among subcortical telencephalic areas, those that form the basal forebrain are clearly implicated in AD. They include the gray matter masses located deep to the neostriatum and globus pallidus and those that converge along the midline at the base of the septum pellucidum. Structures such as the septum, the nuclei of the horizontal and vertical limbs of the diagonal bands of Broca, the substantia innominata and its associated nucleus basalis of Meynert, and the amygdala are major parts. Anatomically these are characterized by reciprocal connections with at least one part of the preoptic–hypothalamic area and reciprocal connections with at least one part of the cerebral cortex. In this sense they serve as intermediaries between those parts of the brain that largely subserve and interact with the internal environment and those that more prominently interact with the external environment.

Nucleus Basalis of Meynert

The nucleus basalis of Meynert is a dispersed group of hyperchromatic neurons that lies in a position ventral to the striatum and globus pallidus. The neurons are multipolar and fusiform in shape and are distributed broadly in both mediolateral and anterior–posterior directions. In the mediolateral plane they occupy a position a few millimeters from the midline anteriorly to a position lying beneath the temporal limb of the anterior commissure posteriorly, where the neurons are situated dorsal to the amygdala and ventral to the globus pallidus. In the anterior–posterior plane they extend from the septum anteriorly to the substantia nigra posteriorly. At some levels, scattered neurons of the nucleus basalis may be noted within the internal and external medullary laminae of the globus pallidus and within the lateral hypothalamic area. Although the neurons of the nucleus basalis of Meynert are dispersed, clustering does occur and can be observed in certain loci (Mesulam, Mufson, Levey, & Wainer, 1983). Some of the larger clusters lie within the so-called substantia innominata.

The nucleus basalis of Meynert has attracted attention because of several factors. During the 1980s, with the advent of retrograde tracing procedures, several investigators observed that the neurons that form the nucleus basalis send axons to much of the cerebral cortex and especially to the somatomotor cortices, including Brodmann's areas 6, 4, 3, 1, 2, and 5 (Divac, 1975; Jones, Burton, Saper, & Swanson, 1976; Kievet & Kuypers, 1975; Mesulam & Van Hoesen, 1976; Pearson, Gatter, Bratal, & Powell, 1983). Using combined retrograde labeling and histochemical methods, Mesulam and Van Hoesen (1976) demonstrated that many of the neurons that form the nucleus basalis of Meynert contain cholinergic enzymes. Subsequent studies using antibodies directed against choline acetyltransferase left little doubt that nucleus basalis neurons provide the major source of cholinergic input to the cerebral cortex (Mesulam et al., 1983). Thus it was of interest to find that some neurons of the basal forebrain are greatly diminished in certain patients with AD (Arendt, Bigl, Arendt, & Tennstedt, 1983; Candy et al., 1983; Whitehouse, Price, Clark, Coyle, & DeLong, 1981; Wilcock, Esiri, Bowen, & Smith, 1983). This pathological change offered a convenient structural correlate for the results of previous neurochemical studies revealing decreased levels of cortical acetylcholine in cerebral cortex in AD (Davies & Maloney, 1976). Moreover, on first impression this association seemed compatible with the memory impairments of AD because of the well-known effects of anticholinergic drugs on memory (Bartus, Dean, Beer, & Lippa, 1982; Coyle, Price, & DeLong, 1983; Drachman, 1977; Smith & Swash, 1978).

There is little doubt that the loss of neurons in the nucleus basalis of Meynert is a notable feature in some cases of AD. Nevertheless, the extent of pathology in this region can be as variable as that in other vulnerable brain areas (Arendt et al., 1983; Mann, Yates, & Marcyniuk, 1984; Pearson et al., 1984), and many cases show no change. It may range from mere shrinkage of perikaryon (Pearson et al., 1985; Pearson, Gatter, & Powell, 1983; Sofroniew, Pearson, Eckenstein, Cuello, & Powell, 1984), to minimal cell loss, to extensive cell loss (Saper, German, & White, 1985). Neurofibrillary tangles may be present or absent, and the number of neuritic plaques can vary widely. The issues here are not unlike those raised for any other affected brain region: What contribution does the loss or diminution of cholinergic input to the cerebral cortex make to the cognitive changes in AD, and why are these neurons targeted when their immediate neighbors survive? The latter is of special interest because of the cholinergic nature and connections of these neurons and the fact that neighboring striatal neurons and brain stem and spinal cord motor neurons, also acetylcholine positive, do not seem affected in AD.

It is important to consider nucleus basalis pathology from a neural systems viewpoint, because it figures prominently in many networks that undoubtedly participate in a wide range of cognitive processes. Virtually nothing is known about the subcortical projections of the nucleus basalis, although work in non-human primates suggests that these may be widespread (Divac, 1975). The cortical projections of this nucleus raise even greater questions. These projections are organized topographically so that they innervate functionally diverse parts of the cortex (Mesulam et al., 1983). Focal pathological changes in the nucleus basalis might be correlated with one cognitive change more than another. However, some of the larger, more conspicuous clusters of nucleus basalis neurons project largely to somatosensory and motor cortices (Jones et al., 1976). These areas are some of the last cortices to be affected in AD; moreover, their destruction in other neurological diseases is not associated with changes in other than somatomotor performance. Additionally, insofar as a relation to cognitive systems is concerned, the large hyperchromatic neurons that partially form the vertical limb of the diagonal band of Broca also are magnocellular basal forebrain nerve cells similar to if not identical to those that form the nucleus basalis of Meynert (Jones et al., 1976). As is the case for the closely related cholinergic neurons of the medial septum, they have projections directed not to the isocortex but preferentially to the proisocortex, periallocortex, and allocortex of the limbic lobe. An especially strong input is directed toward the hippocampal formation via the fimbria fornix and forms the well-known septohippocampal cholinergic system. Evidence suggests that this pathway is affected in AD (Arendt et al., 1983; Nakano & Hirano, 1982, 1983), and in such cases the hippocampal formation would be deprived of another major afferent source. This is of special interest because infarcts in this region cause a specific impairment of memory (Damasio, 1985; Volpe & Hirst, 1983).

Unlike many neural systems of the cortex, direct reciprocity of connections does not characterize the nucleus basalis. Although the nucleus has extremely widespread and topographically organized cortical projections, it receives input from only a subset of the cortical areas to which it projects. These inputs are largely derived from those parts of the limbic lobe that are located in the temporal lobe, anterior insula, and medial and orbital parts of the frontal lobe (Mesulam & Mufson, 1984). Thus, for instance, nucleus basalis output, or feedback, to the visual cortex is reciprocated only after the entire feedforward sequence of corticocortical outflow from sensory cortex to the limbic lobe is traced.

Amygdala

The amygdala is the largest basal forebrain structure. The various nuclei of the amygdala receive powerful cortical projections from all types of cortex including the visual and auditory association cortex along the lateral part of the temporal lobe. Other nuclei are more closely associated with proisocortices of the limbic lobe. The superficial nuclei, the so-called cortical amygdaloid nuclei, receive prominent projections from the olfactory and hippocampal allocortices. Periallocortical projections exist but have a limited distribution (Van Hoesen, 1981). In nearly all instances, these consist of reciprocal connections that feed back to parts of the cortex that originally projected to individual amygdaloid nuclei (Amaral & Price, 1984; Porrino et al., 1981). Prominent subcortical input arises from the hypothalamus, periaqueductal gray, peripeduncular nucleus, ventral tegmental area, supramammillary nucleus, and various midline thalamic nuclei.

The involvement of the amygdala in AD has been studied by several researchers (Burger, 1983; Herzog & Kemper, 1980; Kemper, 1983), although little emphasis has been given to the patterns of pathology with regard to individual amygdaloid nuclei. Neutritic plaques can be found in at least some parts of the structure, as can neurofibrillary tangles. Major cell loss has been noted in the superficial amygdaloid nuclei. It would be desirable to correlate the distribution of Alzheimer pathology with the neural systems that enter and leave the amygdala. The cortical elements of these pathways are partially understood in nonhuman primates. The origins of subcortical afferents are known, but their terminal patterns are not yet fully defined. The subcortical efferent projections of the amygdala have been well studied in many mammals, and a substantial amount is known regarding intrinsic amygdaloid connections. The role that amygdaloid pathology plays in the cognitive defects of AD is not known, but this structure is certainly related to memory at least in animals (Mishkin, 1978, 1982) and unquestionably is involved in many types of motivated and emotional behavior. The knowledge of amygdaloid anatomy in higher mammals invites correlative studies with the patterns of pathology in AD to gain insight into the altered behavior of the victims of this disorder. A host of putative transmitters and modulators has been localized in the amygdala, but little is known about their fate in AD.

Basal Ganglia
Other subcortical components of the telencephalon (the caudate nucleus, putamen, and claustrum) do not escape the pathological processes of AD (Rudelli, Ambler, & Wisniewski, 1984). For example, claustrum abnormalities in the form of both neurofibrillary tangles and neuritic plaques have been noted by several investigators. Recent studies have demonstrated that the caudate nucleus and putamen contain neuritic plaques in AD. These occur in a mosaiclike pattern that is reminiscent of the pattern of certain afferents to these structures as well as the distribution of some receptors.

Diencephalic Structures

Unlike most other components of the neuraxis, the diencephalon has been thought to be relatively spared in AD. It is difficult to assess the accuracy of this opinion, because few systematic investigations have addressed the issue. Moreover, of those reports in which these areas have been examined, it is difficult to appreciate the relative density of the associated abnormalities. In the absence of more evidence to the contrary, apparently both the hypothalamus and thalamus are generally spared in AD. Abnormalities may affect these structures but almost certainly in lesser density than in limbic and cortical areas. When structural changes do affect the diencephalon in AD, they are distributed in a nonrandom pattern confined to certain cells in selective nuclei.

In the hypothalamus only a subset of the many hypothalamic nuclei has been implicated, including the tuberal, anterior, paraventricular, dorsal, and lateral nuclei. The mammillary complex and lateral preoptic area have also been implicated (Ishii, 1966; Mann et al., 1985). A similar selectivity occurs for the thalamus. Included are the ventral anterior, reticular, ventral lateral, dorsomedial, lateral posterior, lateral dorsal, centromedian, parafascicular, paracentral, and central lateral nuclei (Rudelli et al., 1984). This array of nuclei is interesting from many viewpoints. First, the changes entirely spare the major lemniscal relay nuclei such as the medial and lateral geniculate nuclei and the ventral posterior complex. Second, several nuclei that are damaged have direct and reciprocal connections with the limbic cortices. Third, the intralaminar and midline thalamic nuclei seem affected, as does the reticular nucleus, the major association nucleus of the thalamus.

Mesencephalic and Myelencephalic Structures

Brain stem abnormalities involving the mesencephalon and myelencephalon have been reported in some individuals with AD (Ishii, 1966; Rossor, 1981). The changes include reduced cell numbers and neurofibrillary tangles in selected nuclei known to give rise to major monoaminergic neural systems that innervate cerebral cortex.

Raphe Nuclei

Several investigations report abnormalities affecting the raphe complex, the principal source of central serotonergic projections, with a sixfold increase in neurofibrillary tangles when compared with age-matched controls (Curcio & Kemper, 1984). At least in the dorsal raphe nucleus, it appears that these changes may not be paralleled by a corresponding reduction of serotonin-producing neurons. The percentage of raphe neurons invested with neurofibrillary tangles appears to be less than 5%, although somewhat larger estimates have been obtained (Yamamoto & Hirano, 1985).

Locus Coeruleus

The locus coeruleus, a major focus of noradrenergic neurons for the CNS, is also damaged in some individuals with AD (Bondareff, Mountjoy, & Roth, 1982; Forno, 1978; Mann, Yates, & Hawkes, 1982; Mann et al., 1984; Tomlinson, Irving, & Blessed, 1981). This small pigmented nucleus, located in the pontine tegmentum, has widespread cortical and subcortical projections; the cortical projections have an especially broad distribution. Both the loss of noradrenergic neurons and the presence of neurofibrillary tangles have been noted in the nucleus locus coeruleus and are thought to correlate closely with a reduction in noradrenergic cortical markers in AD (Perry & Perry, 1986). A recent report of special interest shows that the locus coeruleus is not uniformly affected in AD except for that part which projects to the temporal lobe (Marcyniuk, Mann, & Yates, 1986).

CONCLUSIONS

Recent interest in the neuroanatomical correlates of AD has revealed many new facts. Clearly, the pathological correlates of this disorder are multicentric and are not found entirely in cortical areas. Discrete subcortical areas are affected but, curiously, they (locus coeruleus, raphe complex, and nucleus basalis of Meynert) are those nuclei that have close connectional relationships with the cortex. The sensory relay and motor nuclei of the thalamus are exceptions in this regard and are not affected, but some association and midline nuclei are. The latter in fact are those thalamic nuclei that project to the hippocampus and to other areas of the limbic lobe.

Additionally, the pathological changes in AD are not distributed randomly in all parts of the cortex. Instead, the association and limbic cortical areas are targeted. The temporo-occipital and temporoparietal cortices and nearly the entirety of the limbic lobe except area 24 are especially vulnerable. Within these areas there is a further refinement such that only selected laminae and fields of the cortex contain evidence of pathology. For example, in the allocortices such as the hippocampal formation, the dentate gyrus, CA3 pyramids, and the pre-subicular cortices are largely spared, whereas the subicular and parasubicular cortices are heavily damaged. In the periallocortex, like the entorhinal area, layers II and IV contain abundant neurofibrillary tangles, whereas other layers are spared. In the proisocortex and isocortex, layers III and V are targeted and in many instances show alterations in Nissl-stained material. In contrast, other cortical areas and laminae are seldom affected. There appears to be a strong likelihood that the affected neurons give rise to corticocortical and corticolimbic neural systems.

The results reviewed here reiterate the fact that AD is largely a disease of the cerebral cortex and related subcortical systems connected intimately with it. However, the cerebral cortex is by no means a uniform and homogeneous structure. Differential projections in relation to cytoarchitecture have been known for decades and in recent years it has become clear that different laminae give rise to different association and corticofugal neural systems. This focuses a new light on the cortical pathology of AD and offers opportunities to view these changes in the perspective of behavioral abnormalities as well as experimental studies regarding cortical connectivity in higher primates.

In AD the most persistent, and perhaps earliest, changes occur in the hippocampal formation and parahippocampal gyrus. In fact, there is abundant evidence from a variety of methods to suggest that the temporal lobe is targeted early in the disease and perhaps overall more heavily than others, excluding, of course, the limbic lobe. Later in the illness the parietal and frontal lobes develop pathology consistent with AD.

In many regards the initial focus and pathological course of AD correlate well with the behavioral changes observed in this disorder. For example, one of the earliest changes in AD occurs in the hippocampus, particularly its subicular subdivision. Other changes early in the illness affect the anterior parahippocampal cortices such as the entorhinal cortex. These lesions disconnect the hippocampal formation from the association cortices and probably underlie the early signs of AD such as changes in the anterograde compartments of episodic and contextual memory. Later changes that affect the lateral temporal, posterior parahippocampal, temporopolar, and anterior insular cortices further exacerbate the problem and contribute to retrograde memory abnormalities in the episodic and contextual memory realms. The involvement of the multimodal association cortices would seem to mark the point in AD when generic and semantic memory decline and where even self-identity is lost. Thus it is suggested that AD does indeed dissect human memory into distinct compartments. It is, as many laymen can tell us, a disease of memory and it highlights the cortical and subcortical neural systems that play a fundamental role in this cognitive ability. Since its cellular correlates can be identified readily, it provides a rare opportunity to understand the neural correlates of a human behavior in cellular terms.

Acknowledgment

Supported by NS 14944, PO NS 19632, and the Mathers Foundation.

REFERENCES

Aggleton, J. P., Burton, J. J., & Passingham, R. E. (1980). Cortical and subcortical afferents to the amygdala of the rhesus monkey *(Macaca mulatta)*. *Brain Research, 190,* 347–368.
Alzheimer, A. (1907). Über eine eigenartige Erkrankung der Hirnrinde. *Allgemeine Zeitschrift für Psychiatrie, 64,* 146–148.
Amaral, D. G. (1987). Memory: Anatomical organization of candidate brain regions. In F. Plum, (Ed.), *Handbook of physiology: Sec. 1. The nervous system* (pp. 211–294). Bethesda, Md.: American Physiological Society.
Amaral, D. G., Insausti, R., & Cowan, W. M. (1983). Evidence for a direct projection from the superior temporal gyrus to the entorhinal cortex in the monkey. *Brain Research, 275,* 263–277.
Amaral, D. G., & Price, J. L. (1984). Amygdalo-cortical projections in the monkey *(Macaca fascicularis)*. *Journal of Comparative Neurology, 230,* 465–496.
Andersen, R. A., Asanuma, C., & Cowan, W. M. (1985). Callosal and prefrontal association projecting associational projecting cell populations in area 7a of the macaque monkey: A study using retrogradely transported fluorescent dyes. *Journal of Comparative Neurology, 232,* 443–455.
Arendt, T., Bigl, V., Arendt, A., & Tennstedt, A. (1983). Loss of neurons in the nucleus basalis of Meynert in Alzheimer's disease, paralysis agitans and Korsakoff's disease. *Acta Neuropathologica, 61,* 101–108.
Armstrong, D. M., Le Roy, S., Shields, D., & Terry, R. D. (1985). Somatostatin-like immunoreactivity within neuritic plaques. *Brain Research, 338,* 71–79.
Ball, M. J. (1976). Neurofibrillary tangles and the pathogenesis of dementia: A quantitative study. *Neuropathology and Applied Neurobiology, 2,* 395–410.
Ball, M. J. (1977). Neuronal loss, neurofibrillary tangles and granulovacuolar degeneration in the hippocampus with ageing and dementia. *Acta Neuropathologica, 37,* 11–18.
Ball, M. J. (1978). Topographic distribution of neurofibrillary tangles and granulovacuolar degeneration in hippocampal cortex of ageing and demented patients: A quantitative study. *Acta Neuropathologica, 42,* 73–80.
Bartus, R. T., Dean, R. L., III, Beer, B., & Lippa, A. S. (1982). The cholinergic hypothesis of geriatric memory dysfunction. *Science, 217,* 408–4173.
Bondareff, W., Mountjoy, C. Q., & Roth, M. (1982). Loss of neurons of adrenergic projection to cerebral cortex (nucleus locus ceruleus) in senile dementia. *Neurology, 32,* 164–169.
Braak, H., & Braak, E. (1985). On areas of transition between entorhinal allocortex and temporary isocortex in the human brain. Normal morphology and lamina-specific pathology in Alzheimer's disease. *Acta Neuropathologica, 68,* 325–332.

Brun, A., & Englund, E. (1981). Regional pattern of degeneration in Alzheimer's disease: Neuronal loss and histopathological grading. *Histopathology, 5,* 549–564.

Brun, A., & Englund, E. (1986). Brain changes in dementia of Alzheimer's type relevant to new imaging diagnostic methods. *Progress in Neuropsychopharmacology and Biological Psychiatry, 10,* 297–308.

Brun, A., & Gustafson, L. (1976). Distribution of cerebral degeneration in Alzheimer's disease. *Acta Psychiatrica Nervenkrankheiten, 223,* 15–33.

Bugbee, N. M. & Goldman-Rakic, P. S. (1983). Columnar organization of corticocortical projections in squirrel and rhesus monkeys: Similarity of column width in species of differing cortical volume. *Journal of Comparative Neurology, 220,* 355–364.

Burger, P. C. (1983). The limbic system in Alzheimer's disease. In R. Katzman (Ed.), *Banbury report. Biological aspects of Alzheimer's disease* (Vol. 15, pp. 37–44). Cold Spring Harbor, N.Y.: Cold Spring Harbor Laboratory.

Candy, J. M., Perry, R. H., Perry, E. K., Irving, D., Blessed, G., Fairbairn, A. F., & Tomlinson, B. E. (1983). Pathological changes in the nucleus of Meynert in Alzheimer's and Parkinson's diseases. *Journal of Neurological Sciences, 59,* 277–289.

Chavis, D. A., & Pandya, D. N. (1976). Further observations on corticofrontal connections in the rhesus monkey. *Brain Research, 117,* 369–386.

Corsellis, J. A. N. (1976). Aging and the dementias. In W. Blackwood & J. A. N. Corsellis (Eds.), *Greenfield's neuropathology* (pp. 796–848). London: Edward Arnold.

Corwin, J., Serby, M., Conrad, P., & Rotrosen, J. (1985). Olfactory recognition deficit in Alzheimer's and Parkinsonian dementias. *IRCS Medical Science Library Compendium, 13,* 260.

Coyle, J. T., Price, D. L., & DeLong, M. R. (1983). Alzheimer's disease: A disorder of cortical cholinergic innervation. *Science, 219,* 1184–1190.

Curcio, C. A., & Kemper, T. (1984). Nucleus raphe dorsalis in dementia of the Alzheimer type: Neurofibrillary changes and neuronal packing density. *Journal of Neuropathology and Experimental Neurology, 43,* 359–368.

Damasio, A. R. (1984). The anatomic basis of memory disorders. *Seminars in Neurology, 4,* 223–225.

Damasio, A. R. (1985). The frontal lobes. In K. Heilman & E. Valenstein (Eds.), *Clinical neuropsychology* (pp. 339–375). New York: Oxford University Press.

Damasio, A. R., Eslinger, P. J., Damasio, H., Van Hoesen, G. W., & Cornell, S. (1985). Multimodal amnesic syndrome following bilateral temporal and basal forebrain damage. *Archives of Neurology, 42,* 252–259.

Damasio, A. R., Graff-Radford, N., Eslinger, P. J., Damasio, H., & Kassell, N. (1985). Amnesia following basal forebrain lesions. *Archives of Neurology, 42,* 263–271.

Davies, P., & Maloney, A. J. F. (1976). Selective loss of central cholinergic neurons in Alzheimer's disease (letter to the editor). *Lancet, 2,* 1403.

Divac, I. (1975). Magnocellular nuclei of the basal forebrain project to neocortex, brain stem, and olfactory bulb: Review of some functional correlates. *Brain Research, 93,* 385–398.

Doty, R. L., Reyes, P. F., & Gregor, T. (1987). Presence of both odor identification and detection deficits in Alzheimer's disease. *Brain Research Bulletin, 18,* 597–600.

Drachman, D. A. (1977). Memory and cognitive function in man: Does the cholinergic system have a specific role? *Neurology, 27,* 783–790.

Esiri, M. M., & Wilcock, G. K. (1984). The olfactory bulbs in Alzheimer's disease. *Journal of Neurology Neurosurgery and Psychiatry, 47,* 56–60.

Eslinger, P. J., & Damasio, A. R. (1986). Preserved motor learning in Alzheimer's disease. *Journal of Neuroscience, 6,* 3006–3009.

Forno, L. S. (1978). The locus coeruleus in Alzheimer's disease. *Journal of Neuropathology and Experimental Neurology, 37,* 614.

Galaburda, A. M., & Pandya, D. N. (1983). The intrinsic architectonic and connectional organization of the superior temporal region of the rhesus monkey. *Journal of Comparative Neurology, 221,* 169–184.

Gibson, P. H. (1983). Form and distribution of senile plaques seen in silver impregnated sections in the brains of intellectually normal elderly people and people with Alzheimer-type dementia. *Neuropathology and Applied Neurobiology, 9,* 379–389.

Goldman-Rakic, P. S. (1987). Circuitry of the primate prefrontal cortex and the regulation of behavior by representational memory. In F. Plum (Ed.), *Handbook of physiology: Sec. 1. The nervous system: Vol. 5. Higher functions of the brain* (pp. 373–417). Bethesda, Md.: American Physiological Society.

Goldman-Rakic, P. S., & Schwartz, M. L. (1982). Interdigitation of contralateral and ipsilateral columnar projections to frontal association cortex in primates. *Science, 216,* 755–757.

Goldman-Rakic, P. S., Selemon, L. D., & Schwartz, M. L. (1984). Dual pathways connecting the dorsolateral prefrontal cortex with the hippocampal formation and parahippocampal cortex in the rhesus monkey. *Neuroscience, 12,* 719–743.

Goodman, L. (1953). Alzheimer's disease. A clinicopathologic analysis of twenty-three cases with a theory on pathogenesis. *Journal of Nervous and Mental Disease, 117,* 97–130.

Herzog, A. G., & Kemper, T. L. (1980). Amygdaloid changes in aging and dementia. *Archives of Neurology, 37,* 625–629.

Herzog, A. G., & Van Hoesen, G. W. (1976). Temporal neocortical afferent connections to the amygdala in the rhesus monkey. *Brain Research, 115,* 57–69.

Hirano, A., & Zimmerman, H. M. (1962). Alzheimer's neurofibrillary changes. *Archives of Neurology, 7,* 73–88.

Hyman, B. T., Damasio, A. R., Van Hoesen, G. W., & Barnes, C. L. (1984). Alzheimer's disease: Cell specific pathology isolates the hippocampal formation. *Science, 225,* 1168–1170.

Hyman, B. T., Van Hoesen, G. W., & Damasio, A. R. (1987). Alzheimer's disease: Glutamate depletion in the hippocampal perforant pathway zone. *Annals of Neurology, 22,* 37–40.

Hyman, B. T., Van Hoesen, G. W., Kromer, L. J., & Damasio, A. R. (1985). The subicular cortices in Alzheimer's disease: Neuroanatomical relationships and the memory impairment. *Society for Neuroscience Abstracts, 11,* 458.

Hyman, B. T., Van Hoesen, G. W., Kromer, L. J., & Damasio, A. R. (1986). Perforant pathway changes and the memory impairment of Alzheimer's disease. *Annals of Neurology, 20,* 472–481.

Ishii, T. (1966). Distribution of Alzheimer's neurofibrillary changes in the brain stem and hypothalamus of senile dementia. *Acta Neuropathologica, 6,* 181–187.

Jamada, M., & Mehrain, P. (1968). Verteilungsmuster der senilen Veranderunger in Gehirn. *Archive für Psychiatrie and Nervenkrankheiten, 211,* 308–324.

Jones, E. G. (1981). Anatomy of cerebral cortex: Columnar input–output organization. In F. O. Schmitt, F. G. Worden, G. Adelman, & S. G. Dennis (Eds.), *The organization of the cerebral cortex* (pp. 199–236). Cambridge, Mass.: MIT Press.

Jones, E. G. (1984). Laminar distribution of cortical efferent cells. In A. A. Peters & E. G. Jones (Eds.), *Cerebral cortex: Vol. 1. Cellular components of the cerebral cortex* (pp. 521–548). New York: Plenum.

Jones, E. G., Burton, H., Saper, C. B., & Swanson, L. W. (1976). Midbrain, diencephalic and cortical relationships of the basal nucleus of Meynert and associated structures in primates. *Journal of Comparative Neurology, 167,* 385–420.

Jones, E. G., & Powell, T. P. S. (1970). An anatomical study of converging sensory pathways within the cerebral cortex of the monkey. *Brain, 93,* 793–820.

Katzman, R. (1976). The prevalence and malignancy of Alzheimer's disease: A major killer. *Archives of Neurology, 33,* 217–218.

Katzman, R. (1986). Alzheimer's disease. *New England Journal of Medicine, 314,* 964–973.

Kemper, T. L. (1978). Senile dementia: A focal disease in the temporal lobe. In K. Nandy (Ed.), *Senile dementia: A biomedical approach* (pp. 105–113). New York: Elsevier/North-Holland.

Kemper, T. L. (1983). Organization of the neuropathology of the amygdala in Alzheimer's disease. In R. Katzman (Ed.), *Banbury report: Vol. 15. Biological aspects of Alzheimer's disease* (pp. 31–35). Cold Spring Harbor, N.Y.: Cold Spring Harbor Laboratory.

Kievet, J., & Kuypers, H. G. J. M. (1975). Basal forebrain and hypothalamic connections to the frontal and parietal cortex in the rhesus monkey. *Science, 187,* 660–662.

Knopman, D. S., & Nissen, M. J. (1987). Implicit learning in patients with probable Alzheimer's disease. *Neurology, 37,* 784–788.

Kosel, K. C., Van Hoesen, G. W., & Rosene, D. L. (1982). Nonhippocampal cortical projections from the entorhinal cortex in the rat and rhesus monkey. *Brain Research, 244,* 201–214.

Lewis, D. A., Campbell, M. J., Terry, R. D., & Morrison, J. H. (1987). Laminar and regional distributions of neurofibrillary tangles and neuritic plaques in Alzheimer's disease: A quantitative study of visual and auditory cortices. *Journal of Neuroscience, 7,* 1799–1808.

Mann, D. M. A. (1985). The neuropathology of Alzheimer's disease: A review with pathogenetic, aetiological and therapeutic considerations. *Mechanisms of Ageing and Development, 31,* 213–255.

Mann, D. M. A., Yates, P. O., & Hawkes, J. (1982). The noradrenergic system in Alzheimer and multi-infarct dementias. *Journal of Neurology Neurosurgery and Psychiatry, 45,* 113–119.

Mann, D. M. A., Yates, P. O., & Marcyniuk, B. (1984). A comparison of changes in the nucleus basalis and locus coeruleus in Alzheimer's disease. *Journal of Neurology Neurosurgery and Psychiatry, 47,* 201–203.

Mann, D. M. A., Yates, P. O., & Marcyniuk, B. (1985). Some morphometric observations on the cerebral cortex and hippocampus in presenile Alzheimer's disease, senile dementia of Alzheimer type and Down's syndrome in middle age. *Journal of the Neurological Sciences, 69,* 139–159.

Marcyniuk, B., Mann, D. M. A., & Yates, P. O. (1986). Loss of nerve cells from locus coeruleus in Alzheimer's disease is topographically arranged. *Neuroscience Letters, 64,* 247–252.

Maunsell, J. H. R., & Van Essen, D. C. (1983). The connections of the middle temporal visual area (MT) and their relationship to a cortical hierarchy in the macaque monkey. *Journal of Neuroscience, 3,* 2563–2586.

Mesulam, M.-M., & Mufson, E. J. (1984). Neural inputs into the nucleus basalis of the substantia innominata (CH4) in the rhesus monkey. *Brain Research, 107,* 253–274.

Mesulam, M.-M., Mufson, E. J., Levey, A. I., & Wainer, B. H. (1983). Cholinergic innervation of cortex by the basal forebrain: Cytochemistry and cortical connections of the septal area, diagonal band nucleus basalis (substantia innominata), and hypothalamus in the rhesus monkey. *Journal of Comparative Neurology, 214,* 170–197.

Mesulam, M.-M., & Van Hoesen, G. W. (1976). Acetylcholinesterase-rich projections from the basal forebrain of the rhesus monkey to neocortex. *Brain Research, 109,* 152–157.

Mesulam, M.-M., Van Hoesen, G. W., Pandya, D. N., & Geschwind, N. (1977). Limbic and sensory connections of the inferior parietal lobule (area PG) in the rhesus monkey: A study using a new method for horseradish peroxidase. *Brain Research, 136,* 393–414.

Mishkin, M. (1978). Memory in monkeys severely impaired by combined but not by separate removal of the amygdala and hippocampus. *Nature, 273,* 297–298.

Mishkin, M. (1982). A memory system in the monkey. *Philosophical Transactions of the Royal Society (London), 298,* 85–95.

Morel, F., & Wildi, E. (1955). Contribution a la connaissance des differentes alterations cerebrales du grand age. *Schweizer Archiv Neurologie und Psychiatrie, 76,* 195–223.

Nakano, I., & Hirano, A. (1982). Loss of large neurons of the medial septal nucleus in an autopsy case of Alzheimer's disease. *Journal of Neuropathology and Experimental Neurology, 41,* 341.

Nakano, I., & Hirano, A. (1983). Neuron loss in the nucleus basalis of Meynert in parkinsonism-dementia complex of Guam. *Annals of Neurology, 13,* 87–91.

Pandya, D. N., & Kuypers, H. G. J. M. (1969). Cortico-cortical connections in the rhesus monkey. *Brain Research, 13,* 13–36.

Pandya, D. N., & Seltzer, B. (1982a). Association areas of the cerebral cortex. *Trends in Neurosciences, 5,* 386–390.

Pandya, D. N., & Seltzer, B. (1982b). Intrinsic connections and architectonics of posterior parietal cortex in the rhesus monkey. *Journal of Comparative Neurology, 204,* 196–210.

Pandya, D. N., Van Hoesen, G. W., & Mesulam, M.-M. (1981). The cortico-cortical projections of the cingulate cortex in the rhesus monkey. *Experimental Brain Research, 42,* 319–330.

Pandya, D. N., & Yeterian, E. H. (1985). Architecture and connections of cortical association areas. In A. Peters & E. G. Jones (Eds.), *Cerebral cortex: Vol. 4. Association and auditory cortices* (pp. 3–61). New York: Plenum.

Pearson, R. C. A., Esiri, M. M., Hiorns, R. W., Wilcock, G. K., & Powell, T. P. S. (1985). Anatomical correlates of the distribution of the pathological changes in the neocortex in Alzheimer disease. *Proceedings of the National Academy of Sciences USA, 82,* 4531–4534.

Pearson, R. C. A., Gatter, K. C., Brodal, P., & Powell, T. P. S. (1983). The projection of the basal nucleus of Meynert upon the neocortex in the monkey. *Brain Research, 259,* 132–136.

Pearson, R. C. A., Gatter, K. C., & Powell, T. P. S. (1983). Retrograde cell degeneration in the basal nucleus in monkey and man. *Brain Research, 261,* 321–326.

Pearson, R. C. A., Sofroniew, M. V., Cuello, A. C., Powell, T. S., Eckenstein, F., Esiri, M. M., & Wilcox, G. K. (1984). Persistence of cholinergic neurons in the basal nucleus in a brain with senile dementia of the Alzheimer's type demonstrated by immunohistochemical staining for choline acetyltransferase. *Brain Research, 289,* 375–379.

Perry, E. K., & Perry, R. H. (1986). A review of neuropathological and neurochemical correlates of the Alzheimer's disease. *Danish Medical Bulletin, 32* (Suppl. 1), 27–34.

Porrino, L. J., Crane, A. M., & Goldman-Rakic, P. S. (1981). Direct and indirect pathways from the amygdala to the frontal lobe in rhesus monkeys. *Journal of Comparative Neurology, 198,* 121–136.

Rockland, K. S., & Pandya, D. N. (1979). Laminar origins and terminations of cortical connections of the occipital lobe in the rhesus monkey. *Brain Research, 179,* 3–20.

Rockland, K. S., & Pandya, D. N. (1981). Cortical connections of the occipital lobe in the rhesus monkey: Interconnections between areas 17, 18, 19 and the superior temporal gyrus. *Brain Research, 212,* 249–270.

Rogers, J., & Morrison, J. H. (1985). Quantitative morphology and regional and laminar distributions of senile plaques in Alzheimer's disease. *Journal of Neuroscience, 5,* 2801–2808.

Rosene, D. L., & Van Hoesen, G. W. (1977). Hippocampal efferents reach widespread areas of the cerebral cortex and amygdala in the rhesus monkey. *Science, 198,* 315–317.

Rossor, M. N. (1981). Parkinson's disease and Alzheimer's disease as disorders of the isodendritic core. *British Medical Journal, 283,* 1588–1590.

Rudelli, R. D., Ambler, M. W., & Wisniewski, H. M. (1984). Morphology and distribution of Alzheimer neuritic (senile) and amyloid plaques in striatum and diencephalon. *Acta Neuropathologica, 64,* 273–286.

Saper, C. B., German, D. C., & White, C. L., III, (1985). Neuronal pathology in the nucleus basalis and associated cell groups in senile dementia of the Alzheimer's type: Possible role in cell loss. *Neurology, 35,* 1089–1095.

Schwartz, M. L., & Goldman-Rakic, P. S. (1982). Single cortical neurones have axon collaterals to ipsilateral and contralateral cortex in fetal and adult primates. *Nature, 299,* 154–155.

Scoville, W. B., & Milner, B. (1957). Loss of recent memory after bilateral hippocampal lesions. *Journal of Neurology Neurosurgery and Psychiatry, 20,* 11–21.

Seltzer, B., & Pandya, D. N. (1976). Some cortical projections to the parahippocampal area in the rhesus monkey. *Experimental Neurology, 50,* 146–160.

Shipley, M. T., & Sorensen, K. E. (1975). Some afferent and intrinsic connections in the guinea pig hippocampal region and a new pathway from subiculum feeding back to parahippocampal cortex. *Experimental Brain Research* (Suppl. 1), 188–190.

Smith, C. M., & Swash, M. (1978). Possible biochemical basis of memory disorder in Alzheimer disease. *Annals of Neurology, 3,* 471–473.

Sofroniew, M. V., Pearson, R. C. A., Eckenstein, R., Cuello, A. C., & Powell, T. P. S. (1984). Retrograde changes in cholinergic neurons in the basal forebrain of the rat following cortical damage. *Brain Research, 289,* 370–374.

Sorenson, K. E., & Shipley, M. T. (1979). Projections from the subiculum to the deep layers of the ipsilateral presubicular and entorhinal cortices in the guinea pig. *Journal of Comparative Neurology, 188,* 313–314.

Squire, L. R. (1986). Mechanisms of memory. *Science, 232,* 1612–1619.

Squire, L. R. (1987). Memory: Neural organization and behavior. In F. Plum (Ed.), *Handbook of physiology: Sec. 1: The nervous system* (pp. 295–372). Bethesda, Md.: American Physiological Society.

Struble, R. G., Cork, L. C., Whitehouse, P. J., & Price, D. L. (1982). Cholinergic innervation in neuritic plaques. *Science Washington, DC, 216,* 413–415.

Swanson, L. W., & Cowan, W. M. (1975). Hippocampo-hypothalamic connections: Origin in subicular cortex, not Ammon's horn. *Science, 189,* 303–304.

Swanson, L. W., & Cowan, W. M. (1977). An autoradiographic study of the organization of the efferent connections of the hippocampal formation in the rat. *Journal of Comparative Neurology, 172,* 49–84.

Terry, R. D. (1983). Cortical morphometry in Alzheimer's disease. In R. Katzman (Ed.), *Banbury report. Biological aspects of Alzheimer's disease* (Vol. 15, pp. 95–103). Cold Spring Harbor, N.Y.: Cold Spring Harbor Laboratory.

Terry, R. D., & Katzman, R. (1983). Senile dementia of the Alzheimer type. *Annals of Neurology, 14,* 497–506.

Terry, R. D., Peck, A., DeTeresa, R., Schechter, R., & Horoupian, D. S. (1981). Some morphometric aspects of the brain in senile dementia of the Alzheimer type. *Annals of Neurology, 10,* 184–192.

Tomlinson, B. E., Blessed, G., & Roth, M. (1968). Observations on the brains of demented old people. *Journal of the Neurological Sciences, 7,* 331–356.

Tomlinson, B. E., & Corsellis, J. A. N. (1984). Ageing and the dementias. In J. Hume Adams, J. A. N. Corsellis, & L. W. Duchen (Eds.), *Greenfield's neuropathology* (pp. 951–1025). New York: Wiley.

Tomlinson, B. E., Irving, D., & Blessed, G. (1981). Cell loss in the locus coeruleus in senile dementia of Alzheimer type. *Journal of the Neurological Sciences, 49,* 419–428.

Tulving, E. (1987). Multiple memory systems and consciousness. *Human Neurobiology, 6,* 67–80.

Turner, B. H., Mishkin, M., & Knapp, M. (1980). Organization of the amygdalopetal projections from modality-specific cortical association areas in the monkey. *Journal of Comparative Neurology, 191,* 515–543.

Van Essen, D. C., & Maunsell, J. H. R. (1983). Hierarchical organization and functional streams in the visual cortex. *Trends in Neurosciences, 6,* 370–375.

Van Hoesen, G. W. (1981). The differential distribution, diversity and sprouting of cortical projections to the amygdala in the rhesus monkey. In Y. Ben Ari (Ed.), *The amygdaloid complex* (pp. 77–90). Amsterdam: Elsevier.

Van Hoesen, G. W. (1982). The primate parahippocampal gyrus: New insights regarding its cortical connections. *Trends in Neurosciences, 5,* 345–350.

Van Hoesen, G. W. (1985). Neural systems of the non-human primate forebrain implicated in memory. In S. Corkin, E. Gramzu, & D. Olton (Eds.), *Memory dysfunctions* (pp. 97–112) (Annals of the New York Academy of Sciences, Vol. 444). New York: New York Academy of Sciences.

Van Hoesen, G. W., & Damasio, A. R. (1987). Neural correlates of cognitive impairment in Alzheimer's disease. In F. Plum (Ed.), *Handbook of physiology: Sec. 1: The nervous system* (pp. 871–898). Bethesda, Md.: American Physiological Society.

Van Hoesen, G. W., Hyman, B. T., & Damasio, A. R. (1986). Cell-specific pathology in neural systems of the temporal lobe in Alzheimer's disease. In D. Swaab (Ed.), *Progress in brain research* (Vol. 70, pp. 361–375). Amsterdam: Elsevier.

Van Hoesen, G. W., & Pandya, D. N. (1975a). Some connections of the entorhinal (area 28) and perirhinal (area 35) cortices in the rhesus monkey. I. Temporal lobe afferents. *Brain Research, 95,* 1–24.

Van Hoesen, G. W., & Pandya, D. N. (1975b). Some connections of the entorhinal (area 28) and perirhinal (area 35) cortices of the rhesus monkey. III. Efferent connections. *Brain Research, 95,* 39–59.

Van Hoesen, G. W., Pandya, D. N., & Butters, N. (1972). Cortical afferents to the entorhinal cortex of the rhesus monkey. *Science, 175,* 1471–1473.

Van Hoesen, G. W., Pandya, D. N., & Butters, N. (1975). Some connections of the entorhinal (area 28) and perirhinal (area 35) cortices in the rhesus monkey. II. Frontal lobe afferents. *Brain Research, 95,* 25–38.

Vogt, B. A., & Miller, M. W. (1983). Cortical connections between rat cingulate cortex and visual, motor and postsubicular cortices. *Journal of Comparative Neurology, 216,* 192–210.

Volpe, B. T., & Hirst, W. (1983). Amnesia following the rupture and repair of an anterior communicating artery aneurysm. *Journal of Neurology Neurosurgery and Psychiatry, 46,* 704–709.

von Cramon, D. Y., Hebel, N., & Schuri, U. (1985). A contribution to the anatomic basis of thalamic amnesia. *Brain, 108,* 993–1008.

Warner, M. D., Peabody, O. A., Flattery, J. J., & Tinklenberg, J. R. (1986). Olfactory deficits and Alzheimer's disease. *Biological Psychiatry, 21,* 116–118.

Whitehouse, P. J., Price, D. L., Clark, A. W., Coyle, J. T., & DeLong, M. R. (1981). Alzheimer disease: Evidence for selective loss of cholinergic neurons in the nucleus basalis. *Annals of Neurology, 10,* 122–126.

Whitlock, D. G., & Nauta, W. J. H. (1956). Subcortical projections from the temporal neocortex in *Macaca mulatta. Journal of Comparative Neurology, 106,* 183–212.

Wilcock, G. K. (1983). The temporal lobe in dementia of Alzheimer's type. *Gerontology, 29,* 320–324.

Wilcock, G. K., & Esiri, M. M. (1982). Plaques, tangles and dementia, a qualitative study. *Journal of the Neurological Sciences, 56,* 343–356.

Wilcock, G. K., Esiri, M. M., Bowen, D. M., & Smith, C. C. T. (1983). The nucleus basalis in Alzheimer's disease—Cell counts and cortical biochemistry. *Neuropathology and Applied Neurobiology, 9,* 175–179.

Yamamoto, T., & Hirano, A. (1985). Nucleus raphe dorsalis in Alzheimer's disease. Neurofibrillary tangles and loss of large neurons. *Annals of Neurology, 17,* 573–577.

COMMENTARIES AND
ALTERNATIVE PERSPECTIVES

12

The Neocortex and Memory Storage

HERBERT P. KILLACKEY

In this brief chapter, I will outline some of the major themes appearing in neocortical research since the early 1960s, how these themes are currently being modified, and how they relate to the involvement of the neocortex in learning and memory. The focus will be on memory processes. I use this term in the lay sense of facts or data about the everyday world that one can (consciously or unconsciously) store and recall on demand. Good examples are telephone or social security numbers or, most wondrously, the name to match the face of a colleague seen but once a year at a scientific meeting.

I will begin with a rather naive statement. In my opinion, memory processing of the sort just referred to is both central to the human experience and carried out at the cortical level (i.e., the neocortex is a major memory storage site). Such memory processes remove each of us from the precarious immediacy of our environment and connect us to a wealth of direct and indirect experiences with which we can interpret environmental events. Indeed, some of the major inventions of human civilization can be regarded chiefly as devices that both greatly extend and externalize our neocortical memory-processing abilities. The most obvious of these are the development of written language, which made possible a permanent and transferable record of events; the printing press and movable type, which together assured an increase in accuracy of written records and resulted in the much wider dissemination of written records than was previously possible; and the computer, which has been with us for a relatively short time but will most likely further extend these processes in ways that cannot be entirely foreseen.

What is the evidence that memory processing of this sort is particularly dependent on the neocortex? First, there is a large body of literature from the neurological clinic. One particularly relevant disorder is Alzheimer's disease, in which memory loss is a major symptom and there are specific and devastating effects on neocortical morphology. Second, there have been experimental studies of the effects of neocortical lesions on behavior in a variety of nonhuman mammalian species. Together, these bodies of literature provide strong circumstantial, if not definitive, evidence for neocortical involvement in memory processes. As a comparative neuroanatomist, I would also advance the following somewhat convoluted argument. The cerebral hemispheres are the portion of the vertebrate brain which have undergone the greatest expansion in the course of evolution. A major part of this expansion can be attributed to the portion of the cerebral hemispheres known as the neocortex. In higher primates, particularly humans, the six-layered neocortex has greatly increased in surface area relative to the other portions of the cerebrum and is its dominant feature. I would assume that this greatly expanded neocortex is correlated with the expanded behavioral repertoire of the human species, including our extensive memory abilities. At a more prosaic level, I would submit that it is only this expanded neocortex that can possibly provide the expanded physical substrate necessary to meet the storage requirements of human memory.

There is, of course, nothing novel in the suggestion that memories are stored in the neocortex. Such an idea has played some role in theories of cortical function going back to the pioneering studies of cortical localization in the late nineteenth century. With the early broad functional characterization of neocortical areas as either sensory, motor, or associational also comes the suggestion that memories are stored in association areas. Such a view was also implicit in the attempts of physiologists early in this century to view neocortical function in terms of conditioned reflex circuits. At the cortical level, such circuits stretched from sensory cortex through association cortex to motor cortex. It was also generally assumed that it was only in association cortex that such a circuit could be modified. For example, Herrick could state in 1926 that

> quite apart from such speculative considerations it is clear that the mnemonic functions of the association cortex are fundamental. The impressionability of this cortex and its retentiveness of patterns once impressed upon it underlie all of its mysterious capacities which are clearly recognizable in the anthropoid apes and which are probably incipient in dogs. (1926/1963, p. 244)

It was in this intellectual context that Lashley set out on his search for the engram, the locus of the memory trace. On the basis of a lifetime of experiments, he concluded not only that association areas of cortex are not specific storehouses for specific memories but also that it was not possible to localize memory traces anywhere within the nervous system (Lashley, 1950). From today's perspective it is clear that the experimental approach used by Lashley was more limited than he recognized, and considerable progress has been made in relating specific parts of the nervous system to memory processes in a number of species. However, the conclusion that no specific cortical area serves as a memory storage site is still valid. In this light, memory storage is probably best regarded as an integral part of more general processing operations, and as such inseparable from these operations and distributed throughout the neocortex. Since Lashley, experimental investigations of the neocortex have been largely approached from a different intellectual vantage.

Since the early 1960s, the dominant approach to the study of neocortical organization has been made through the major sensory systems (the visual system, in particular, but also the somatosensory and auditory systems). At a functional level, the analysis of receptive field properties of neurons at a number of levels along the neural axis, as well as within multiple cortical areas, has greatly expanded our knowledge of the way sensory information is processed within the brain. In the visual system, processing of information is clearly multifaceted. On the one hand, there is evidence for the serial and hierarchical processing of visual information; on the other hand, there is compelling evidence for parallel processing of visual information in the sense that different functional categories of visual information may be processed in separate but overlapping channels at both the subcortical and cortical levels. Similarly, anatomical studies carried out with recently introduced methods of great sensitivity have significantly increased our knowledge of cortical connectivity. For example, it was once assumed that major regions of neocortex, particularly association areas, did not receive afferent input from the dorsal thalamus. Association areas were thought to be dependent on sensory cortical areas for their afferent inputs. It is now clear that this is not the case. Indeed, it has become clear that the classical notions of a primary cortical sensory area for the analysis of sensation and of cortical association areas subserving more complex perceptual functions are at best almost too simplistic to be useful. The use of the term association area in the classical sense has almost disappeared from the current literature and has been replaced by either neutral terms or terms that relate a given cortical area to a major sensory system on the basis of the neural response properties in this area. For example, in the rhesus monkey over a dozen cortical areas which are largely devoted to visual function have been identified, and undoubtedly future investigations will uncover still more cortical areas that can be characterized as visual (Van Essen & Maunsell, 1983).

There has also been some progress in our understanding of the general functional properties of the neocortex. While much of the research referred to in the preceding paragraphs focused on defining discrete and different cortical areas in both a functional and morphological sense, there is increasing evidence that neocortex may follow the same general operational and computational principles across cortical areas. At the morphological level, the similarities in organization across cortical areas far outweigh the differences. There are overall similarities across cortical areas in the distribution of cell types, patterns of afferent input, and distribution of efferent output neurons. Further, it has been hypothesized that there is a basic functional unit of neocortical organization composed of a vertically oriented column of neurons extending across all cortical layers (Mountcastle, 1978). Thus it seems reasonable to suggest that similar processing operations may be performed in diverse cortical areas. If this is indeed the case, the task of understanding neocortical organization is potentially much simpler.

This hypothesis receives some general support from two very different approaches to neocortical organization. First, there have been experimental developmental studies in which visual input was diverted into the subcortical somatosensory system and the response properties of neurons in the adult soma-tosensory cortex was assayed (Frost & Metin, 1985). Under these circumstances, some neurons in the somatosensory cortex respond to visual stimulation and their response properties are similar to normal visual cortex neurons. This sug-gests that cortical processing operations are somewhat independent of sensory modality and specific cortical area. Second, it has been reported that the absolute number of neurons in a small volume of neocortex extending from the surface to the white matter is invariant across both cortical areas and species as diverse as rat, cat, and humans (Rockel, Hiorns, & Powell, 1980).

These findings have significant implications for our understanding of neocor-tical phylogeny. First, the fundamental unit of cortical information processing may be quite conservative and have remained relatively unchanged in the course of mammalian evolution. Second, the phylogenetic expansion of mam-malian neocortex may have been accomplished by the straightforward addition of basic vertical processing units. Thus the varying number of cortical areas seen in different mammalian species may be composed of the same basic functional units which in different species are grouped into different cortical areas on the bases of the adaptive pressures acting in a given species.

A major component of any such cortical processing unit must be the pyram-idal cell, the most common neocortical neuron and the only one with an axon leaving the neocortex. This neuron with its vertically organized apical dendrite stretching across the cortical layers between its cell body and the cortical surface is positioned to sample afferent inputs from diverse sources and richly encrusted with dendritic spines. A single pyramidal cell may have as many as 30,000 of these postsynaptic specializations. This is particularly important to bear in mind as most conceptions of the neural basis of learning and memory are couched in terms that seem to regard the neuron as being involved in a single, or at best a few synapses. The reality, far more complicated, was perhaps hinted at by Lash-ley (1950) in another of the conclusions he reached in "In Search of the Engram":

> From the numerical relations involved, I believe that even the reservation of indi-vidual synapses for special associative reactions is impossible. The alternative is, per-haps, that the dendrites and cell body may be locally modified in such a manner that the cell responds differentially, at least in the timing of its firing, according to the pattern of combination of axon feet through which excitation is received. (p. 482)

As outlined above, the major heuristic approach to the understanding of neo-cortical organization has been based on the sensory systems. Further, the approach can be characterized as one that begins at the periphery, at the sensory receptor, and then proceeds inward station by station in an attempt to unravel both processing operations and sequence. This approach has been very valuable and has greatly increased our knowledge of neocortical organization. At the same time, this focus on sensory-based information, and consequently the dorsal thalamus, has overshadowed other major afferent sources to the neocortex.

Indeed, it was often assumed until fairly recently that the dorsal thalamus was the only source of afferent input to the neocortex. It is now clear that there are a number of major nonthalamic afferent systems to the neocortex (Foote & Morrison, 1987). Each of these extrathalamic afferent systems arises in a different site and is associated with a different putative neurotransmitter. The best characterized to date are noradrenergic afferents from the locus coeruleus, serotonergic afferents from the raphe nuclei, dopaminergic projections from the ventral tegmental area, and acetylcholinergic afferents from the nucleus basalis. Each of these afferent systems projects to the neocortex in a distinct areal and laminar fashion, although as a whole their projection patterns are more widespread and less highly organized than thalamic projections. The functional role played by these systems in neocortical processing is still obscure, but it is likely to differ significantly from the highly topographically organized thalamic system. The functions of these systems are broadly viewed as modulatory but in a local, not a global, sense. That is, these systems are organized in such a fashion that they may regulate activity in small groups of neurons during particular stages in information processing. Whether these afferent systems play any particular role in memory processing remains to be determined. The developmental gating mechanisms discussed by Singer (Chapter 10, this volume) point to one area where thalamic and extrathalamic afferent systems to the cortex may overlap.

Our sensory system–based orientation toward neocortical organization has also influenced how we view patterns of connections within the neocortex. Analyses of corticocortical connections have mainly focused on projections that arise in sensory cortical areas. Such studies are aimed largely at outlining the major flow of information within the neocortex, which is presumed to begin in sensory cortex and then continue in other cortical areas. Such assumptions are made explicit in the terms "feed forward," which characterizes projections originating from a primary sensory cortical area or a cortical area that is assumed to be lower in a hierarchical processing sequence, and "feed backward," which characterizes projections in the opposite direction. Again, there has been much heuristic value in such an approach but the time may have come to take a wider approach, recognizing other major influences besides sensory systems on neocortical processing. Van Hoesen (Chapter 11, this volume) and Rolls (Chapter 9, this volume) stress the largely ignored projections from other telencephalic regions onto major portions of the neocortex, including primary sensory areas. Although many of the details of such projections have not yet been studied nearly as well as other neocortical inputs, they include direct and indirect projections from both the hippocampus and amygdala to most regions of the neocortex. The model presented by Rolls is particularly noteworthy in that it postulates several specific functions for these projections, including the recall of memories stored in the neocortex. Such hypotheses will undoubtedly be tested by future research and further enrich our still evolving ideas of neocortical organization.

REFERENCES

Foote, S. L., & Morrison, J. H. (1987). Extrathalamic modulation of cortical function. *Annual Review of Neuroscience, 10,* 67–95.

Frost, D. O., & Metin, C. (1985). Induction of functional retinal projections to the somatosensory system. *Nature, 317,* 162–164.

Herrick, C. J. (1963). *Brains of rats and men.* New York: Hafner. (Original work published in 1926)

Lashley, K. S. (1950). In search of the engram. *Symposium of the Society for Experimental Biology, 4,* 454–482.

Mountcastle, V. B. (1978). An organizing principle for cerebral function: The unit module and the distributed system. In G. M. Edelman (Ed.), *The mindful brain* (pp. 7–50). Cambridge, Mass.: MIT Press.

Rockel, A. J., Hiorns, R. W., & Powell, T. P. S. (1980). The basic uniformity in structure of the neocortex. *Brain, 103,* 221–244.

Van Essen, D. C., & Maunsell, J. H. R. (1983). Hierarchical organization and functional streams in the visual cortex. *Trends in Neuroscience, 6,* 370–375.

13

A Network Model for Learned Spatial Representation in the Posterior Parietal Cortex

RICHARD A. ANDERSEN
DAVID ZIPSER

Anatomists and neurophysiologists who study the cerebral cortex generally believe that they are studying a hard-wired, genetically determined circuitry. It is usually assumed that it is only during brief "critical periods" that the cortex is amenable to changes dictated by exposure to the environment which fine tune its structure. However, recent evidence suggests that the cortex is very plastic and that this plasticity extends into adult life (see Merzenich, Recanzone, Jenkins, Allard, & Nudo, in press, for review). In the experiments described in this chapter, combined neurophysiological and computational approaches were used to investigate how the posterior parietal cortex of macaque monkeys represents the location of visual stimuli in craniotopic coordinates (Andersen & Zipser, 1988; Zipser & Andersen 1988). A computer-generated network model was designed to learn stimulus locations in craniotopic space based on eye and retinal position inputs that were modeled on similar signals derived from the recording data and are assumed to be inputs to the posterior parietal cortex. The units in the network that map from input to output were found to develop the same response properties as a large subset of cells found in area 7a of the posterior parietal cortex. These experiments suggest that the spatial representation found in area 7a is in fact learned by associating eye position with retinal inputs.

SPATIAL REPRESENTATIONS AND THE ROLE OF THE POSTERIOR PARIETAL CORTEX

There are several reasons to believe that the brain uses representations of visual space that are nonretinotopic and are framed in head- or body-centered coordinates. One can reach accurately to the location of visual targets without visual feedback and independent of eye position, head position, or the location of the image on the retinas. Thus the motor system appears to use representations of visual stimuli mapped in body-centered rather than retinal coordinates. There is substantial evidence that the planning of eye movements involves a stage in which the target of the eye movement is represented in craniotopic coordinates (Hallet & Lightstone, 1976; Mays & Sparks, 1980; Robinson, 1975). We know by introspection that the visual world appears perceptually stable in spite of the fact that we are constantly making eye movements and subsequently shifting the location of images on the retinas. All these results suggest that there exist neural representations of space that are head or body centered.

A likely area of the brain to find nonretinotopic representations of visual space is the posterior parietal cortex. Lesions in this area in humans and monkeys produce visual disorientation, a syndrome in which the subjects cannot reach accurately to visual targets and have difficulty navigating around seen obstacles (see Andersen, 1987, for review). The patients are not blind and when tested often have normal visual field functions. However, they appear to be unable to associate what they see with the positions of their bodies.

RECORDING DATA FROM AREA 7

We examined the coordinate frame for visual space used by the posterior parietal cortex by mapping visual receptive fields in this area with animals looking in different directions (Andersen, Essick, & Siegel, 1985). The animals' heads were fixed to simplify the coordinate space examined to a head-centered coordinate frame. We reasoned that if the receptive fields moved with the eyes, then the coordinate frame was retinotopic; if they remained static in space, then they were coding in at least craniotopic coordinates. Figure 13.1 shows an example of this experiment. The receptive field is first mapped with a flashed visual stimulus while the animal fixates a small fixation spot located straight ahead at 0,0 in screen coordinates. Figure 13.1B shows a typical receptive field mapped in this way where the axes represent screen coordinates and the contour lines different levels of neural response. Once the receptive field has been mapped, the stimulus is then presented at the retinotopic location that gave the maximum

---

$\longrightarrow$

FIGURE 13.1. (A) Method of determining spatial gain fields of area 7a neurons. The animal fixates point f at different locations on the screen with his head fixed. The stimulus, s, is always presented in the center of the receptive field, rf. (B) Receptive field of a neuron plotted in coordinates of visual angle determined with the animal always fixating straight ahead (screen coordinates 0,0). The contours represent the mean increased response rates in spikes per second. (C) Spatial gain field of the cell in (B). The poststimulus histograms are positioned to correspond to the locations of the fixations on the screen at which the responses were recorded for retinotopically identical stimuli presented in the center of the receptive field (histogram ordinate, 25 spikes per division, and abscissa, 100 msec per division; arrows indicate onset of stimulus flash). (From Andersen et al., 1985)

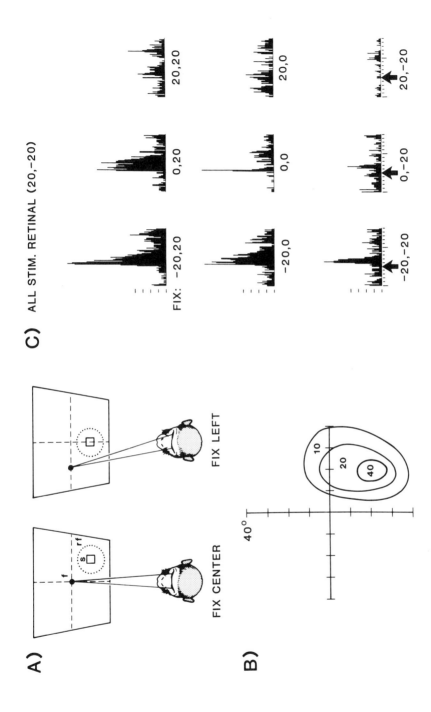

response, but with the animal gazing in different directions. If the response changes with eye position for retinotopically identical stimuli, then the cells are not coding in strictly retinotopic coordinates. Figure 13.1A shows how the visual response is tested at different eye positions. The dashed line *rf* delineates the receptive field that was mapped in Figure 13.1B. Stimulus *s* is presented at the most responsive location in the receptive field, in this case the approximate center of the response zone. On the left the animal is first required to fixate straight ahead at 0,0 in screen coordinates. On the right the animal has been required to fixate to the left of straight ahead by 20° at −20,0 in screen coordinates. Since the head is fixed the eyes are now in different positions in the orbits. The target is again flashed in the same retinotopic location; however, since the eyes have moved 20° to the left the stimulus has also been moved 20° to the left such that the stimulus falls on the same retinotopic location.

In these experiments nine eye positions are tested in this manner. Results from this cell are seen in Figure 13.1C. Each histogram is plotted at the corresponding fixation location. The cell was most active for fixations up 20° and left 20°, less active for looking straight ahead, and not active at all when looking down 20° and right 20°. The activity of the cell for retinotopically identical stimuli varied as a function of the angle of gaze. Plots for the nine fixation positions as shown in Figure 13.1C are called spatial gain fields. Notice that the shape of this particular gain field can be described by a plane tilted down and to the right.

We recorded complete spatial gain fields for 86 area 7a cells. The mean evoked responses of these gain fields were further analyzed using a first-order linear model with independent variables of horizontal and vertical eye position to determine how many of these gain fields could be fit with a plane. The evoked activity was obtained by subtracting the background activity before the stimulus flash from the overall activity during and just after the stimulus flash. Three types of gain fields were obtained by this analysis. Thirty-one percent of the gain fields had a significant planar component and no significant lack of fit, indicating that a plane was the best model for the data. Another 32% showed a planar component but also a significant lack of fit, indicating that although a plane could be fit to the data a plane was not the optimal model. Fully 75% of these neurons looked very planar. Finally, another 37% showed no planar component and a significant lack of fit. Thus a majority of cells showed planar or largely planar gain fields (55%), but a significant number of gain fields (45%) are not planar. When the same cells were analyzed for their overall activity rather than just the evoked activity, it was found that a larger proportion of the cells (78%) had planar or largely planar gain fields. Thus the total signal of background activity and evoked activity shows a greater degree of planarity than just the evoked response. The total activity is the most likely signal used by the brain for spatial localization since it is the output of the neurons.

A major concern is that the visual background, which is imaged at different locations on the retinas at different angles of gaze, is influencing the responsiveness of the cells to the test flash. Two controls were performed to eliminate this possibility. Many of the recordings were made in complete darkness except for the stimulus and the fixation point so that there was no visual background. The second control was to change the angle of gaze using prisms; this requires the animal to change eye position without changing the retinal locations of the imaged background or visual stimulus. The cells showed the same gain fields whether the eye positions were changed with prisms or without prisms by moving the fixation point. Thus we can conclude that the effect of eye position on visual responses was not a result of background shifts.

EYE POSITION–DEPENDENT SPATIAL TUNING

The change in visual responses for retinotopically identical stimuli with eye position could be a result of two mechanisms. First, the cells could have been coding locations of targets in space independent of eye position. In this situation the cells' receptive fields remain static in space and the retinal addresses of the receptive fields change with eye movements to remain constant for spatial location. Second, the receptive fields could remain retinotopic, with only the responsiveness of the cells varying as a function of eye position. In other words, eye position gates the activity of the retinal receptive fields. To distinguish between these two possibilities we mapped entire axes through the center of the receptive fields. It was found that the responsiveness of neurons varies as a function of eye position, but the peaks and symmetry of their receptive fields do not change. Thus the receptive fields remain retinotopic and it is only the responsiveness of the cells that is modulated by eye position.

The activity of parietal neurons was modeled as a multiplicative interaction of eye position and retinal position using the equation $A = G(e_x, e_y) \times R(r_x, r_y)$ where A is the cells' firing rate, G is a gain factor that is a function of horizontal (e_x) and vertical (e_y) eye position, and R is the visual stimulus response profile, which is a function of horizontal (r_x) and vertical (r_y) retinal locations. This multiplicative interaction produced a tuning for the location of visual stimuli in craniotopic space, but it was dependent on eye position. A simple example of this would be a cell that has a gain of 0 for all eye positions except looking 10° to the right, in which case the gain is 1. This cell also has a narrow receptive field centered at 10° to the right of the fovea. This cell will then be tuned to a location 20° to the right in craniotopic coordinates, but only when the animal is looking 10° to the right.

PROBLEMS TO BE ADDRESSED BY MODELS OF SPATIAL REPRESENTATION IN AREA 7a

Cells have never been found that are spatially tuned in an eye position–independent manner. From these experiments it must be concluded that the neural representation of space in an eye position–independent manner is distributed. This distributed coding presents a problem: How do you determine eye position–independent spatial location from the population response? One way would be to map spatial location tuning systematically across the tangential dimension of area 7a. Recording experiments have so far not revealed any obvious topography for spatial tuning, indicating that if such a map for craniotopic space does exist, it will likely be crude. Moreover, the very large receptive fields and spatial tuning fields would tend to mitigate against high-resolution mapping like that found for retinotopy in V1.

Another unusual feature of the receptive fields of area 7a neurons is their complexity. The fields are large, have approximately equal weighting to the fovea and periphery, and can have multiple peaks. The fields generally have smoothly varying levels for response for nearby sample points. No topographic organization for retinal location of the receptive fields has been found. Any model for spatial representation in area 7a should reproduce these unusual visual receptive fields.

Another interesting aspect of the area 7a neurons is that the background activity of the cells also often varies as a function of eye position. In many cases the background activity varies in the same direction as the gain on the visual response. This result is not unexpected since the eye position input could increase the visual response by depolarizing the membrane and in some cases this depolarization would not only lower the cell's threshold to visual stimulation but may also fire the cell, leading to an increase in its background activity. However, other cells showed background effects that went in the opposite direction to the gain of the visual response. Again, any model of spatial coding in area 7a would need to explain this behavior.

NETWORK MODEL FOR SPATIAL REPRESENTATION

Zipser and Andersen created a parallel network model that learns to map inputs of retinotopic position and eye position to an output of location in head-centered space (Andersen & Zipser, 1988; Zipser & Andersen, 1988). This network consists of three layers and uses the backpropagation learning algorithm (Rumelhart, Hinton, & Williams, 1986). The units in the middle layer that accomplish the spatial transformation show the same eye position–dependent spatial tuning properties that are found for area 7a neurons. This model also generates retinal receptive fields similar to those found for area 7a neurons and reproduces similar background activities. The remarkable correspondence between the model and experiment suggests that the distributed spatial coding discovered in area 7a neurons is indicative of spatial transformations carried out using the same computational algorithm discovered by the backpropagation learning technique.

Figure 13.2 presents a schematic diagram of the network. The input layer consists of a 10 by 10 retinal array and four eye position units. The retinal receptive fields are Gaussian in shape with $1/e$ widths of 15°. This input is designed to be similar to the receptive fields that are found in area 7a that do not show eye position effects and are assumed to be the retinal inputs to area 7a. The centers of the 100 receptive fields are equally spaced over the 10 by 10 grid with 8° spacings. The four eye position units consist of two units coding vertical position and two horizontal position using opposite, symmetrical slopes. Each unit used either a linear or, in later simulations, a squared function to approximate the signal coming from eye position cells. The rationale for using a squared function is to approximate the cumulative response of a group of eye position cells. Eye position inputs are assumed to be those cells in area 7a that have only eye position signals and no visual response. These cells generally code horizontal and/ or vertical position in a linear fashion (Andersen & Zipser, 1988). We ran simulations with both square functions and simple linear functions and got indistinguishable results, indicating that the exact representation of the eye position does not appear to be crucial as long as it is a monotonically increasing function.

The intermediate layer receives inputs from all 104 input units and in turn projects to two or four output units. The output units code position in head-

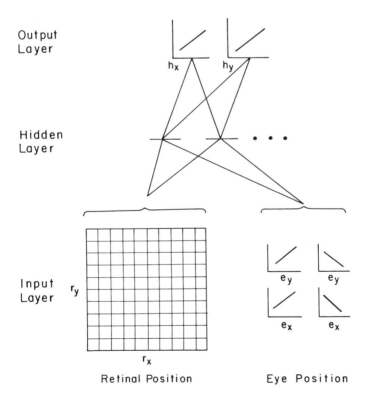

FIGURE 13.2. Backpropagation network used to model area 7a. The input to the network consists of retinal position and eye position information. The activity of the output units is a monotonic function of the location of the visual stimulus in craniotopic coordinates. The middle or "hidden" layer units map input to output. The details of the network are explained in the text.

centered space as a linear function of spike rate. There are four output units with pairs of opposite slope for horizontal and vertical position. As in the case with the eye position inputs, the exact form of the function did not appear to matter as long as it was monotonically increasing; also, whether only one unit of positive slope or two units of opposite slope were used did not seem to be important. The rationale for using a monotonic function for the output was that the eye position cells could be used as a teaching signal if the animal saccaded to fixate the stimulus. In later experiments we also tried mapping to Gaussian representations of head-centered location; the interesting results are listed below.

The output of each cell in the network is calculated by first summing all inputs, both inhibitory and excitatory, and then calculating the output as a sigmoidal function of the input. A sigmoid is chosen as an output function since it is similar to the operation performed by actual nerve cells that sum inputs, have a threshold, and saturate at high levels of activity. There is also a threshold term that can be either trained or set, and simulations using both of these options will be discussed.

The network begins training with all the connections set to random weights and completes training when the output units accurately indicate positions in head-centered space for any pair of arbitrary retinal and eye position inputs. The network learns by subtracting the output vector from the desired output vector for each input pattern to generate an error. This error signal is then propagated back through the network to change the weights in the network. The backpropagation algorithm ensures that the weights will change to reduce error in the performance of the network. The actual equations and derivation of the backpropagation procedure are discussed in Rumelhart et al. (1986). This cycle is repeated until the network reduces error to desired levels. The spatial transformation network learns quickly and always settles to very low error values. Within 1000 trials the network shows accuracy that is better than the spacing of the distance between the centers of the retinal receptive fields. For large numbers of trials the network continues to show improvement to vanishingly small errors.

After training is complete the middle-layer units have receptive fields that remain retinotopic, but their activity becomes modulated by eye position in a manner similar to that seen in the recording data from area 7a neurons. The receptive fields remain retinotopic but the responsiveness changes with eye position. The change in responsiveness is roughly planar and similar to a majority of the gain fields recorded from area 7a neurons. Moreover, the receptive fields are large and can have peculiar shapes, not unlike the cells in area 7a.

In Figure 13.3 the retinotopic visual receptive fields from recording experiments are compared with retinotopic receptive fields generated by the model. It should be emphasized that these comparisons are intended to be qualitative and show only that they are similar; obviously they will not be exactly the same, just as no two area 7a neuron receptive fields will ever be identical. Surfaces have been fit to the recording and model data using a Gaussian interpolation algorithm. Each receptive field is 80° in diameter. The fields have been categorized

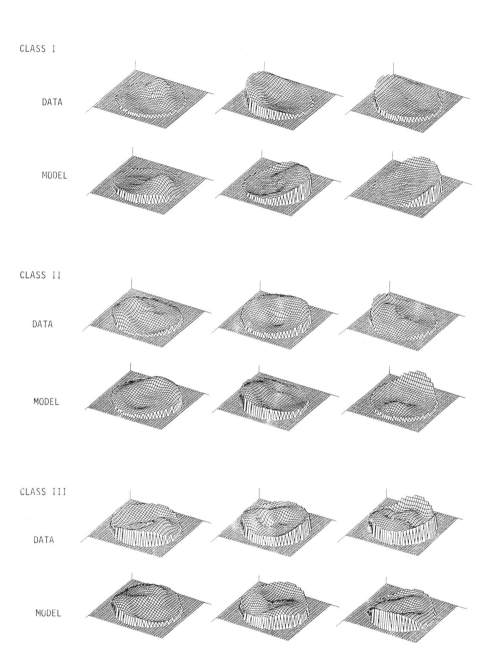

FIGURE 13.3. Visual receptive fields from the data and the model compared. The receptive fields were divided into three classes: class I cells have a single, smooth peak of activity; class II cells have one peak of activity but also other smaller peaks or depressions in the receptive field; class III cells have multiple peaks of activity. Note the close correspondence between model- and data-receptive fields.

by complexity into three classes: class I has the simplest receptive fields with each having a single peak of activity; class II fields are of intermediate complexity with each field having a single greatest peak of activity and one or more smaller peaks of activity; class III receptive fields are the most complex with each having multiple peaks of greatest activity. The most complex fields are similar to fields of the untrained model. The trained model seldom produces such complex fields.

Next we compared gain fields generated by the model with data gain fields. Figure 13.4 shows gain fields from recording data and Figure 13.5 gain fields

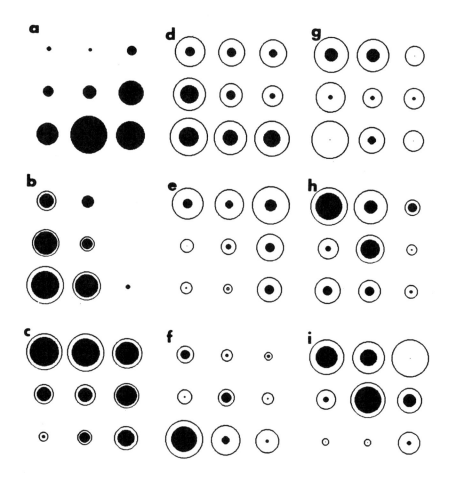

FIGURE 13.4.   The spatial gain fields of nine cells recorded from area 7a using the technique shown in Figure 13.1. The diameter of the inner, dark circle is proportional to the magnitude of the visually evoked response. The outer circle diameter is proportional to the total rate (visual response and background activity). The white annulus represents the firing rate in the absence of visual stimulation.

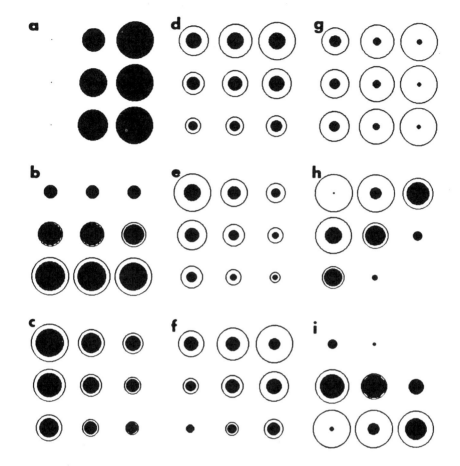

FIGURE 13.5.   Hidden unit spatial gain fields generated by the network model, in the same format as Figure 13.4. All the fields illustrated resulted from 10,000 training trials. Units g, h, and i are from runs in which the craniotopic Gaussian format for the output layer was used. The remainder of the cells were using a craniotopic monotonic format.

generated by the model's hidden unit. The nine pairs of circles for each data or model unit represent the activity for the same retinotopic stimulus delivered at nine different eye positions. The dark inner circle's diameter is proportional to the response to the visual stimulus alone, and the outer circle's diameter is proportional to the entire activity, both background and evoked.

Three basic types of planar gain fields were found from the recording data. For 28%, the background and evoked activities changed in a parallel fashion (Figure 13.4b,e,f). In the largest proportion of cells (43%), the evoked activity changed while the background activity, if any, remained constant (Fig. 13.4a,c,d); 75% of these cells had low rates of background activity. For the remaining 28% of the neurons the background and evoked activities changed in different directions, so the activity of either alone was grossly nonplanar, but the overall activity was planar (Fig. 13.4g,h,i).

Figure 13.5 shows gain fields generated by the model; the arrangement shows the close correspondence between recording and model gain fields. Both monotonic and Gaussian output representations were used in the training that generated these fields. Either output representation generates total response gain fields that are planar. However, when the training is made to monotonic output function the visual response gain fields are generally planar (67%; Fig. 13.5a–f), whereas training to the Gaussian format produces only 13% in this class. These figures compare to the 55% found in the experimental data. If the thresholds are trained along with the synaptic weights for monotonic outputs, then the background and evoked activities almost always change in a parallel fashion. However, if the threshold is held constant and at high values, the background activity is low and does not change with eye position, similar to the largest proportion of parietal cells. Finally, if training is done using a Gaussian format output, then the visual evoked response is usually grossly nonplanar but the combination of background and evoked responses is planar (Fig. 13.5g,h,i).

DISCUSSION OF THE MODEL

The simulation results show that training a parallel network to perform coordinate transformations produces the same type of distributed code that is found in area 7a. This similarity should be pursued to determine if it represents a fundamental outcome of using parallel networks to perform coordinate transformations. One line of research would be to make the model more complex by incorporating features analogous to those found in the brain such as Hebb learning and reciprocal pathways for error feedback. It will be interesting to see if these more complex and brainlike ·models still produce the same distributed code. Another avenue would be to see if this model generalizes to three-dimensional space- and body-centered coordinates by collecting data under these conditions for parietal neurons and comparing the results to predictions made from the model.

These results suggest that the posterior parietal cortex learns to associate body position with respect to visual space. Thus the parietal lobe appears to form associative memories for performing spatial transformations. A learning theory for parietal spatial functions seems in order, since it would not be practical to hard-wire spatial representations during development when the body is changing size. Moreover, distortions of space with prisms lead to rapid recalibration in adults, suggesting that, unlike ocular dominance, there is no critical period for spatial representations and they remain plastic in adults.

It is important to note that the model by definition does not have a topographic organization. Thus there is no requirement for topographic organization in the brain. The reason topography is not necessary is that the organization of the network is distributed and the information is contained in the weights in the synapses. It would be interesting to determine whether putting a crude topography into the connections of the network would accelerate learning.

If the spatial representation in area 7a lacks topography, this does not of course mean that there is not topographic organization in this area. We imagine that learning spatial localization can occur within the dimensions of a typical cortical column, 1 mm^2. Recordings made within an area of parietal cortex of this size contain a complete complement of receptive fields, eye position signals, and gain fields necessary for a complete representation of craniotopic space (Andersen, Essick, & Siegel, unpublished observation, 1985). Thus spatial location can be mapped over and over again in many repeating units in the cortex and may overlie some as yet unknown functional repetitive architecture that would need in each of its modules the complete machinery for coordinate transformations.

The rather large receptive fields suggest that every posterior parietal neuron has access to the entire retina and the particular shape of each receptive field is a result of competitive learning. This competition produces in both the parietal neurons and the model units receptive fields that, although they are complex, tend to coalesce so that they are smoothly varying rather than random in structure. The large receptive fields are presumably due to the cascading divergence that occurs in the multistage corticocortical projections from V1 to area 7a.

The fact that many fewer eye position synapses than retinal synapses were requried at the convergence onto the hidden units in the model has interesting parallels to the anatomy of the parietal lobe connections. It is believed that the source of eye position information comes from lower brain stem centers and is relayed through the intralaminar nuclei (Schlag-Rey & Schlag, 1984). However, these nuclei are small compared to the cortical areas relaying visual information to area 7a.

There is the question of where the output units of the model might exist in the brain. Cells showing the expected eye position–independent behavior have not been found in area 7a. Another possibility is that this distributed coding is used throughout all brain regions that need spatial representations. The final spatial output might be seen only in the eventual motor output. The final spatial output may be pointing the eye or a finger accurately to a location in space and no single cell in the brain might be found that codes the location of visual space in an eye position–independent fashion.

Finally, there is the question of whether this form of model of distributed coding in parallel networks, which appears to explain the parietal data rather well, will be useful in other brain regions. Recently the response of area V4 cells was examined in a task in which the monkey must match the orientation of a visual or somatosensory cue grating with the orientation of a visual test grating (Haenny, Maunsell, & Schiller, in press). They find cells that respond to the cue that are orientation tuned, cells that respond to the test stimulus that are orientation tuned, and cells that show facilitated activity for a particular combination of cue and test stimulus. Thus the activity of some V4 neurons shows a multiplicative interaction between two inputs that is similar to the interaction for eye and retinal inputs for area 7a neurons. It would be useful to construct a similar network in which the inputs were the cue and test stimuli and the output the correct match. Would the hidden units develop properties like those of V4 neurons?

Acknowledgments

We thank Carol Andersen for editorial assistance. R.A.A. was supported by grants EY05522 and EY07492 from the National Institutes of Health, the Sloan Foundation, and the Whitaker Health Sciences Foundation. D.Z. was supported by grants from the System Development Foundation, ONR contract N0014-87K-0671, and the AFOSR.

REFERENCES

Andersen, R. A. (1987). Inferior parietal lobule function in spatial perception and visuomotor integration. In F. Plum (Ed.), *Handbook of physiology* (pp. 483–518). Bethesda, Md.: American Physiological Society.

Andersen, R. A., Essick, G. K., & Siegel, R. M. (1985). Encoding of spatial location by posterior parietal neurons. *Science, 230,* 456–458.

Andersen, R. A. & Zipser, D. (1988). The role of the posterior parietal cortex in coordinate transformations for visual-motor integration. *Canadian Journal of Physiology and Pharmacology, 66,* 488–501.

Haenny, P. E., Maunsell, J. H. R., & Schiller, P. H. (in press). State dependent activity in monkey visual cortex. *Experimental Brain Research.*

Hallet, P. E., & Lightstone, A. D. (1976). Saccadic eye movements toward stimuli triggered by prior saccades. *Vision Research, 16,* 99.

Mays, L. E., & Sparks, D. L. (1980). Dissociation of visual and saccade-related responses in superior colliculus neurons. *Journal of Neurophysiology, 43,* 207–232.

Merzenich, M. M., Recanzone, G., Jenkins, W. M., Allard, T. T., & Nudo, R. J. (in press). Cortical representational plasticity. In P. Rakic & W. Singer (Eds.), *Neurobiology of neocortex. Dahlem konferenze.* Chichester: Wiley.

Robinson, D. A. (1975). Oculomotor control signals. In P. Bach-y-Rita & G. Lernerstrand (Eds.), *Basic mechanisms of ocular motility and their clinical implications* (pp. 337–374). London: Pergamon.

Rumelhart, D. E., Hinton, G. E., & Williams, R. J. (1986). Learning internal representations by error propagation. In D. E. Rumelhart, J. L. McClelland, & PDP Research Group (Eds.), *Parallel distributed processing: Explorations in the microstructure of cognition: Vol. 1. Foundations* (pp. 318–362). Cambridge, Mass.: Bradford Books/MIT Press.

Schlag-Rey, M., & Schlag, J. (1984). Visuomotor functions of central thalamus in monkey. I. Unit activity related to spontaneous eye movements. *Journal of Neurophysiology, 51,* 1149–1174.

Zipser, D., & Andersen, R. A. (1988). A back propagation programmed network that simulates response properties of a subset of posterior parietal neurons. *Nature. 331,* 679–684.

14

Cortical Localization
of Working Memory

PATRICIA S. GOLDMAN-RAKIC

WORKING MEMORY

Working memory is the term applied by cognitive psychologists and theorists to the type of memory that is relevant only for a short period of time, usually on the scale of seconds. This criterion—relevant only transiently—distinguishes working memory from almost every other form of memory in which the contents are stable over time. Thus working memory can be distinguished easily from what has been termed reference memory (Olton, Becken, & Handelmann, 1979), declarative memory (Squire & Cohen, 1984), semantic memory (Tulving, 1972), procedural memory (Squire & Cohen, 1984), and habit (Mishkin, Malamut, & Bachevalier, 1984)—all of which have in common that their contents do not depend on current experience or where or when the information was learned.

A major idea about working memory is that it is a single common resource with a limited capacity. Indeed, Baddeley (1986) argued that there is a process of general working memory (his WMG) that can be used concurrently by a range of cognitive tasks: learning, reading, comprehension, and so on. A significant issue in current research on the psychology of working memory is whether there may, in fact, be multiple memory systems, each dedicated to different information-processing domains, or just one central executive system that is shared by all concurrent tasks (Baddeley, 1986; Squire, 1987). As will be discussed later, neuroscience has much to contribute toward elucidating this issue.

The distinction between working and other forms of memory has been invoked less frequently by physiological psychologists. Olton can be credited as the researcher who brought this distinction to the attention of neuroscientists and demonstrated its usefulness in studies of maze behavior in rats (Olton et al., 1979). Otherwise, the concept has not been given prominence in reviews of the neuropsychological literature on the role of the limbic or diencephalic structures in memory (Mishkin et al., 1984; Squire, 1982, 1986) and correspondingly little has been said about the neural structures or mechanisms underlying working memory. This is surprising because several of the tasks used to study memory in human and nonhuman primates have strong working memory components; that is, matching-to-sample and nonmatching-to-sample tasks engage working memory for object features.

In this chapter I will review old and new evidence that the brain obeys the distinction between working and associative forms of memory and I will argue that the prefrontal cortex has a specialized, perhaps even preeminent, role in working memory processes. Moreover, there is already considerable evidence to suggest that more than one working memory system exists in prefrontal cortex and that still others may be disclosed. Perhaps through the study of experimental animals more can be learned about the neurobiological principles underlying these fundamental processes which govern our behavior and which decompose in numerous neurological diseases.

DELAYED-RESPONSE TASKS: TESTS OF WORKING MEMORY

The delayed-response tests were designed and introduced to psychology by the comparative psychologist Walter Hunter (1913). His intention was to devise a test that would differentiate among animals (including humans) on their relative ability to respond to situations on the basis of stored information, rather than on the basis of "immediate" stimulation. The classical version of the delayed-response test is essentially a hiding task in which the subject is shown the location of a food morsel that is then hidden from view by an opaque screen (Fig. 14.1). Following a delay period of several seconds, the subject chooses the correct location out of two or more choices. In this situation the subject must remember where the bait had been placed a few seconds earlier. In a variation of this task, spatial delayed alternation, the subject is required to alternate between left and right foodwells on successive trials that are separated by delay periods (Fig. 14.1). Since in the latter task the animal is not permitted to observe the experimenter baiting the foodwells in the delay periods, to be correct on any given trial the subject must keep track of which response was made last. A crucial feature of these tests is the lack of a fixed relationship between stimuli and correct responses. Unlike the procedure employed in associative learning or conditioning paradigms, although the stimulus arrangement at the time of response is identical on each trial, the correct response varies depending on information presented several seconds earlier. Thus the correct response is different on every trial and information relevant to the response on one trial is irrelevant on the next trial and actually best forgotten, lest it interfere with the current response. The same underlying principle operates in other commonly used behavioral paradigms: object alternation and match-to-sample or nonmatch-to-sample paradigms.

Delayed-response function has been associated with prefrontal cortex since the early discovery that monkeys with prefrontal cortex damage were severely

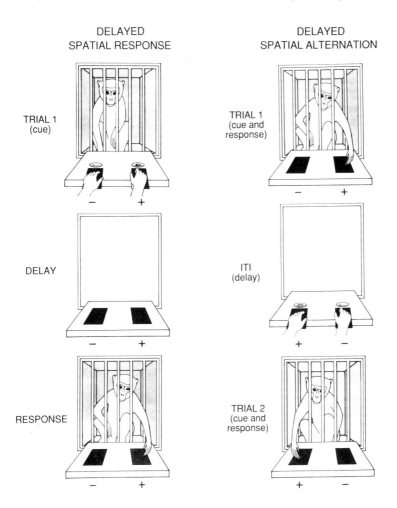

FIGURE 14.1. Two working memory tests, delayed spatial response and delayed-spatial alternation. Dorsolateral prefrontal lesions produce impairments on these tasks, but not on associative memory tasks such as visual pattern discriminations. (Modified from Friedman and Goldman-Rakic, in press; see Goldman-Rakic, 1987b, for review.)

impaired on this and related tasks (Jacobsen, 1936). Although the association between the capacity to perform delayed-response tasks and the functional integrity of the dorsolateral prefrontal cortex is firmly established, the nature of the process(es) tapped by these tasks has been the subject of continuing discussion and seemingly contradictory interpretations. Jacobsen stressed the mnemonic or temporal–sequential processes required by delayed-response tasks (and hence mediated by prefrontal cortex), but this explanation somehow did not take hold. In retrospect, it seems evident that in the thirties, and for several decades later, memory was considered a unitary mechanism thought to have a single location.

As patients and monkeys with prefrontal lesions displayed surprisingly adequate performance on discrimination learning, object reversal, and conditional memory tasks and, in addition, patients displayed remarkably normal scores, at least on conventional IQ tests, the impairment produced by prefrontal damage was not global enough to fit the neuropsychologist's midcentury concept of a mnemonic deficit. Thus various investigators sought other explanations—for example, spatial perception and/or spatial orientation (e.g., Pohl, 1973; Pribram & Mishkin, 1956), attentional functions (Bartus & LeVere, 1977; Malmo, 1942), and motor control functions (Teuber, 1972)—and some considered disturbance in the central representations of kinesthesis (Konorski, 1967) or proprioception (Gentile & Stamm, 1972) as basic to the prefrontal deficit.

NEUROPHYSIOLOGICAL EVIDENCE FOR WORKING MEMORY

A major development in our understanding of delayed-response tasks and prefrontal cortex came in the early seventies when unit recording studies were performed for the first time in awake behaving monkeys trained on delayed-response tasks (Fuster & Alexander, 1970; Kubota & Niki, 1971). These studies revealed that neurons in the prefrontal cortex became activated during the delay period of a delayed-response trial. It was difficult to resist the hypothesis that these prefrontal neurons were the cellular expression of a mnemonic process. A similar conclusion had been reached in a paper that H. E. Rosvold and I published one year earlier on the cortical localization of delayed-response deficits and the nature of the difficulty experienced by monkeys with bilateral lesions on delayed-response tasks. We suggested that cortex around the principal sulcal cortex was involved in what we termed at the time "modality-specific" memory (Goldman & Rosvold, 1970). In a series of studies (Goldman & Rosvold, 1970; Goldman, Rosvold, Vest, & Galkin, 1971), we compared monkeys with various circumscribed prefrontal lesions on spatial tasks (delayed-response and delayed alternation) which contained temporal delays between spatial cues and spatial responses and on other tasks (conditional position response and go–no go alternation) which removed the delay or the spatial feature, respectively, from the behavioral task. Our goal in these studies was to determine the importance of the delay relative to the spatial features of tasks on which monkeys with prefrontal lesions were impaired. The results were clear-cut. Monkeys with principal sulcus lesions were impaired only on tasks that contained *both* spatial cues/responses *and* a delay, but they performed well on tasks that contained only a delay or only a spatial cue/response. The full significance of our experiments and conclusions are clearer now than they were in the early seventies, for they provided evidence of a working memory system dedicated to spatial vision—that did not overlap with memory mechanisms for other (e.g., nonspatial) domains of knowledge.

The evidence from neurophysiological studies of prefrontal neurons has been steadily accumulating since 1970. Since that time, numerous studies have provided evidence that certain classes of prefrontal neurons are particularly activated during delay periods (for review, see Fuster, 1980). Yet the interpretation that such activity reflected a memory process was still not widely appreciated outside of a narrow circle of scientists working on the primate prefrontal cortex. Perhaps one reason was that neurons activated during the delay of a delayed-response trial were not necessarily coding specific information, but rather were engaged in some sort of preparatory or motor set to respond. Further, preparation to respond could invoke postural mechanisms rather than central processes. Whatever the reason, scientists did not seem to be impressed with the delay-related activation of prefrontal neurons. However, some recent evidence from studies that I have been conducting with Shintaro Funahashi and Charles Bruce have provided the most convincing evidence yet of mnemonic processing in prefrontal cortex. We have been using an oculomotor delayed-response paradigm to study prefrontal function (Funahashi, Bruce, & Goldman-Rakic, 1989). The advantage of this paradigm over other methods of studying delayed-response performance is that we require the animal to fixate a spot of light on a television monitor and maintain fixation during the brief (0.5-sec) presentation of a light followed by a delay period of variable length. Visual targets can be presented in any part of the visual field and, importantly, we have complete control over the specific information that the animal has to remember on any given trial. The fixation point is turned off only at the end of the delay period and its offset is our instruction to the animal to break fixation and direct its gaze to wherever the target had been presented. Under these circumstances high levels of performance can be attained only if the monkey uses mnemonic processing. In the oculomotor task, as in manual delayed-response tasks, prefrontal neurons increase (or often decrease) their discharge rate during the delay period of a trial. The neuron displayed in Figure 14.2. is an example: its activity rises sharply at the end of the stimulus, remains tonically active, and then ceases rather abruptly at the end of the delay.

The activation of prefrontal neurons when a stimulus disappears from view and the maintenance of that activation until a response is executed is highly suggestive of a working memory process. However, other interpretations are possible. For example, it could still be argued that the delay period activity reflects simply the motor set of the animal to respond at the end of the delay, as has been described for neurons in premotor fields (Mauritz and Wise, 1986; Tanji, 1985). However, we and others showed that prefrontal neurons have directional delay-period activity, that is, they exhibit increased or decreased discharge only for specific targets. Our own studies testing behavioral performance and single neuron activity with stimuli presented in eight different locations showed that prefrontal neurons have "memory fields." Monkeys performed this task with proficiency for *every* target location, but most neurons that we recorded in prefrontal cortex altered their discharge rate only for one or a few specific target locations. A general motor set explanation cannot easily account for this result.

If prefrontal neurons are involved in mnemonic processing, one would expect their activity to be sensitive to changes in the duration of the delay period. Indeed, it has been shown that the activity of prefrontal neurons in the delay

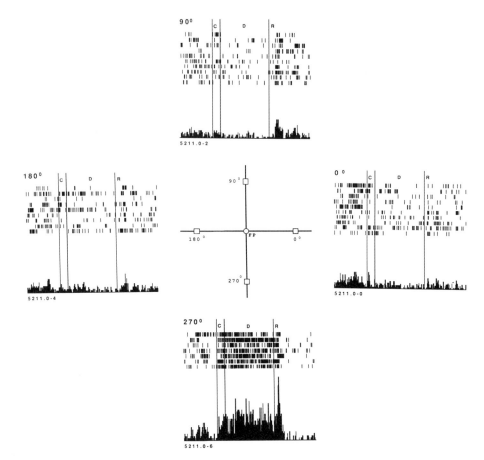

FIGURE 14.2.   Single unit activity of a prefrontal neuron recorded during performance on an oculomotor delayed-response task. The neuron's "memory field" is for the target at 270°. Activity was enhanced during the delay period only when the target to be remembered was at that location and not at any other tested. (Modified from Funahashi et al., 1989)

period expands and contracts as the delay duration is lengthened or foreshortened (Kojima & Goldman-Rakic, 1982). Again, this would be expected if the neuron is coding information that is to be retained until the end of the delay period.

ANATOMICAL EVIDENCE

The principal sulcus in the prefrontal cortex is the anatomical focus for spatial delayed-response function and knowledge of its connections with other structures is helping researchers to understand the circuit and cellular basis of working memory. It has become clear that this prefrontal subdivision has reciprocal connections with more than a dozen distinct association regions, with premotor centers, with the caudate nucleus, superior colliculus, and brain stem centers (for review see Goldman-Rakic, 1987b). One major goal of research in my laboratory is to relate the different connections of prefrontal cortex to its capacity to mediate delayed-response performance by decomposing the task into its composite subfunctions. For this purpose, my colleagues and I proposed that in general the ability to guide behavior by working memory requires mechanisms for (1) selecting or accessing pertinent information; (2) holding that information "on-line" for the temporal interval over which a decision or operation is to be performed; and (3) executing motor commands. In the case of the delayed-response task, the animal at a minimum must (1) attend to the relevant visuospatial coordinates; (2) remember the most recent preceding event (where the bait was placed or which response was made last); and (3) select and execute the appropriate manual or oculomotor response while inhibiting the inappropriate response. Each of these component processes is presumably mediated by different pathways that comprise the neural circuitry of the principal sulcus. I have suggested that the parietoprefrontal projection system is one that may supply the sensory–representational information to the prefrontal cortex, and connections with the caudate and superior colliculus, among other motor centers, play a role in relaying motor commands (Goldman-Rakic, 1987b). However, the mechanism for holding information in the short-term memory buffer is a total mystery at this point and the role in this process of any connections that the prefrontal cortex has with other centers, including memory centers, is not clear. The parietoprefrontal circuit described above may be crucial. At the same time, we described several multisynaptic connections between the prefrontal cortex and the hippocampal formation and speculated that these connections imply a cooperative functional relationship between the hippocampus and the prefrontal cortex (Goldman-Rakic, Selemon, & Schwartz, 1984). As described below, our recent examination of metabolic rate in the dentate gyrus and hippocampus in monkeys performing working memory tasks supports this line of thinking (Friedman & Goldman-Rakic, 1988).

METABOLIC STUDIES OF WORKING AND ASSOCIATIVE MEMORY

One strategy that we have been using to test the functional significance of various prefrontal connections is the 2-deoxyglucose method of functional mapping. We used this method to examine the metabolic rate in the dentate gyrus and hippocampal subfields as well as other neural structures in monkeys trained to perform working memory tasks and compared their brain metabolism with that of monkeys performing other types of memory and/or control tasks. We showed that metabolic rate increases about 20% in specific parts of the trisynaptic path in monkeys performing a variety of working memory tasks including delayed-response as compared with those performing visual pattern or sensorimotor tasks (Friedman & Goldman-Rakic, 1988).

Our results not only implicate the hippocampus and dentate gyrus in a cooperative relationship with the prefrontal cortex; they also allowed us to identify other parts of the neural system or circuitry engaged by working memory. For example, we recently showed that the mediodorsal nucleus and anterior nuclei are selectively driven in terms of enhanced metabolic rate by working memory requirements. However, the amygdala (Friedman & Goldman-Rakic, 1988) and mammillary bodies (Friedman, Janas, & Goldman-Rakic, 1987) exhibit the same metabolic rate for associative memory and sensorimotor tasks as they do for working memory tasks. The 2-deoxyglucose studies in normal monkeys performing tasks that vary in their mnemonic requirements should shed light on the components of a neural system that are (or are not) crucial for selective memory processes. Our preliminary results indicate that there is a network of interconnected cortical and subcortical areas and hence an elaborate network of structures that is activated by the working memory requirement in many mnemonic tasks. Although the precise mechanisms are unknown, it seems that this anatomical system includes at minimum the dorsolateral prefrontal cortex, the trisynaptic pathway of the hippocampus, and selected medial and anterior thalamic nuclei.

SIGNIFICANCE OF WORKING MEMORY: REGULATION OF BEHAVIOR BY REPRESENTATIONAL KNOWLEDGE VERSUS REGULATION BY IMMEDIATE STIMULATION

The significance of working memory for higher cortical function is widely recognized and attested to by cognitive psychologists. However, one reason it may not have received the attention it deserves among neuroscientists is that its importance is not self-evident. Perhaps even the quality of its transient nature misleads us into thinking it is somehow less important than the more permanent archival nature of long-term memory. However, the working memory function of our brains may be its most inherently flexible mechanism and its evolutionarily most significant achievement. Thus working memory confers the ability to guide behavior by representations of the outside world rather than by immediate stimulation. It is the cornerstone of the human capacity to base behavior on ideas and thoughts and is critical for linguistic processing.

This capacity is not easily won: prosimian primates have much greater difficulty learning delayed-response tasks than do rhesus monkeys, and some normal galagos even fail to learn this task (Preuss & Goldman-Rakic, unpublished observation, 1988). Cats and dogs have not been shown to perform a delayed-response task given in the same manner as it is given to monkeys. Only if the animals are allowed to keep the hidden object in view during the delay period, as in a Nencki test apparatus, is delayed-response performance attained (Warren, Warren, & Akert, 1972). One may even question whether rhesus monkeys are using working memory processes if allowed to keep the to-be-remembered object in view during a delay period. The opportunity to view the target during the delay period could obviate the whole purpose of the delayed-response task.

As working memory is the process that allows behavior to be regulated by representations, it may underlie our ability to form concepts—representations of *classes* of stimuli of particular color, size, or form. It is significant, therefore, that the neuropsychological deficit most widely recognized as being associated with prefrontal dysfunction in humans is that revealed by a test of categorization, the Wisconsin Card Sort Test. In this task, the subject is asked to sort a deck of cards which bear stimuli that vary in number, color, and shape. As each card in the stack comes up, the subject has to match it to a set of reference cards on the basis of one dimension that is arbitrarily selected by the experimenter (e.g., color). The experimenter then informs the subject if he or she is "right" or "wrong" and the patient tries to get as many correct matches as possible. After the patient achieves a specified number of consecutive correct matches, the sorting principle is shifted without warning (e.g., to shape or number) and the patients must modify their responses accordingly. Patients with right or left hemisphere prefrontal damage exhibit difficulty in switching from one category to another (Milner, 1963, 1964).

At first glance there would seem to be little similarity between the Wisconsin Card Sort Test used with frontal lobe patients and the delayed-response task used with lesioned monkeys. Commonalities between these two tasks have rarely been claimed. However, the Wisconsin Card Sort Test does resemble the delayed-response tasks in one essential respect. Although the relevant features of the stimuli (color, size, shape) are all present at the time of response, there is nevertheless no information given about the correct response; it must be provided from representational memory, perhaps in this case a second-order representation (representation of a representation), that is, a concept for guiding response choice. Although the capacity for this type of second-order representational system appears to be a unique acquisition of human intelligence, undoubtedly linked to the emergence of language, it clearly must be built on a first-order representational capacity shared with other mammals.

Another concept that may depend on working memory is object permanence: the capacity to recognize that an object has continuity in time and space when out of view. It may not be coincidental, therefore, that Piaget's Stage IV Object Permanence Test (OPT) is formally similar to delayed-response. As in delayed response, the child watches as a reward is hidden in one of two spatially separated locations; then, after a delay of a few seconds, the child is allowed to find the reward. We have shown that the performance of adult rhesus monkeys with dorsolateral prefrontal lesions on the Piagetian test is remarkably similar to that of human infants on the same test (Diamond & Goldman-Rakic, 1989). In monkeys, moreover, the capacity to perform the OPT has been shown to develop concomitantly with the emergence of delayed-response ability during the first half-year of life (Diamond & Goldman-Rakic, 1989). On the basis of their common dependence on prefrontal cortex and on what we know and can theorize about prefrontal cortex, we conclude that both tasks measure a common process. If our reasoning has merit, this process may be considered a building block of concept development in humans. In any event, the elemental capacity to form representations of the outside world and especially to base responses on those representations in the absence of the objects they represent is a nontrivial achievement of the mammalian cortex.

In addition to the Wisconsin Card Sort Test and Piaget's Object Permanence Test, a variety of other tests may depend to some extent on working memory and thus reflect prefrontal cortical function. These include the Stroop Test, in which the names of colors are printed in the ink of another color (the word *yellow* is printed in red) and subjects are instructed to report the color of the word while suppressing the natural or prepotent tendency to report the written content of the word. Here again subjects must guide their response by a representational memory, in this case the memory of an instruction. Patients with prefrontal lesions are impaired on the Stroop Test (Perret, 1974) and on tasks in which they must keep track of the recency or order of their previous responses (Petrides & Milner, 1982) as well as project sequences of future responses on "look-ahead" puzzles, like the Tower of London test (Shallice, 1982). In the latter task, a goal has to be decomposed into subgoals and the subgoals must be tackled in the correct order. Such tasks, like delayed-response tasks, require an ability to base current responses on representations of past or future events. Finally, patients with prefrontal damage have difficulty in generating new responses. Their well-documented impairments in generating word lists (Milner, 1964; Perret, 1974) and in inventing abstract designs (Jones-Gotman & Milner, 1977) and reproducing gestures might be expected and predicted if they suffer an impoverished ability to guide behavior on the basis of representations or ideas, and if this ability itself depends on working memory. Thus it may be that a seemingly diverse set of measures, rather than tapping into diverse processes, shares a common neurobiological mechanism—working memory.

EVOLUTIONARY SIGNIFICANCE OF WORKING MEMORY

The type of behavioral regulation subserved by prefrontal cortex can be contrasted with the formation of stimulus–response associations, which depend in an obligatory manner on the repeated association of stimulus–response pairings and/or the amplitude, duration, and frequency of stimuli in the environment. Indeed, the evolution of a capacity for representational knowledge may provide a mechanism for overriding the governance of behavior by conditioned, reflexive, or innate prepotent responses, particularly when such behavior could be maladaptive for the organism. The fact that delayed-response impairments produced by prefrontal lesions are absent at nil delays between stimulus and response, yet are nearly as severe at delays of 1 to 2 sec as at much longer delays (Goldman, 1971), suggests a sharp dissociation in the neural mechanisms that mediate representational and strictly sensory guidance of behavior. Working memory, as previously indicated, allows information coming in at one point in time to be *transiently* associated with information encountered at a later time. In contrast, the mechanisms of associative memory are precisely designed to preserve or "stamp in" lasting relationships between stimuli and responses.

Finally, efficient representational memory requires information to be dismissed as efficiently as it is accessed; this type of memory demands a flexible, nonbinding relationship between a given stimulus and a given response. Thus the memory mechanisms of prefrontal cortex could be expected to differ from those that mediate associative learning.

The functional dissociation of working and associative memory mechanisms is supported by anatomical localization studies. Decortication spares certain forms of conditioned responses, and many classically conditioned responses have been localized to the amygdala, diencephalon, brain stem, and spinal cord (for review see Thompson, 1986). However, associative learning is completely spared by prefrontal and also hippocampal lesions (for reviews see Goldman-Rakic, 1987a; Squire, 1986). It therefore seems possible that the type of behavior which utilizes memory in the representational, working memory, sense requires participation of the prefrontal cortex, whereas that involving associative learning may rely more heavily on subcortical structures and/or other areas of neocortex. The evolution of a capacity to guide behavior on the basis of representations of the outside world rather than on the trigger of immediate stimulation introduces the possibility that concepts and plans may govern our behavior. One way they may do so is by regulating, facilitating, or inhibiting the associatively conditioned or reflexly organized responses of motor centers to which the prefrontal cortex projects (Goldman-Rakic, 1987c).

Although the mechanisms of working and associative memory are undoubtedly different, their contributions to behavior can be thought of as complementary. Associative mechanisms are the basis of our vast store of experience and knowledge; those of working memory provide a means for *utilizing* that knowledge in a flexible manner. Thus a complete understanding of behavioral regulation would entail a detailed analysis of the relationships and interconnections between mechanisms of associative and working memory.

THOUGHT DISORDERS: LOSS OF WORKING MEMORY

Consider what happens when working memory is lost, as it may be, in patients and in experimental animals with prefrontal cortex damage. Studies of the loss of this capacity may help researchers understand certain well-established features of behavior expressed both by patients and by monkeys with prefrontal lesions. One such feature is distractibility. In a hypothetical delayed-response trial, a normal animal would form an internal representation of the position of the bait during the cue period and maintain reference to that representation for as long as is necessary to guide its response. Access to this knowledge during the delay period bridges the temporal gap between cue and response and enables the animal to select and execute the correct response; at the same time, inappropriate responses to irrelevant or distracting external stimuli that may command the animal's attention at the moment of response are, of necessity, suppressed. Deprived of access to representational knowledge, the opposite would be true: an animal would almost be forced to rely on external stimuli present at the time

296 REGULATION OF CORTICAL FUNCTION IN MEMORY

of response; it would be at the "mercy" of environmental cues. Indeed, a dominant feature of the frontal lobe syndrome in both human and nonhuman primates is an excessive dependence on, or sensitivity to, external cues (e.g., humans: Lhermitte, 1986; Woods & Knight, 1986; monkey: Bartus & LeVere, 1977; Malmo, 1942). The monkey with prefrontal lesions seems to respond to the first foodwell that catches its eye or to the just previously reinforced side rather than to recently stored information about the location of the reward. The description "out of sight, out of mind" (Jacobsen, 1936) or "animal of the moment" (Bartus & LeVere, 1977) applies very well to the mindless performance observed in prefrontally lesioned patients and experimental animals. Thus it is possible that the capacity to guide behavior on the basis of internalized representations marvelously accomplishes the dual task of initiating the correct response and perforce disallowing or inhibiting the incorrect one that is presumably mediated by lower centers. Although the mechanisms for issuing both facilitatory and inhibitory motor commands may be expected to be complex, the prefrontal cortex has multiple connections with the motor centers by which these complementary control functions could be exerted (Goldman-Rakic, 1987c).

Loss of a mechanism for guiding behavior by representational knowledge might also explain the perseveration of incorrect responses that is so characteristic of animals and patients with prefrontal lesions. If they are destined to respond to situations on the basis of information available at the time of response, they would be subject not only to control by external stimuli but to conditioning by adventitious pairing of stimuli and responses. If a response on any given delayed-response trial happened to be reinforced, there would be a strong tendency to repeat that response, even in the face of intervening information indicating that the same response is no longer appropriate. Perseveration of previously rewarded responses is exactly what prefrontally damaged subjects do. The integrity of the prefrontal cortex and access to representational memories may be necessary to *override* the tendency to behave strictly on the basis of reinforcement contingencies or on the basis of stimulation present at the moment of response and hence may enable the normal monkey to suppress such tendencies. Viewed in this way, perseveration and distractibility are consequences rather than primary causes of a more basic defect in the regulation of behavior by representations. Since these are common symptoms of numerous neurological conditions, understanding of the neural mechanisms subserving working memory may be expected to shed light on human diseases that affect cognition.

REFERENCES

Baddeley, A. D. (1986). *Working memory.* New York: Oxford University Press.
Bartus, R. T., & LeVere, T. E. (1977). Frontal decortication in rhesus monkeys: A test of the interference hypothesis. *Brain Research, 119,* 223–248.

Diamond, A., & Goldman-Rakic, P. S. (1989). Evidence for involvement of prefrontal cortex in cognitive changes during the first year of life: Comparison of human infants and rhesus monkeys on Piaget's AB task. *Experimental Brain Research, 74,* 24–40.

Friedman, H., & Goldman-Rakic, P. S. (1988). Activation of the hippocampus by working memory: A 2-deoxyglucose study of behaving rhesus monkeys. *Journal of Neuroscience, 8,* 4693–4706.

Friedman, H., Janas, J., & Goldman-Rakic, P. S. (1987). Metabolic activity in the thalamus and mammillary bodies of the monkey during spatial memory performance. *Society for Neuroscience Abstracts, 13,* 206.

Funahashi, S., Bruce, C., & Goldman-Rakic, P. S. (1989). Mnemonic coding of visual space by neurons in the monkey's dorsolateral prefrontal cortex revealed by an oculomotor delayed-response task. *Journal of Neurophysiology, 61,* 1–19.

Fuster, J. M. (1980). *The prefrontal cortex.* New York: Raven.

Fuster, J. M., & Alexander, G. E. (1970). Delayed-response deficit by cryogenic depression of frontal cortex. *Brain Research, 20,* 85–90.

Gentile, A. M., & Stamm, J. S. (1972). Supplementary cues and delayed-alternation performance of frontal monkeys. *Journal of Comparative and Physiological Psychology, 80,* 230–237.

Goldman, P. S. (1971). Functional development of the prefrontal cortex in early life and the problem of neuronal plasticity. *Experimental Neurology, 32,* 366–387.

Goldman, P. S., & Rosvold, H. E. (1970). Localization of function within the dorsolateral prefrontal cortex of the rheusus monkey. *Experimental Neurology, 27,* 291–304.

Goldman-Rakic, P. S. (1987a). Circuitry of the primate prefrontal cortex and the regulation of behavior by representational memory. In F. Plum (Ed.), *Handbook of physiology: Sec. 1. The nervous system: Vol. 5. Higher functions of the brain* (pp. 373–417). Bethesda, Md.: American Physiological Society.

Goldman, P. S., Rosvold, H. E., Vest, B., & Galkin, T. W. (1971). Analysis of the delayed alternation deficit produced by dorsolateral prefrontal lesions in the Rhesus monkey. *Journal of Comparative and Physiological Psychology, 77,* 212–220.

Goldman-Rakic, P. S. (1987b). Development of cortical circuitry and cognitive function. *Child Development, 58,* 642–691.

Goldman-Rakic, P. S. (1987c). Motor control functions of the prefrontal cortex. In R. Porter (Ed.), *Motor areas of the cerebral cortex* (CIBA Foundation Symposium, No. 132, pp. 187–200). Chichester: Wiley.

Goldman-Rakic, P. S., Selemon, L. D., & Schwartz, M. L. (1984). Dual pathways connecting the prefrontal cortex with the hippocampal formation and parahippocampal cortex in the rhesus monkey. *Neuroscience, 12,* 719–743.

Hunter, W. S. (1913). The delayed reaction in animals and children. *Behavioral Monographs, 2,* 1–86.

Jacobsen, C. F. (1936). Studies of cerebral function in primates. *Comparative Psychology Monographs, 13,* 1–68.

Jones-Gotman, M., & Milner, B. (1977). Design Fluency: The invention of nonsense drawings after focal lesions. *Neuropsychologia, 15,* 653–674.

Just, M. A., & Carpenter, P. A. (1985). Cognitive coordinate systems: Accounts of mental rotation and individual differences in spatial ability. *Psychological Review, 92,* 137–172.

Kojima, S., & Goldman-Rakic, P. S. (1982). Delay-related activity of prefrontal cortical neurons in rhesus monkeys performing delayed-response. *Brain Research, 248,* 43–49.

Konorski, J. (1967). *Integrative activity of the brain.* Chicago: University of Chicago Press.

Kubota, K., & Niki, H. (1971). Prefrontal cortical unit activity and delayed cortical unit activity and delayed alternation performance in monkeys. *Journal of Neurophysiology, 34,* 337–347.

Lhermitte, F. (1986). Human anatomy and the frontal lobes. II. Patient behavior in complex and social situations: The "environmental dependency syndrome." *Annals of Neurology, 19,* 335–343.

Malmo, H. P. (1942). Interference factors on delayed response in monkeys after removal of frontal lobes. *Journal of Neurophysiology, 5,* 295–308.

Mauritz, M. H., & Wise, S. P. (1986). The premotor cortex of Rhesus monkeys: Neuronal activity before predictable environmental events. *Experimental Brain Research, 61,* 229–244.

Milner, B. (1963). Effects of different brain lesions on card sorting. *Archives of Neurology, 9,* 100–110.

Milner, B. (1964). Some effects of frontal lobectomy in man. In J. M. Warren & K. Akert (Eds.), *The frontal granular cortex and behavior* (pp. 313–334). New York: McGraw-Hill.

Mishkin, M., Malamut, B., & Báchevalier, J. (1984). Memories and habits: Two neural systems. In G. Lynch, J. L. McGaugh, & N. M. Weinberger (Eds.), *Neurobiology of learning and memory* (pp. 65–67). New York: Guilford.

Olton, D. S., Becken, J. T., & Handelmann, G. E. (1979). Hippocampus, space and memory. *Behavioral Brain Science, 2,* 313–365.

Perret, E. (1974). The left frontal lobe of man and the suppression of habitual responses in verbal categorical behaviour. *Neuropsychologia, 12,* 323–330.

Petrides, M., & Milner, B. (1982). Deficits on subject-ordered tasks after frontal- and temporal-lobe lesions in man. *Neuropsychologia, 20,* 249–262.

Piaget, J. (1954). *The construction of reality in the child.* New York: Basic Books.

Pohl, W. (1973). Dissociation of spatial discrimination deficits following frontal and parietal lesions in monkeys. *Journal of Comparative Psychology, 82,* 227–239.

Pribram, K. H., & Mishkin, M. (1956). Analysis of the effects of frontal lesions in monkey: III. Object alternation. *Journal of Comparative and Phsyiological Psychology, 49,* 41–45.

Shallice, T. (1982). Specific impairments in planning. *Philosophical Transactions of the Royal Society of London B, 298,* 199–209.

Squire, L. R. (1982). The neuropsychology of human memory. *Annual Review of Neuroscience, 5,* 241–273.

Squire, L. R. (1986). Mechanisms of memory. *Science, 232,* 1612–1619.

Squire, L. R. (1987). *Memory and brain.* New York: Oxford University Press.

Squire, L. R., & Cohen, N. J. (1984). Human memory and amnesia. In G. Lynch, J. L. McGaugh, & N. M. Weinberger (Eds.), *Neurobiology of memory and learning* (pp. 3–77). New York: Guilford.

Tanji, J. (1984). The neuronal activity in the supplementary motor area of primates. *Trends in Neuroscience, 7,* 282–285.

Tanji, J. (1985). Comparison of neuronal activities in monkey supplementary and precentral motor areas. *Behavioural Brain Research, 18,* 137–142.

Teuber, H.-L. (1972). Unity and diversity of frontal lobe functions. *Acta Neurobiologia Experimentalis, 32,* 615–656.

Thompson, R. D. (1986). The neurobiology of learning and memory. *Science, 233,* 941–947.

Tulving, E. (1972). Episodic and semantic memory. In E. Tulving & W. Donaldson (Eds.), *Organization of memory* (pp. 381–403). New York: Academic Press.

Warren, J. M., Warren, H. B., & Akert, K. (1972). The behavior of chronic cats with lesions in the frontal association cortex. *Acta Neurobiologia. Experimentalis, 32,* 345–392.

Woods, D. L., & Knight, R. I. (1986). Electrophysiologic evidence of increased distractibility after dorsolateral prefrontal lesions. *Neurology, 36,* 212–216.

III

Representations:
Beyond the Single Cell

Introduction

GORDON L. SHAW

Theoretical studies of the brain have been under way for several decades. For example, the pioneering works of Turing (1936), McCulloch and Pitts (1943), Hebb (1949), MacKay and McCulloch (1952), Cragg and Temperley (1954), Beurle (1956), von Neumann (1956), Lettvin, Maturana, McCulloch, and Pitts (1959), Rochester, Holland, Haibt, and Duda (1956), Caianiello (1961), Farley and Clark (1961), Rall (1962), Rosenblatt (1962), and Uttley (1962) all were published over 25 years ago. Over the years since, there have been relatively few brain theorists, doing their research in a somewhat isolated fashion and publishing in a range of journals (see Shaw & Palm, 1988). These factors kept brain theory from playing as important a role as it should have.

An explosion occurred in the early 1980s as physicists, engineers, mathematicians, computer scientists, and biologists from other fields started working in theoretical neurobiology (or, perhaps more accurately, mostly in artificial intelligence). At the same time, experimental neurobiologists became critically aware that in going "beyond the single cell" there needed to be a close, continuing interplay of theory and experiment. That is not to say that theorists and experimentalists had not spoken to each other, but they certainly had not in any formal setting.

In some ways, brain theory has been ahead of its time. The brilliant conceptual principle for correlated pre–post synaptic plasticity put forward by Hebb in his remarkable 1949 book, *The Organization of Behavior,* was almost immediately incorporated into mathematical models of memory in neural networks and then into computer simulations of these models. The pioneering neurophysiology experiments of Hubel and Wiesel in visual cortex were recognized and referred to by brain theorists in the early 1960s (e.g., Uttley, 1962).

To understand memory and cortical function, I believe we will need to discover the fundamental principles of cortical function and incorporate them into mathematical models. Studies connecting networks of "neurons" with a Hebb-type learning rule, which contributed to large advances in the past, are clearly not sufficient. Some of my favorite candidate principles of cortical function are given below.

HEBB SYNAPSE

Although there is increasing experimental evidence that the synaptic plasticity dependent on correlated pre–post synaptic firing activity as predicted by Hebb in 1949 is present, many questions remain to be answered: What are the exact rules of this plasticity with respect to pre–post timing relations? Can the strength of the synapse increase only as postulated by Hebb, or can it also decrease as required by certain classes of mathematical models? What is the role of the network? Interesting results related to this point are discussed by Singer (Chapter 10, this volume). What are the time scales of the changes? Do these Hebb-synaptic changes occur after 50 msec, as suggested by Malsburg (Chapter 18) as being crucial for short-term memory? What is the role of modulator neuropeptides?

MOUNTCASTLE COLUMNAR ORGANIZATIONAL PRINCIPLE

Mountcastle (1978) proposed that the well-established cortical column (Goldman-Rakic, 1984), roughly 500 μ in diameter, is the basic network in the cortex and is comprised of small irreducible processing subunits (perhaps minicolumns, roughly 100 μ in diameter). The subunits are connected into columns or networks that have the capability of being excited into complex spatial–temporal firing patterns. The assumption is that higher, complex mammalian processes involve the creation and transformation of complex spatial-temporal neuronal firing patterns. This is in contrast to the assumption that the "code" for information processing and memory recall involves only sets of neurons firing with high frequency (the "grandmother" cell code). Perhaps there are several codes in the CNS for communication among various regions, depending on the sophistication of the information being analyzed and its urgency. In simple terms, what are the next spatial and temporal scales for information processing and memory recall beyond those associated with the single neuron? I suggest that this next spatial scale is rough 100 μ (corresponding to roughly 100 neurons), and the temporal scale is roughly 50 msec (corresponding to firing bursts of these spatial subunits). In Chapter 14, Goldman-Rakic has presented some exciting new results on the complex, highly specific connections from prefrontal and from posterior parietal cortex to many other cortical areas in correlated columnar fashion.

EDELMAN SELECTION PRINCIPLE FOR LEARNING

Edelman (1978) argues that a network has a basic repertoire of firing patterns inherently built into it. Through experience or learning, associations between patterns and stimuli are made, and these patterns are enhanced and "selected" out (via Hebb-type synaptic changes). Several mathematical models can be used to implement this idea. The selection principle for learning should be contrasted with models in which a network would learn from "scratch" or have a "teacher."

STATISTICAL FLUCTUATIONS

The reality of statistical fluctuations being present in neuronal spike trains and in postsynaptic potentials has been clear for many years. The very early, brilliant work of Katz (1969) and collaborators on the statistical nature of the release of neurotransmitters from vesicles in the synapses was completely confirmed. These synaptic fluctuations apparently play a crucial role in the functioning of neural networks and are not simply a fact of nature that the brain must live with. Cragg and Temperley (1954) took from physics the ideas of cooperative phenomena among groups of atoms to give magnetism, and the role of temperature T and interaction energy E in the Boltzmann probability distribution [proportional to $\exp(-E/k\mathrm{T})$] in determining the state of the material. They suggested the neuronal analogy of cooperativity in the dynamical interactions of a network of neurons and that a Boltzmann-like expression determined the time evolution of the network firing behavior. Although they had no biological analogues for E and T, and they did not develop their ideas mathematically, their work contained many important concepts.

Some 20 years later, Little (1974), unaware of Cragg and Temperley's work, developed his mathematical model of neuronal network firing behavior based on an analogy with the modern statistical mechanics spin systems developments used in understanding magnetism (and other strongly interacting many-body systems such as the highly successful Bardeen, Cooper, and Schrieffer theory of superconductivity). Vasudevan and I (Shaw & Vasudevan, 1974) showed that the physiological basis for the "temperature" and the Boltzmann-like probability equations in Little's model followed from the statistical fluctuations in synaptic transmission found by Katz.

Present physical spin system analogies used to model neural networks, for example, that of Hopfield (1982), derive from Little (1974). The full implications of the current, very popular theoretical neuronal models are yet to be determined and experimentally tested. It will be very interesting to see if, indeed, statistical fluctuations as found in synaptic operation play an important role in cortical function and memory on the more "global" level.

BALANCE BETWEEN EXCITATION AND INHIBITION

It has been made clear from many neurophysiological experiments that the balancing effects of excitation and inhibition play a vital role in determining neuronal firing behavior in the CNS. For example, "lateral" inhibition shapes the receptive fields of many sensory neurons with excitatory center and inhibitory surround. Wilson and Cowan (1972) in their theoretical analysis showed interesting effects of interacting populations of excitatory and inhibitory neurons. Key questions that need to be settled concern (1) spatial and strength distributions of excitory and inhibitory synaptic connections and (2) temporal scales for excitatory and inhibitory postsynaptic potentials. Both of these points have crucially important global network implications as well as obvious local neuronal relevance. For example, consider the fact that inhibitory PSPs have considerably longer time constants than excitatory PSPs. This can effectively translate in models with discrete time steps to the network firing behavior being dependent on the firing state of (at least) two previous time steps rather than (in most models) just the previous network firing state. The possible "big payoff" here is that second-order difference equations in time easily generate sophisticated, oscillating firing solutions for the network.

Many more "potential cortical principles" could be added that are relevant for brain theorists. Others might include the role of the layers in cortex and the role of the many neurotransmitters. In my recent work I have concentrated on building a testable mathematical model that incorporates the first five principles listed above (Shaw, Silverman, & Pearson, 1985) in a specific manner. Clearly there are many choices and many possible models. The excitement of the future lies in close, interactive, collaborative efforts between theorists and experimentalists to understand the neurobiology of learning and memory. The principles of cortical function are there to be discovered.

REFERENCES

Beurle, R. L. (1956). Properties of a mass of cells capable of regenerating pulses. *Philosophical Transactions of the Royal Society (London) B,240,* 55–94.

Caianiello, E. R. (1961). Outline of a theory of thought processes and thinking machines. *Journal of Theoretical Biology, 2,* 204–235.

Cragg, B. G., & Temperley, H. N. V. (1954). The organisation of neurones: A cooperative analogy. *Electroencephalography and Clinical Neurophysiology, 6,* 85–92.

Edelman, G. M. (1978). Group selection and phasic reentrant signaling: A theory of higher brain function. In G. M. Edelman & V. B. Mountcastle (Eds.), *The mindful brain* (pp. 51–100). Cambridge, Mass.: MIT Press.

Farley, B. G., & Clark, W. A. (1961). Activity in networks of neuron-like elements. In C. Cherry (Ed.), *Information theory* (pp. 242–251). Washington, D.C.: Butterworths.

Goldman-Rakic, P. S. (1984). The frontal lobes: Uncharted provinces of the brain. *Trends in Neuroscienses, 7,* 425–429.

Hebb, D. O. (1949). *The organization of behavior.* New York: Wiley.

Hopfield, J. J. (1982). Neural networks and physical systems with emergent collective computational abilities. *Proceedings of the National Academy of Sciences USA, 79,* 2554–2558.

Katz, B. (1969). *The release of neural transmitter substances.* Springfield, Ill.: Charles C. Thomas.

Lettvin, Y. J., Maturana, H. R., McColluch, W. S., & Pitts, W. H. (1959). What the frog's eye tells the frog's brain. *Proceedings of the IRE, 47,* 1940–1951.

Little, W. A. (1974). The existence of persistent states in the brain. *Mathematical Biosciences, 19,* 101–120.

MacKay, D. M. & McCulloch, W. S. (1952). The limiting information capacity of a neuronal link. *Bulletin of Mathematical Biophysics, 14,* 127–135.

McCulloch, W. S., & Pitts, W. (1943). A logical calculus of the ideas immanent in nervous activity. *Bulletin of Mathematical Biophysics, 5,* 115–133.

Mountcastle, V. B. (1978). An organizing principle for cerebral function: The unit module and the distributed system. In G. M. Edelman & V. B. Mountcastle (Eds.), *The mindful brain* (pp. 7–50). Cambridge, Mass.: MIT Press.

Rall, W. (1962). Electrophysiology of a dendritic neuron model. *Biophysical Journal, 2,* 145–167.

Rochester, N., Holland, J. H., Haibt, L., & Duda, W. L. (1956). Tests on a cell assembly theory of the action of the brain, using a large digital computer, *IRE Transactions, IT-2,* 80–93.

Rosenblatt, F. (1962). A comparison of several perception models. In M. C. Yovitts, G. T. Jacobi, & G. D. Goldstein (Eds.), *Self-organizing systems* (pp. 463–484). Washington, D.C.: Spartan Books.

Shaw, G. L., & Palm, G. (Eds.). (1988). *Brain theory reprint volume.* Singapore: World Scientific Press.

Shaw, G. L., Silverman, D. J., & Pearson, J. C. (1985). Model of cortical organization embodying a basis for a theory of information processing and memory recall. *Proceedings of the National Academy of Sciences USA, 82,* 2364–2368.

Shaw, G. L., & Vasudevan, R. (1974). Persistent states of neural networks and the random nature of synaptic transmission. *Mathematical Biosciences, 21,* 207–218.

Turing, A. M. (1936). On computable numbers with an application to the entscheidungsproblem. *Proceedings of the London Mathematical Society, 42,* 230–265.

Uttley, A. M. (1962). Properties of plastic networks. *Biophysics Journal, 2* (Suppl.), 169–188.

von Neumann, J. (1956). Probabilistic logics and the synthesis of reliable organisms from unreliable components. In C. E. Shannon & J. McCarthy (Eds.), *Automata studies* (pp. 43–98). Princeton, N.J.: Princeton University Press.

Wilson, H. R., & Cowan, J. D. (1972) Excitatory and inhibitory interactions in localized populations of model neurons. *Biophysics Journal, 12,* 1–24.

15

Neural Networks: Test Tubes to Theorems

LEON N. COOPER
MARK F. BEAR
FORD F. EBNER
CHRISTOPHER SCOFIELD

When interest in neural networks revived around 1970, few people believed that such systems would ever be of any use. Computers worked too well; it was felt that they could be programmed to perform any desired task. But limitations of current computers in solving many problems involving difficult to define rules or complex pattern recognition now are widely recognized; if anything, expectations for neural networks may be too high. The problem is no longer to convince anyone that neural networks might be useful but rather to incorporate such networks into systems that solve real-world problems economically.

Neural networks are inspired by biological systems where large numbers of neurons, which individually function rather slowly and imperfectly, collectively perform tasks that even the largest computers have not been able to match. They are made of many relatively simple processors connected to one another by variable memory elements whose weights are adjusted by experience. They differ from the now standard Von Neumann computer in that they characteristically process information in a manner that is highly parallel rather than serial, and that they learn (memory element weights and thresholds are adjusted by experience) so that to a certain extent they can be said to program themselves. They differ from the usual artificial intelligence systems in that (since neural networks learn) the solution of real-world problems requires much less of the expensive and elaborate programming and knowledge engineering required for such artificial intelligence products as rule-based expert systems.

To properly function, neural networks must learn in order that vast arrays of memory elements (synapses) are assigned the proper strengths. A basic problem becomes how this learning occurs: how these synapses adjust their weights so that the resulting neural network shows the desired properties of memory storage and cognitive behavior.

306

The problem can be divided into two parts. First, what type of modification is required so that in the course of actual experience the neural network arrives at the desired state? The answer to this question can be illuminated by mathematical analysis of the evolution of neural networks using various learning hypotheses. The second part of this problem is to find experimental justification for any proposed modification algorithm. A question of extraordinary interest is: What are the biological mechanisms that underlie the nervous system modification that results in learning, memory storage, and eventually cognitive behavior?

One experimental model that appears to be well suited for the purpose of determining how neural networks modify is the cat visual cortex. The modification of visual cortical organization by sensory experience is recognized to be an important component of early postnatal development (Sherman & Spear, 1982). Although much modifiability disappears after the first few months of life, some of the underlying mechanisms are likely to be conserved in adulthood to provide a basis for learning and memory. We have approached the problem of experience-dependent synaptic modification by determining theoretically what is required of a mechanism in order to account for the experimental observations in visual cortex. This process has led to the formulation of hypotheses, many of which are testable with currently available techniques. In this chapter we illustrate how the interaction between theory and experiment suggests a possible molecular mechanism for the experience-dependent modifications of functional circuitry in the mammalian visual cortex.

THE EXPERIMENTAL MODEL

Neurons in the primary visual cortex, area 17, of normal adult cats are sharply tuned for the orientation of an elongated slit of light and most are activated by stimulation of either eye (Hubel & Wiesel, 1962). Both of these properties—orientation selectivity and binocularity—depend on the type of visual environment experienced during a critical period of early postnatal development. We believe that the mechanisms underlying the experience-dependent modification of both receptive field properties are likely to be identical. However, for the sake of clarity, we concentrate primarily on the modification of binocular connections in striate cortex.

The majority of binocular neurons in the striate cortex of a normal adult cat do not respond with equal vigor to stimulation of either eye; instead they typically display an eye preference. To quantify this impression, Hubel and Wiesel (1962) originally separated the population of recorded neurons into seven ocular dominance (OD) categories. The OD distribution in a normal kitten or adult cat shows a broad peak at group 4, which reflects a high percentage of binocular neurons in area 17. This physiological assay of ocular dominance has proved to be an effective measure of the state of functional binocularity in the visual cortex.

Monocular deprivation (MD) during the critical period (extending from approximately 3 weeks to 3 months of age in the cat [Hubel & Wiesel, 1970]) has profound and reproducible effects on the functional connectivity of striate cortex. Brief periods of MD will result in a dramatic shift in the OD of cortical neurons such that most will be responsive exclusively to the open eye. The OD shift after MD is the best known and most intensively studied type of visual cortical plasticity.

When the MD is begun early in the critical period, the OD shift can be correlated with anatomically demonstrable differences in the geniculocortical axonal arbors of the two eyes (LeVay, Wiesel, & Hubel, 1980; Shatz & Stryker, 1978). However, MD initiated late in the critical period (Presson & Gordon, 1982) or after a period of rearing in the dark (Mower, Caplan, Christen, & Duffy, 1985) will induce clear changes in cortical OD without a corresponding anatomical change in the geniculocortical projection. Long-term recordings from awake animals also indicate that ocular dominance changes can be detected within a few hours of monocular experience, which seems too rapid to be explained by the formation or elimination of axon terminals. Moreover, deprived-eye responses in visual cortex may be restored within minutes under some conditions (such as during intracortical bicuculline administration (Duffy, Snodgrass, Burchfiel, & Conway, 1976]), which suggests that synapses deemed functionally "disconnected" are nonetheless physically present. Therefore, it is reasonable to assume that changes in function binocularity are explained not only by adjustments of the terminal arbors of geniculocortical axons, but also by changes in the efficacy of individual cortical synapses.

The consequences of binocular deprivation (BD) on visual cortex stand in striking contrast to those observed after MD. Whereas 7 days of MD during the second postnatal month leave few neurons in striate cortex responsive to stimulation of the deprived eye, most cells remain responsive to visual stimulation through either eye after a comparable period of BD (Wiesel & Hubel 1965, 1965). Thus it is not merely the absence of patterned activity in the deprived geniculocortical projection that causes the decrease in synaptic efficacy after MD.

Work over the past several years has led to a theoretical solution to the problem of visual cortical plasticity (Cooper, 1973). According to Cooper, Liberman, and Oja (1979), when a visual cortical neuron is depolarized beyond a "modification threshold," θ_M, synaptic efficacies change along lines envisaged by Hebb (1949). However, when the level of postsynaptic activity falls below θ_M, synaptic strengths decrease. Thus in this model the sign of a synaptic change is a function primarily of the level of postsynaptic activity. Analysis by Cooper et al. (1979) confirmed that such a modification scheme could lead to the development of selectivity that is appropriate for the input environment. However, these authors also noted that a fixed modification threshold leads to certain technical problems. For instance, if the postsynaptic response to *all* patterns of input activity slipped below θ_M (as might occur during binocular deprivation), then the efficacy of *all* synapses would decrease to zero. Bienenstock, Cooper, and Munro (1982) solved this problem by allowing the modification threshold to float as a function of the averaged activity of the cell. With this feature, the theory can successfully account for virtually all the types of modification that have been observed in kitten striate cortex since 1970. This theory is outlined in more detail in the next section; then we shall return to the question of possible mechanisms.

THEORETICAL ANALYSIS

Cortical neurons receive synaptic inputs from many sources. In layer IV of visual cortex the principal afferents are those from the lateral geniculate nucleus (LGN) and from other cortical neurons. This leads to a complex network that has been analyzed in several stages. In the first stage, consider a single neuron with inputs from both eyes (Fig. 15.1A). Here **d** represents the level of presynaptic geniculocortical axon activity, **m** the synaptic transfer function (synaptic strength or weight), and c the level of postsynaptic activity of the cortical neuron. The output of this neuron (in the linear region) can be written

$$c = \mathbf{m}^l \cdot \mathbf{d}^l + \mathbf{m}^r \cdot \mathbf{d}^r \qquad (1)$$

which means that the neuron firing rate (or dendritic depolarization) is the sum of the inputs from the left eye multiplied by the left-eye synaptic weights plus the inputs from the right eye multiplied by the right-eye synaptic weights. Thus the signals from the left and right eyes are integrated by the cortical neuron and determine its level of depolarization (output) at any instant.

The crucial question becomes: How does **m** change in time according to experience? According to Bienenstock et al. (1982), **m** modifies as a function of local, quasi-local, and golbal variables. Consider the synaptic weight of the jth synapse on a neuron, m_j (Fig. 15.1B). This synapse is affected by *local* variables in the form of information available only through the jth synapse, such as the presynaptic activity levels d and the efficacy of the synapse at a given instant in time mj (t). *Quasi-local* variables represent information that is available to the jth synapse through intracellular communication within the same cell. These include the instantaneous firing rate (or dendritic depolarization) of the cell c, the time-averaged firing rate $\bar{c}$, and the potentials generated at neighboring synaptic junctions $(dm)k,\ l,\ m,\ \dots$ Finally, *global* variables represent information that is available to a large number of cortical neurons, including the neuron receiving the jth synapse. These variables might include the presence or absence of "modulatory" neurotransmitters such as acetylcholine and norepinephrine.

We can delay consideration of the global variables by assuming that they act to render cortical synapses modifiable or nonmodifiable by experience. In the

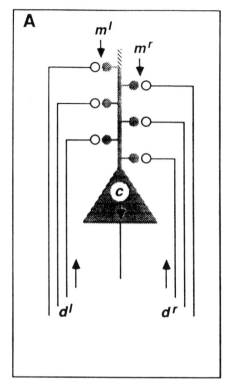
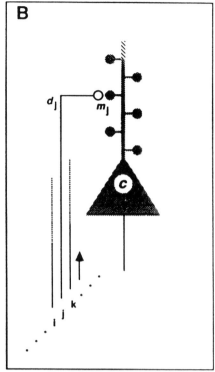

FIGURE 15.1.   Pyramidal shaped cortical neurons and the proximal segments of their apical dendrites. The shaded circles attached to the dendrites represent dendritic spines. (A) In the first stage of the theoretical analysis, we consider only the inputs to the cell from the lateral geniculate nucleus. The signals conveyed along these afferents arise from either the left retina (d^l) or the right retina (d^r) and are transferred to the cortical neuron by the synaptic junctions m^l and m^r. The output of the cortical neuron, as measured by the firing rate or the dendritic depolarization, is represented as c, which is the sum of $d^l \cdot m^l$ and $d^r \cdot m^r$. (B) The central question is how one of these afferent synapses, m_j, modifies in time as a function of both its level of presynaptic activity d_j and the level of postsynaptic depolarization.

"plastic state," the Bienenstock et al. algorithm for synaptic modification is written

$$dm_j/dt = \phi(c, \bar{c}) \, d_j \qquad (2)$$

so that the strength of the jth synaptic junction m_j changes its value in time as a function ϕ of the quasi-local states c and $\bar{c}$, and as a linear function of the local variable d_j. The crucial function, ϕ, is seen in Figure 15.2.

One significant feature of this model is the change of sign of ϕ at the modification threshhold, θ_M. When the input activity of the jth synapse d and ϕ are both concurrently greater than zero, then the sign of the synaptic modification is positive and the strength of the synapse increases; $\phi > 0$ when the output of the cell exceeds the modification threshold (this type of synaptic modification is "Hebbian"). When dj is positive and ϕ is less than zero, then the synaptic efficacy weakens; $\phi < 0$ when $c < \theta_M$. Thus "effective" synapses will be strengthened and "ineffective" synapses will be weakened, where synaptic effectiveness is determined by whether the presynaptic pattern of activity is accompanied by the simultaneous depolarization of the target dendrite beyond θ_M. Since the depolarization of the target cell beyond θ_M normally requires the synchronous

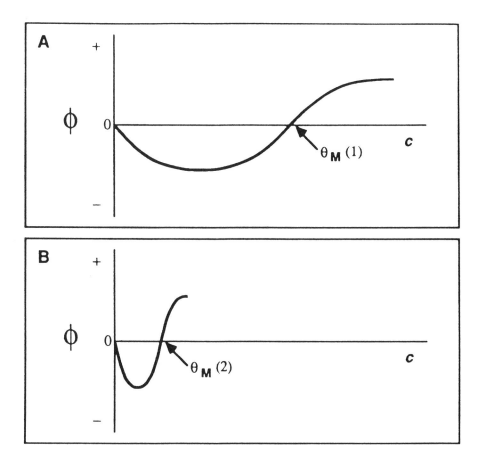

FIGURE 15.2.   The ϕ function at two values of the modification threshold θ_M. According to Bienenstock et al. (1982), active synapses ($d > 0$) are strengthened when ϕ is positive and are weakened when ϕ is negative. ϕ is positive when c, the postsynaptic depolarization, is greater than θ_M. The modification threshold, where ϕ changes sign, is a nonlinear function of the average activity of the postsynaptic neuron ($\bar{c}$). Hence in this example θ_M (1) would be expected when cortical neurons have experienced a normal visual environment (A) while $\theta_M(2)$ would result from a prolonged period of binocular deprivation (B).

activation of converging excitatory synapses, this type of modification will "associate" those synapses that are concurrently active by increasing their effectiveness together.

Another significant feature of this model is that the value of θ_M is not fixed but instead varies as a nonlinear function of the average output of the cell, c. In a simple situation

$$\theta_M = (c)^2 \qquad (3)$$

By allowing θ_M to vary with the average response in a faster-than-linear fashion, the response characteristics of a neuron evolve to maximum selectivity starting at any level within the range of the input environment. It is also this feature that provides the stability properties of the model so that, for instance, simultaneous presynaptic and postsynaptic activity at a continued high level does not continue to increase the synaptic strength.

Now consider the situation of reverse suture where the right, formerly open eye is closed and the left, formerly sutured eye is reopened. The output of a cortical neuron in area 17 approaches zero just after the reversal, since its only source of patterned input is through the eye whose synapses had been functionally disconnected as a consequence of the prior MD. However as c diminishes, so does the value of θ_M. Eventually the modification threshold attains a value below the small output that is evoked by the stimulation of the weak left-eye synapses. Now the efficacy of these "functionally disconnected" synapses will begin to increase because even their low response values exceed θ_M. As these synapses strengthen and the average output of the cell increases, θ_M again slides out until it overtakes the new left-eye response values. At the same time, the efficacy of the right-eye synapses continually decreases because their response values remain below the modification threshold. In its final stable state, the neuron is responsive only to the newly opened eye, and the maximum output to stimulation of this eye equals θ_M. One particular consequence is that if θ_M does not adjust to the new average firing rate too rapidly, in the course of the rearrangement of response, the cell's response to the previously open eye will diminish before its response to the newly opened eye increases.

Thus far the discussion has been limited to an idealized single neuron whose inputs arise only from the lateral geniculate nucleus. The second stage of the theoretical analysis requires that relevant intracortical connections be incorporated into the model (Cooper & Scofield, 1988). Input from other regions of cortex are considered part of a background excitation or inhibition contributing to the spontaneous activity of the cell. In addition, the various time delays that result in structure in the poststimulus time histogram are assumed to be integrated over periods of the order of a second for purposes of synaptic modification. This leads to a circuit as shown in Figure 15.3.

The output of the cells of the full network can be written

$$c = c^*(Md + Lc) \qquad (4)$$

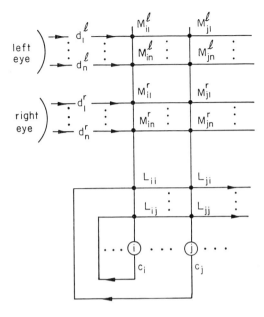

FIGURE 15.3. Network with inputs from left and right eyes, with LGN-cortical and corticocortical synapses.

where c^* is a sigmoidal response function,

$$c = (c_1 \dots c_N)^T \qquad (4a)$$

c_i is the output firing rate of the ith cortical cell, and

$$M = (M_{is}^l, M_{is}^r) \qquad (4b)$$

where M_{is}^l and M_{is}^r are the sth LGN "synapses" from the left and right eye to the ith cortical cell.

$$d = (d^l, d^r)^T \quad \text{and} \quad d_l^{l(r)} \dots d^{l(r)n})^T \qquad (4c)$$

are the time-averaged inputs from the left and right eye as described in Bienenstock, Cooper, and Munro (1982),

$$L = (L_{ij}) \qquad (4d)$$

is the matrix of cortico-cortical synapses and L_{ij} is the synapse from the jth cell to the ith cell. (Notice that italicized boldface symbols always contain left and right eye components.) In the monotonically increasing region above threshold and below saturation, in a linear approximation,

$$c = Md + Lc \qquad (5)$$

We consider a region of cortex for which the neural mapping of the input from the visual field is constant (all of the cells, in effect, look at a given region of the visual field). Under these conditions, for an input d constant in time, the equilibrium state of the network would be

$$c = (1 - L)^{-1}Md \tag{5a}$$

MEAN FIELD APPROXIMATION

For a given LGN–cortical vector of synapses m_i (the ith row of M) and for a given input from both eyes d, Eq. 5 for the firing rate of the ith cortical cell becomes

$$c_i = m_i d + \sum_j L_{ij} c_j \tag{5b}$$

where the first term is due to the input from LGN and the second due to input from other cortical cells. We define $\bar{c}$ as the spatially averaged firing rate of all of the cortical cells in the region defined above:

$$\bar{c} = \frac{1}{N} \sum_i c_i \tag{6}$$

The mean field approximation is obtained by replacing c_j in the sum in Eq. 5 by its average value, so that c_i becomes

$$c_i = m_i d + \bar{c} \sum_j L_{ij} \tag{7}$$

Here, in a manner similar to that in the theory of magnetism, we have replaced the effect of individual cortical cells by their average effect (as though all other cortical cells can be replaced by an "effective" cell). It follows that

$$\bar{c} = \overline{m}d + \bar{c}L_0 = (1 - L_0)^{-1}\overline{m}d \tag{7a}$$

where

$$\overline{m} = \frac{1}{N} \sum_i m_i \tag{8}$$

and

$$L_0 = \frac{1}{N} \sum_{ij} L_{ij}$$

so that

$$c_i = \left[m_i + \left(\frac{\sum_j L_{ij}}{1 - L_0} \right) \overline{m} \right] d$$

If we assume that the lateral connection strengths are a function of $i - j$ only (not dependent on the absolute position of a cell in the network, therefore dependent only on the distance of two cells from one another), L_{ij} becomes a circular matrix so that

$$\sum_i L_{ij} = \sum_j L_{ij} = L_0 = \text{constant} \tag{9}$$

and

$$c_i = \left[m_i + \left(\frac{L_0}{1 - L_0} \right) \overline{m} \right] d \tag{10}$$

In the mean field approximation we can therefore write

$$c_i(\alpha) = (m_i - \alpha)d = (m_i^l - \alpha^l) \cdot d^l + (m_i^r - \alpha^r) \cdot d^r \tag{11}$$

where the mean field

$$\alpha = (\alpha^l, \alpha^r) = -a(\overline{m}^l, \overline{m}^r) \tag{12}$$

with

$$a = |L_0|(1 + |L_0|)^{-1} \tag{12a}$$

and we assume that $L_0 \leq 0$ (the network is, on average, inhibitory).

THE CORTICAL NETWORK

The behavior of visual cortical cells in various rearing conditions suggests that some cells respond more rapidly to environmental changes than others. In monocular deprivation, for example, some cells remain responsive to the closed eye in spite of the very large shift of most cells to the open eye. Singer (1977) found, using intracellular recording, that geniculo-cortical synapses on inhibitory interneurons are more resistant to monocular deprivation than are synapses on pyramidal cell dendrites. In dark rearing some cells become nonresponsive to visual stimuli, although most cells retain some responsiveness (Sherman & Spear, 1982). Recent work suggests that the density of inhibitory GABAergic synapses in kitten striate cortex is also unaffected by MD during the critical period (Bear, Schmechel, & Ebner, 1985; Mower, White, & Rustad, 1986).

These results suggest that some LGN cortical synapses modify rapidly, whereas others modify relatively slowly, with slow modification of some cortico-cortical synapses. Excitatory LGN cortical synapses onto excitatory cells may be those that modify primarily. (Since these synapses are formed exclusively on dendritic spines, this raises the possibility that the mechanisms underlying synaptic modification exist primarily in axospinous synapses.) To embody these facts we introduce two types of LGN cortical synapses: those (m_i) that modify (according to the modification rule discussed in Bienenstock et al., 1982) and those (z_k) that remain relatively constant. In a simple limit we have

$$\dot{m}_i = \phi(c_i, \bar{\bar{c}}_i)d \quad \text{and} \quad \dot{z}_k = 0 \tag{13}$$

where c denotes the spatial average over cortical cells, and $\bar{\bar{c}}_i$ denotes the time-averaged activity of the ith cortical cell. The function ϕ appears in Figure 15.2. We assume for simplicity, and consistent with the foregoing physiological interpretation, that these two types of synapses are confined to two different classes of cells and that both left and right eye have similar synapses (both m_i or both z_k) on a given cell. We therefore can write

$$c_i = m_i d + \sum_j L_{ij} c_j \quad \text{and} \quad c_k = z_k d + \sum_j L_{kj} c_j \tag{14}$$

Further, in what follows, we assume for maximum simplicity that there is no modification of cortico-cortical synapses, although experimental results suggest only that modification of inhibitory cortico-cortical synapses is slow (Bear et al., 1985; Mower et al., 1986). The consequences of a theory including cortico-cortical synapse modification for the full network was briefly discussed in Bienenstock et al (1982) and will be discussed more fully in the mean field approximation elsewhere.

In a cortical network with modifiable and nonmodifiable LGN cortical synapses and nonmodifiable cortico-cortical synapses, the synaptic evolution equations become

$$\dot{m}_i = \phi(c_i, \bar{\bar{c}}_i)d, \quad \dot{z}_k = 0, \quad \text{and} \quad \dot{L}_{ij} = 0 \tag{15}$$

This leads to a very complex set of coupled nonlinear stochastic evolution equations that have been simulated and partially analyzed by Cooper and Scofield (1988). The mean field approximation permits dramatic simplification of these equations, leading to analytic results and a fairly transparent understanding of their consequences in various conditions. In this approximation Eqs. 14 become

$$c_i = m_i d + L_0 \bar{c} \quad \text{and} \quad c_k = z_k d + L_0 \bar{c} \tag{16}$$

So that we can now write

$$c_i(\alpha) = (m_i - \alpha)d = (m_i^l - \alpha^l) \cdot d^l + (m_i^r - \alpha^r) \cdot d^r$$

and

$$c_k(\alpha) = (z_k - \alpha)d = (z_k^l - \alpha^l) \cdot d^l + (z_k^r - \alpha^r) \cdot d^r \tag{17}$$

where $\alpha^{l(r)}$ contains terms from modifiable and nonmodifiable synapses:

$$\alpha^{l(r)} = a(\overline{m}^{l(r)} + \overline{z}^{l(r)}), \ \overline{m}^{l(r)} = N^{-1} \sum_{i=1}^{N_m} m_i^{l(r)}, \ \overline{z}^{l(r)} = N^{-1} \sum_{k=1}^{N_{nm}} z_k^{l(r)} \quad (18)$$

and a is defined in Eq. 12a. ($N = N_m + N_{nm}$, where N_m is the number of cells with modifiable synapses and N_{nm} is the number of cells with nonmodifiable synapses.) Since it is assumed that neither L nor z changes as the network evolves, only $\overline{m}^{l(r)}$ is time dependent.

Having defined a mean field approximation that greatly simplifies the equations for the response and evolution of cortical cells, we have obtained a fundamental result: the stability and position of the fixed points in this network are related to the fixed points in the absence of mean field ($\alpha^{l(r)} = 0$) by

$$m_i^*(\alpha) = m_i^*(0) + \alpha \quad (19)$$

where $m_i^* (\alpha)$ is a fixed point of Eq. 15 in the mean field α and $m_i^* (0)$ is a fixed point of this equation in zero mean field.

Thus if $m_i^* (\alpha)$ is restricted to the first quadrant (positive values for all of its components due to the excitatory nature of LGN cortical synapses), as long as α is large enough and nonspecific (there is sufficient inhibition for all pattern inputs), $m_i(\alpha)$ can still reach all of the fixed points that would have been reached by $m_i(0)$ (not restricted to the first quadrant). This means that if network inhibition is sufficient, the selective stable fixed points can be reached even though LGN cortical synapses are excitatory. Once reached, the fixed points $m_i^*(\alpha)$ have the same stability characteristics as the corresponding $m_i^*(0)$.

We find, consistent with previous theory and with experiment, that most learning can occur in the LGN cortical synapses; inhibitory (cortico-cortical) synapses need not modify and some nonmodifiable LGN cortical synapses are required. It becomes useful to know whether these could be associated with some anatomical feature. (E.g., might these be synapses into shafts rather than spines?)

As in the zero mean field theory, zero cell output is an unstable fixed point. Thus in binocular deprivation the cell output could be on average above or below spontaneous activity (depending on the level of inhibition). Some "nonvisual" cells would reappear if excitation were enhanced or inhibition diminished.

In monocular deprivation the closed-eye response goes to

$$c = (x - \alpha) \cdot d \rightarrow 0 \quad (20)$$

Therefore, LGN cortical synapses do not go to zero. Rather

$$x \rightarrow \alpha \quad (21)$$

Thus if inhibition is suppressed, one would expect some response from the closed eye. This is in agreement with experiment.

A POSSIBLE PHYSIOLOGICAL MECHANISM

One of the consequences of the network theory discussed in the previous section is that the experimental results obtained in visual cortex over the last generation can be explained by modification of excitatory synapses, with minimal changes in intracortical inhibition. The balance of available experimental evidence supports this conclusion. For example, using intracellular recording Singer (1977) found that geniculocortical synapses on inhibitory interneurons are more resistant to monocular deprivation than are synapses on pyramidal cell dendrites. And recent work suggests that the density of inhibitory GABAergic synapses in kitten striate cortex is also unaffected by MD during the critical period (Bear et al., 1985). Taken together, these theoretical and experimental results indicate that the search for mechanisms should be focused on the excitatory synapses that impinge on excitatory cells in visual cortex. Interestingly, this type of synapse is formed exclusively on dendritic spines, a feature that distinguishes it from other types of cortical synapse (Colonier, 1981). This suggests that experience-dependent modifications in striate cortex occur primarily at axospinous synapses.

What mechanisms support the experience-dependent modification of axospinous synapses? Recall that, according to the theory, when the postsynaptic cell is depolarized beyond the modification threshold θ_M, active synapses will be strengthened. Depolarization beyond θ_M minimally requires the synchronous activation of converging excitatory afferents. When postsynaptic activity fails to reach θ_M, the active synapses will be weakened. The identification of the physiological basis of θ_M is therefore central to an understanding of the modification mechanism.

Work on long-term potentiation (LTP) in the hippocampal slice preparation has provided an important insight into the nature of the modification threshold that may be applicable to the visual cortex. LTP is a long-lasting increase in the synaptic strength of excitatory afferents that have been tetanically stimulated. The induction of LTP depends on the coactivation of converging excitatory afferents (input cooperativity [McNaughton, Douglas, & Goddard, 1978]), the depolarization of the postsynaptic neuron (Kelso, Ganong, & Brown, 1986), the activation of NMDA receptors (Collingridge, Kehl, & McLennan, 1983; Harris, Ganong, & Cotman, 1984), and the postsynaptic entry of calcium ions (Lynch, Larson, Kelso, Barrionuevo, & Schottler, 1983). A current working hypothesis is that the synchronous tetanic activation of converging afferents depolarizes the target dendrite beyond the threshold for postsynaptic Ca^{2+} entry through gates linked to the NMDA receptor (Wigstrom & Gustafsson, 1985). Elevated dendritic calcium then triggers the intracellular changes that lead to enhanced synaptic efficacy (Lynch & Baudry, 1984).

NMDA receptors are a subclass of excitatory amino acid receptor, and glutamic acid or a closely related substance is thought to be the transmitter of excitatory axospinous synapses at many locations in the forebrain (Cotman, Foster, & Lanthorn, 1981). These receptors are widely distributed in the cerebral cortex, including the visual areas (Monaghan & Cotman, 1984). It appears that NMDA receptors normally coexist postsynaptically with quisqualate and/or kainate receptors (Foster & Fagg, 1985). The "non-NMDA" receptors are thought to mediate the classical excitatory postsynaptic potential that normally results from electrical stimulation of axospinous synapses. NMDA receptors, on the contrary, appear to be linked to a membrane channel that will pass calcium ions. Dingledine (1983) first reported that NMDA receptor activation leads to calcium flux only when the cell is concurrently depolarized. This is apparently due to a blockage of the NMDA channel by Mg^{2+} ions, which is alleviated only when the membrane is depolarized sufficiently (Nowak, Bregostovski, Ascher, Herbert, & Prochiantz, 1984). Thus calcium entry through channels linked to the NMDA receptor could specially signal presynaptic and postsynaptic coactivation.

Recently Kleinschmidt, Bear, and Singer (1987) obtained results suggesting that NMDA receptor–mediated Ca^{2+} entry also contributes to the synapse modifications that underlie ocular dominance plasticity in striate cortex. Specifically, they found that intracortical infusion of 2-amino-5-phosphonovaleric acid (APV), a selective antagonist of the NMDA receptor (Watkins & Evans, 1981), prevents the ocular dominance shift that would normally occur after MD. Moreover, this pharmacological treatment also resulted in a striking loss of orientation selectivity.

Our theoretical analyses lead us to suggest the following:

1. θ_M is linked to the membrane potential at which NMDA receptor activation by sensory fiber activity results in dendritic calcium entry.
2. Increased calcium flux across the dendritic spine membrane results specifically in an increase in the synaptic gain.
3. Activated synapses accompanied by no postsynaptic calcium signals will be weakened over time.
4. The membrane potential at which Ca^{2+} enters through NMDA channels or the efficacy of the entering Ca^{2+} in producing synaptic enhancement should vary depending on the history of prior cell activity.

This physiological model is consistent with the Bienenstock, Cooper, and Munro (1982) theory. According to the model, the value and sign of ϕ is linked to the calcium ion movement into dendritic spines. Synaptic efficacy will increase when presynaptic activity evokes a large postsynaptic calcium signal ($\phi > 0$). This will occur only when the membrane potential exceeds the level required to open the NMDA receptor–activated calcium channels ($c > \theta_M$). When the amplitude of the evoked Ca^{2+} signal falls below a certain critical level, corresponding to $\phi = 0$ and $c = \theta_M$, then active synapses will be weakened over time. Application of an NMDA receptor blocker theoretically would increase the value of θ_M, such that it would take a greater level of depolarization to achieve the critical calcium concentration. In accordance with the experimental observations of Kleinschmidt et al. (1987), the theoretical consequence would be a loss of orientation selectivity and a prevention of ocular dominance plasticity.

This model makes some explicit predictions about the regulation of the calcium messenger system that is linked to the NMDA receptors on cortical dendrites. Recall that θ_M depends on the average activity of the cell. If the average activity decreases, as it does during binocular deprivation, then θ_M decreases, and it should take less dendritic depolarization to maintain synaptic efficacy. One way this could occur in our model would be to alter the voltage or transmitter sensitivity of the NMDA receptors with the result that less synaptic activity (depolarization) would be required to evoke the necessary calcium signal. It is well documented that receptor supersensitivity occurs as a consequence of postsynaptic inactivity at many locations in the nervous system (Cannon & Rosenblueth, 1949). Alternatively, a weak calcium signal could be amplified at points further downstream, for example, by increasing the activity or genetic expression of calcium-activated enzymes.

CONCLUSIONS

We have presented an algorithm for synaptic modification that reproduces classical experimental results in visual cortex. These include the relation of cell tuning and response to various visual environments experienced during the critical period: normal rearing, binocular deprivation, monocular deprivation, and reverse suture. A molecular model for this form of modification has been proposed based on the NMDA receptors. In this model the Bienenstock et al. (1982) modification threshold θ_M is linked with the voltage-dependent unblocking of the NMDA receptor channels. A consequence of this relationship is that the membrane potential at which Ca^{2+} enters through NMDA channels or the efficacy of the entering Ca^{2+} in producing synaptic enhancement should vary depending on the history of prior cell activity.

Stated in this language, many interesting questions are generated: How long does it take θ_M to adjust to a new average firing rate? What is the molecular basis for this adjustment? How do the putative global modulators of cortical plasticity, such as acetylcholine and norepinephrine, interact with the second-messenger systems linked to NMDA receptors on cortical dendrites? Can we provide direct evidence that those cells that modify are or are not those acted on by the modulators? Are the known morphological features of dendritic spines causally related to the modifiability of synaptic strength? Do the same rules apply to reorganization in adults and in the developmental period?

There has been much discussion in recent years about possible modification of synapses between neurons as the physiological basis of learning and memory storage. Molecular models for learning at the single-synapse level have been presented, various learning algorithms have been proposed that show some indication of appropriate behavior, and a mathematical structure for networks of neurons is rapidly evolving. We have begun a concerted effort to unite these approaches, and we believe that the close interaction between theory and experiment has greatly enriched both endeavors. Theory has been anchored to experimental observations and experiments have been focused onto those issues most relevant to sorting out the various possible hypotheses. Further, this interaction has enabled us to pose new questions with precision and clarity.

Acknowledgment

This work was supported in part by the Office of Naval Research Accelerated Research Initiative on Learning and Memory.

REFERENCES

Andersen, P. O. (1987). Long term potentiation: Outstanding problems. In J.-P. Changeux & M. Konishi (Eds.), *The neural and molecular bases of learning.* (pp. 239–262). New York: Wiley.

Bear, M. F., Schmechel, D. M., & Ebner F. F. (1985). Glutamic acid decarboxylase in the striate cortex of normal and monocularly deprived kittens. *Journal of Neuroscience, 5,* 1262–1275.

Bienenstock, R. L., Cooper, L. N., & Munro, P. W. (1982). Theory for the development of neuron selectivity: Orientation specificity and binocular interaction in visual cortex. *Journal of Neuroscience, 2,* 32–48.

Bliss, T. V. P., & Lomo, T. (1973). Long-lasting potentiation of synaptic transmission in the dentate area of the anaesthetized rabbit following stimulation of the perforant path. *Journal of Physiology (London), 232,* 331.

Cannon, W. B., & Rosenblueth, A. (1949). *The supersensitivity of denervated structures.* New York: Macmillan.

Collingridge, G. L., Kehl, S. L., & McLennan, H. (1983). Excitatory amino acids in synaptic transmission in the Schaffer collateral–commisural pathway of the rat hippocampus. *Journal of Physiology, 334,* 33–46.

Colonier, M. (1981). The electron-microscope analysis of the neuronal organization of the cerebral cortex. In F. O. Schmitt, F. G. Worden, G. Adelman, S. G. Dennis (Eds.), *The organization of the cerebral cortex* (pp. 125–152). Cambridge, Mass.: MIT Press.

Cooper, L. N. (1973). A possible organization of animal memory and learning. In B. Lindquist & S. Lindquist (Eds.), *Proceedings of the Nobel symposium on collective properties of physical systems* (Vol. 24, pp. 252–264). New York: Academic Press.

Cooper, L. N., Liberman, F., & Oja, E. (1979). A theory for the acquisition and loss of neuron specificity in visual cortex. *Biological Cybernetics, 33,* 9–28.

Cooper, L. N., & Scofield, C. (1988). Mean field approximation in neural networks, *Proceedings of the National Academy of Sciences USA, 85,* 1973–1977.

Cotman, C. W., Foster, A., & Lanthorn, T. (1981). In G. DiChiara & G. Gessa (Eds.), *Glutamate as a neurotransmitter* (pp. 1–27). New York: Raven.

Dingledine, R. (1983). N-methylaspartate activates voltage-dependent calcium conductance in rat hippocampal pyramidal cells. *Journal of Physiology, 343,* 385–405.

Duffy, F. H., Snodgrass, S. R., Burchfiel, J. L., & Conway, J. L. (1976). Bicuculline reversal of deprivation amblyopia in the cat. *Nature, 260,* 256–257.

Foster, A. C., & Fagg, G. E. (1985). Amino acid binding sites in mammalian neuronal membranes: Their characteristics and relationship to synaptic receptors. *Brain Research Review, 7,* 103.

Harris, E. W., Ganong, A. H., & Cotman, C. W. (1984). Long-term potentiation involves activation of N-methyl-D-aspartate receptors. *Brain Research, 232,* 132–137.

Hebb, D. O. (1949). *The organization of behavior.* New York: Wiley.

Hubel, D. H., & Wiesel, T. N. (1962). Receptive fields, binocular interactions and functional architecture in the cat's visual cortex. *Journal of Physiology (London), 160,* 106–154.

Hubel, D. H., & Wiesel, T. N. (1970). The period of susceptibility to the physiological effects of unilateral eye closure in kittens. *Journal of Physiology, 206,* 419–436.

Kelso, S. R., Ganong, A. H., & Brown, T. H. (1986). Hebbian synapses in hippocampus. *Proceedings of National Academy Science, USA, 83,* 5326 (1986).

Kleinschmidt, A., Bear, M. F., & Singer, W. (1987). Blockade of "NMDA" receptors disrupts experience-dependent plasticity of kitten striate cortex. *Science, 238,* 355–358.

LeVay, S., Wiesel, T. N., & Hubel, D. H. (1980). The development of ocular dominance columns in normal and visually deprived monkeys. *Journal of Comparative Neurology, 191,* 1–52.

Lømo, T. (1966). Frequency potentiation of excitatory synaptic activity in the dentate area of the hippocampal formation. *Acta Physiologica Scandinavica, 68* (Suppl. 277), 128.

Lynch, G., & Baudry, M. (1984). The biochemistry of memory: A new and specific hypothesis. *Science, 224,* 1057–1063.

Lynch, G., Larson, J., Kelso, S., Barrionuevo, S., Schottler, F. Intracellular injections of EGTA block induction of hippocampal long-term potentiation. (1983). *Nature (London), 305,* 719.

McNaughton, B. L., Doughlas, R. M., & Goddard, G. V. (1978). Synaptic enhancement in fascia dentata: Cooperativity among coactive afferents. *Brain Research, 157,* 277.

Monaghan, D. T., & Cotman, C. W. (1984). Distribution of N-methyl-D-aspartate–sensitive L-[^{3}H] glutamate binding sites in rat brain, *Journal of Neuroscience, 11,* 2909–2919.

Mower, G. D., Caplan, C. J., Christen, W. G., & Duffy, F. H. (1985). Dark rearing prolongs physiological but not anatomical plasticity of the cat visual cortex. *Journal of Comparative Neurology, 235,* 448–466.

Mower, G. D., White, W. F., & Rustad, R. (1986). [^{3}H] Muscimol binding of GABA receptors in the visual cortex of normal and monocularly deprived cats. *Brain Research, 380,* 253–260.

Nicholls, D. G., & Sihra, T. S. (1986). Synaptosomes possess an exocytotic pool of glutamate. *Nature (London), 321,* 772–773.

Nowak, L., Bregostovski, P., Ascher, A., Herbert, A., & Prochiantz, A. (1984). Magnesium gates glutamate-activated channels in mouse central neurones. *Nature (London), 307,* 462–465.

Presson, J., & Gordon, B. (1982). The effects of monocular deprivation on the physiology and anatomy of the kitten's visual system. *Society of Neuroscience Abstracts, 8,* 5–10.

Shatz, C. J., & Stryker, M. P. (1978). Ocular dominance in layer IV of the cat's visual cortex and the effects of monocular deprivation. *Journal of Physiology, 281,* 267–283.

Sherman, S. M., & Spear, P. D. (1982). Organization in visual pathways in normal and visually deprived cats. *Physiological Review, 62,* 738–855.

Singer, W. (1977). Effects of monocular deprivation on excitatory and inhibitory pathways in cat striate cortex. *Experimental Brain Research, 134,* 508–518.

Watkins, J. C., & Evans, R. H. (1981). Excitatory amino acid transmitters. *Annual Review of Pharmacology and Toxicology, 21,* 165–204.

Wiesel, T. N., & Hubel, D. H. (1965). Comparison of the effects of unilateral and bilateral eye closure on cortical unit responses in kittens. *Journal of Neurophysiology, 28,* 1029–1040.

Wigstrom, H., & Gustafsson, B. (1985). *Acta Physiologica Scandinavica, 123,* 59.

16

Notes on Neural Computing and Associative Memory

TEUVO KOHONEN

There is no doubt that the brain consists of discrete operational units (cells or cell groups) that are selectively activated to perform specific functions. Another salient feature is the vast number of feedback loops of local as well as global scale, which gives rise to various kinds of collective effects. A further indisputable fact is that the interconnections (the structures and/or strengths) are adaptive, a property without which learning would be impossible. Any remaining discrepancies then concern the conceptualization and characterization of these properties.

Consider the issue of localization of neural functions. I doubt whether anybody, at least nowadays, wants to suggest that the mental processes are derivable from the intrinsic properties of the neural tissue, or that, for instance, the neural matters of the left and right hemispheres are different, although they respond differently in mental tasks. The specialization of functions results partly from different input and partly from the computations made thereby. The coarse localization of computing functions in sensory, motor, and associative areas may result from the most probable course of ontogenesis in which these functions are specialized, whereas, for instance, in hydrocephalic patients, other parts of the cell mass have become responsible for the same functions. This seems to show that a particular type of localization represents one possible stable state in the developmental process. After that, however, any neural network organization must rely on its components, which are consolidated and confined to some places.

The main difficulties in understanding seem to arise from the fact that in a collectively operating system, the spatial distribution of the activities of the units may vary (temporally, even for constant-stimulus conditions), whereas the material components need not move anywhere from their place. Unless the distinction between function and activity is made, the nature of the internal representations in the brain will remain obscure.

A high-level function that seems to be very difficult to conceptualize and concretize is memory, especially associative memory. Depending on the scientific paradigm, one may thereby understand (1) basic (adaptive, distributed) memory mechanisms, (2) adaptive transformations of signals in a neural network, (3) detailed representations ("coding") of information that are actually stored, (4) dynamic processes or temporal recollections that are synthesized in such a feedback system referring to a global scale, (5) the semantic content and relations between the representations stored in memory, or (6) possibly other aspects. In the scientific tradition, especially in the explanation of basic mechanisms, one has to concentrate on one aspect at a time; if the phenomena are then studied in reduced form, simplification is necessary to quantify the processes, although any claim that the basic models do not explain general mental effects would be unjustified.

This chapter begins with the categorization of neural models, and simple structures and system equations for some of them are suggested. This is followed by an example of a collective effect which shows that neural activity can be localized in a discrete place while neural functions are not; this effect is utilized in self-organization. After that, one possibility for the formation of internal representations is devised. The associative memory connections and associative recall of signal patterns can thereby be related to these representations. Finally, a few issues concerning the extension of modeling to other aspects of the neural functions are considered.

CATEGORIZATION OF NEURAL MODELS

It is obvious that the main purpose of the nervous system is to monitor and control the living conditions of the organism relative to its environment. In other words, sensory functions and motor control are the most basic tasks implemented in all species. In higher animals, including humans, some kind of logic inference and decision making must be involved with sensory and intellectual tasks, but one important question is whether these operations occur at every neuron and in the lowest level neural networks. I am inclined to believe that such inference and decision operations do not result until collective actions in rather large (hierarchical) assemblies of neurons have been realized at the last stages of phylogenesis; at least these are not the functions with which the study of the neural networks should be started.

In an attempt to qualify the basic theoretical models set up to explain the operations of the nervous system, it may be necessary to consider them describing functions at different levels of organization and abstraction. First of all, one may distinguish the following categories of models:

1. *Neuronal-level (decoupled) models,* where the most careful studies concentrate on the dynamic and adaptive properties of each neuron, in order to describe the neuron as a unit that gives selective responses to patterns and has some elementary control and memory functions.
2. *Network-level models,* where identical neurons are interconnected to exhibit

one of the following functions in idealized form: filter function (e.g., projection operator, optimal estimator, or associative memory) or nonlinear feedback, which makes the system activity converge to one of its eigenstates. Because these models are computationally heavier, they must apply simplified neuronal-level models for their basic units and concentrate on the description of the basic collective effects.

3. *Nervous system–level (organizational) models,* in which usually two or more networks of type 2 with different properties are combined to demonstrate more complex or abstract functions of sensory perception, such as automatic classification, concept formation, motor functions, or global stability control. The latter is an important aspect, because the overall system must be kept in a globally stable state all the time, but it must on demand exhibit the control functions identifiable as attention, priming, and other psychological effects. The primary objective is to study more qualified systemic phenomena than those mentioned above.

4. *Mental operation–level models,* which are the most abstract models, usually describing operations, procedures, algorithms, and strategies on the so-called human information processing level. These models are meant to describe the basic processes of cognition, thinking, problem-solving, and the like, and they are very closely related to the approaches made in artificial intelligence research.

STRUCTURES AND FUNCTIONS OF SOME BASIC NEURAL NETWORKS

Elementary Network Structures

The basic structure in most neural networks is the crossbar switch (Fig. 16.1a), which is formed when a bundle of axons or their branches pierces the dendritic trees of a set of neurons and makes synaptic connections with them. The next development of neural functions results from lateral feedback (Fig. 16.1b). This kind of connectivity has long been known in neuroanatomy. Many interesting neural functions are derivable from its behavior, as discussed later in more detail.

In an attempt to devise theoretical operation modules for neural systems, it was found by the mid-1970s that it is useful to define the basic network structure containing adaptive crossbars at input as well as for feedback (Fig. 16.2; see also Kohonen, 1984; Kohonen, Lehtiö, & Rovamo, 1974).

The most natural topology of the network is two-dimensional (Fig. 16.2 shows only a one-dimensional section for simplicity), and the distribution of lateral feedbacks within this subsystem is the same around every neuron; however, the distribution of the interconnections could strongly depend on the distance between two points in the network. Within an artificial module, all unit neurons could receive the same set of input signals in parallel. Effects similar to those

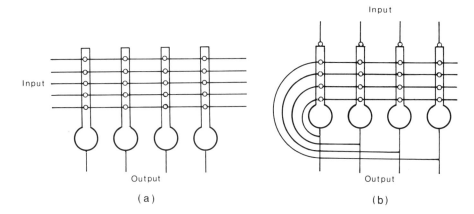

FIGURE 16.1.   Elementary neural network structures. (a) Crossbar switch. (b) Complete feedback matrix; input one-to-one to the neurons.

described below are demonstrable, although the input connections are more random and incomplete. None of these simplifying assumptions is unnatural, however, even when relating to biological structures.

Functional Laws

The system equations for one module of Figure 16.2 may be written in the following general way:

$$dy/dt = f(x, y, M, N) \tag{1a}$$
$$dM/dt = g(x, y, M) \tag{1b}$$
$$dN/dt = h(y, N) \tag{1c}$$

Here x is the vector of all external inputs to the module, y the vector of all output activities, and M and N are two (adaptive) connectivity matrices, respectively. In biological systems, Eq. 1a might be called the relaxation equation, and its time constants are small, on the order of 10 msec; y describes electrical activities, and among other things involves the effect of diffusion of light ions. Equations 1b and 1c have much larger time constants, say, weeks, because M and N describe changes in proteins, other macromolecules, and anatomical structures. Both of these equations are adaptation equations; Eq. 1c further seems to describe the basic function of associative memory.

The transfer properties of individual biological neurons should actually be derived from the so-called membrane-triggering equations. Even in simplified form, physical description of an active cell membrane may contain about two dozen process variables and 15 parameters. Based on certain simplifying arguments, I suggested (Kohonen, 1984) the following differential equation for the electrical activity (average triggering frequency) η_i of neuron i:

$$d\eta_i/dt = \sum_{j=1}^{n} \varphi_{ij}(\xi_{ij}) - \gamma_i(\eta_i) \tag{2}$$

where ξ_{ij} is the activity at the input j of cell i, and $\varphi_{ij}(\xi_{ij})$ represents the effect of input on membrane potential, and thereby on output activity too; $\gamma_i(\eta_i)$ is a non-linear loss term which combines all refractory time, leakage, shunting, and saturation effects taking place at the membranes. The steady-state solution derived from Eq. 2 will then lead to the popular static relation between the signals, called the sigmoidal function $\sigma(\cdot)$. If the synaptic control effects were then linearized, we would have for one type of modeling equation

$$\eta_i = \sigma\left(\sum_{j=1}^{n} \mu_{ij}\xi_{ij} - \theta_i\right) \tag{3}$$

where σ has two saturation limits and θ_i is an offset parameter, often termed "threshold". The μ_{ij} correspond to synaptic efficacies.

For the adaptation equations, a simple but nonetheless theoretically very influential equation could then read (Kohonen, 1984)

$$d\mu_{ij}/dt = \alpha\eta_i\xi_{ij} - \beta(\eta_i)\mu_{ij} \tag{4}$$

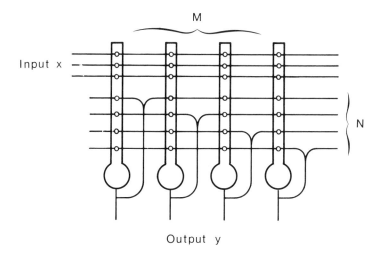

FIGURE 16.2. Operational neural module.

where the first term on the right corresponds to the classical law of Hebb (1949) widely used in modeling, α is a positive constant, and $\beta(\eta_i)$ a scalar function of η_i, with certain rather mild restrictions (e.g., the constant term in its Taylor expansion must be zero). The second term represents active forgetting, being nonzero only for nonzero η_i. This term seems to be necessary to prevent the synaptic strengths increasing monotonically with use, which would soon lead to an inoperative state. The form of this term may be justified in different ways. Active forgetting, of course, would be a natural physical effect caused by, say, turnover of the molecules that are responsible for synaptic efficacy; proportionality to cell activity is a natural feature since the chemical reactions may be facilitated or strongly enhanced at the triggering of the cell. One may notice that an essentially similar form for Eq. 4 results if it is assumed that the synapses compete on postsynaptic resources.

Some experimental evidence for the particular form of Eq. 4 also exists. For instance, Levy and Burger (1987) showed by hippocampal recordings that no changes in synaptic efficacies occur at zero postsynaptic activity; the efficacies are increased at high simultaneous presynaptic and postsynaptic activities and decreased at low presynaptic activity coinciding with high postsynaptic activity.

DYNAMIC LOCALIZATION OF ACTIVITY IN A DISTRIBUTED FEEDBACK NETWORK

The response from a neural network to external stimuli, although seemingly localized at a particular neuron, is actually defined by rather complicated collective interactions resulting from abundant feedback connections. There are many kinds of coupling in nervous systems, but it seems that a commonplace type of local interaction between neighboring neurons is one whereby the closest neighbors (say, up to a distance of 0.5 mm) excite each other, and the neighbors at a somewhat longer distance (say, 1 to 2 mm) inhibit each other, respectively. In the first approximation, interactions beyond this range may be ignored. This type of local interaction is frequently termed the "Mexican hat function." It will first be shown that such a network tends to concentrate its activity into local clusters, "bubbles," and the locations of such bubbles depend on the external signals in a particular way; the signals need not be spatially localized.

Consider again Figure 16.2 in which the ξ_j are components of vector x, η_i are components of vector y, and μ_{ki} are elements of matrix M. The relaxation equation is written in the form

$$d\eta_i/dt = I_i + \sum_{k=1}^{K} \mu_{ki}\eta_k - \gamma_i(\eta_i), \qquad \eta_i \geq 0 \qquad (5)$$

where I_i is the net control effect of all external inputs to cell i, μ_{ki} the interconnection strength or kernel between cells k and i, K the number of cells, and γ_i the nonlinear loss term. We take $\mu_{ki} = \mu(|k - i|)$, which has the form of the Mexican hat (exemplified in Fig. 16.3a), and for simplicity let $\gamma_i(\eta_i) = \text{const. } \eta_i^2$, although the exact form of this function is not important. If the width of the μ function is not much less than the width of the cell array, and if I_i, on average, is a smooth function of i (although a random, even time-variable background input is allowed), then the activity values η_i start to concentrate into a one-dimensional bubble, that is, a stabilized, bounded activity cluster, as seen in Figure 16.3b. Apparently the bubble is formed at a place where the initial activity, due to stimulation I_i, was maximum. (To be more exact, it is the maximum of the smoothed downward curvature of the η_i that defines the position of the bubble.) Remember that the I_i are also proportional to the inner product of x with the various input weights m_i.

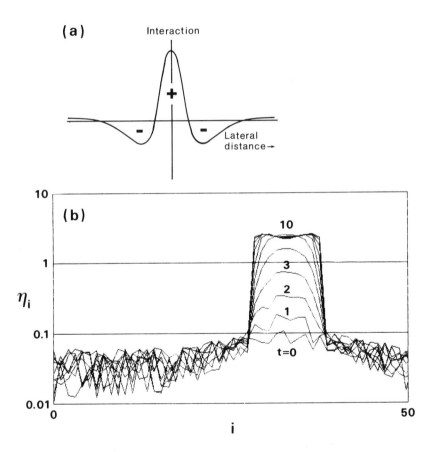

FIGURE 16.3. (a) The "Mexican-hat" interaction kernel. (b) Formation of a bubble of activity over a one-dimensional network, with 51 units (horizontal coordinate) indexed by i. Development of activity η_i as a function of time, $t = 0,1,2, \ldots , 10$.

SELF-ORGANIZED FORMATION OF SENSORY MAPS

The issues about internal representations of abstract knowledge in the brain may be very difficult to treat in any detailed form. This section describes a rather primitive case in which internal representations of primary sensory signals are formed in a basic physical network; even this example, however, is far from trivial and is very difficult to explain theoretically.

It seems that the two essential effects that lead to spatially organized maps are (1) spatial concentration or clustering of the network activity into a bubble whose location depends on the input information and (2) sensitization to the prevailing input of those network units that lie within the bubble.

Simplification of the Clustering Effect for Computer Simulations

For numerical simulations by computer, without essentially losing any of the general physical behavior, we shall "quantitize" the clustering process, or formation of the bubble, in a very mild way. At the same time the basic effect may become more lucid.

Let us recall that in the vector notation $x = [\xi_{i1}, \xi_{i2}, \ldots, \xi_{in}]^T$ is the input vector, which, for notational simplicity and computational efficiency, is assumed to be connected to all the neurons i in this network. The synaptic weight vector of neuron i was denoted by $m_i = [\mu_i, \mu_{i2}, \ldots, \mu_{in}]^T$. Thus finding the best match of x with the m_i on the basis of the simplest measure would be identical to comparing the inner products $m_i^T x$, since they occur as additive terms in the monotonically increasing sigmoidal functions in Eq. 3. The thresholds θ_i must thereby be assumed constant with i. The $m_i^T x$ are also proportional to the I_i terms in Eq. 5, the relative magnitudes of which determined at which location the bubble was formed.

At this time we shall make use of a result that has been justified elsewhere. It seems, that due to the "active forgetting" in Eq. 4 the input weight vectors m_i in the adaptive process tend to become normalized to constant lengths, or norms that are independent of the signal values. Then, instead of using inner products, the matching of x and the m_i can also be based on the comparison of their norms of the vectorial differences $x - m_i$. If this expression is used in the computerized simulation process from the beginning to indicate the match, an even more reliable self-organizing result usually is obtained.

Let us recall that in reality the neurons formed a sheet. The topology of the interactions in the network defines which neurons are neighbors. In the following simulations the neurons were arranged in a two-dimensional hexagonal grid and we can easily define six or more immediate neighbors to each unit. One possible definition of the neighborhood can be seen in Figure 16.4: In the simplest simulations we take it for granted that a bubble is formed corresponding to such a neighborhood N_c and concentrated around the best matching neuron c. For good ordering results it has further been found advantageous that the bubble, or N_c, be large in the beginning and shrink with time. How this corresponds to the physical or physiological reality cannot be discussed here, but it has some-

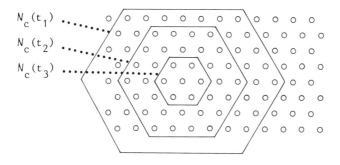

FIGURE 16.4.   The mapping array and examples of topological neighborhood ($t_1 < t_2 < t_3$).

thing to do with the balance between excitatory and inhibitory interconnections (Kohonen, 1984).

Computational Simplification of the Adaptive Process

Each synaptic weight vector m_i, which is a column of the input matrix M in Figure 16.2, is assumed to change in relation to the signals. For the adaptation law we use Eq. 4.

Earlier we referred to a result that further contributes to simplification. We may assume that if the input vector x is changing slowly in time, at least in relation to the electrical relaxation time constants of activity, μ_i attain either the low or the high saturation limit value (inside or outside of the bubble, respectively) whereby $\beta(\mu_i)$ is binary, too. With no loss in generality we can rescale the variables such that $\mu_i \in \{0, 1\}$ and $\beta(\mu_i) \in \{0, \alpha\}$ whereby we obtain, in vector notation,

$$\begin{aligned} dm_i/dt &= \alpha(x - m_i) \quad &\text{inside the bubble} \\ &= 0 &\text{outside the bubble} \end{aligned} \tag{6}$$

The Self-Organizing Algorithm

All the results derived thus far are now collected into a single algorithm that can effectively be computed on general-purpose digital computers, special array processors, or even neural network computers. If the bubble is represented by a neighborhood set N_c, depicted in Figure 16.4, which is centered around the best matching neuron with index $i = c$, and $N_c = N_c(t)$ as well as the factor $\alpha = \alpha(t)$ are both made time variable, as specified later in more detail, we can convert Eq. 6 into the discrete-time formalism ($t = 0, 1, 2, \ldots$):

$$\begin{aligned} m_i(t + 1) &= m_i(t) + \alpha(t)[x(t) - m_i(t)], \quad &i \in N_c(t) \\ &= 0, &i \notin N_c(t) \end{aligned} \tag{7}$$

Here $N_c = N_c(t)$ is centered at cell c, which is defined by the condition

$$\|x(t) - m_c(t)\| = \min_i \{\|x(t) - m_i(t)\|\} \tag{8}$$

During computation, Eqs. 8 and 7 alternate. Notice that x is a stochastic variable with a well-defined statistical density function $p(x)$, from which the successive input values $x(t)$ are drawn. In real-world observations, such as speech recognition, the $x(t)$ can simply be successive samples of the observation x in their natural order of occurrence.

The process may be started by choosing completely random initial values for the $m_i = m_i(0)$, and the only restriction is that they should be different.

No attempt is made to give the mathematical proof of the ordering of the map in this chapter. The problem is extremely difficult and its treatment lengthy. Interested readers can find the proof in the references at the end of this chapter. Numerical examples of efficient process parameters with the simulation examples are given here. It may be helpful to emphasize the following general conditions.

1. Since learning is a stochastic process, the final accuracy of the mapping depends on the number of steps, which must be reasonably large; there is no way to circumvent it. A rule of thumb states that for good statistical accuracy the number of steps needed is at least 500 times the number of network units. On the other hand, the number of components in x has no effect on the number of iteration steps, and if neural computers were used, a very high dimensionality of input might be allowed. Typically up to 100,000 steps are used in simulations, but for "fast learning," as in speech recognition, 10,000 steps may be enough. Notice that the algorithm is computationally extremely light. If only a small number of samples is available, they must be recycled for the wanted total number of steps.

2. During the first 1000 steps or so $\alpha = \alpha(t)$ should start with a value close to unity, thereafter decreasing gradually but staying above 0.1. The ordering of the m_i occurs during this initial period, while the rest of the steps are needed only for the fine adjustment of the map. For final accuracy, $\alpha = \alpha(t)$ should attain small values (e.g., of the order of or less than 0.01) over a long time.

3. A special precaution relates to the choice of $N_c = N_c(t)$. If the neighborhood, or the radius of the bubble, were too small in the beginning, the map would not be ordered globally. Instead one would discern various kinds of parceling of the map at the borders of which the ordering direction would change discontinuously. This phenomenon can be avoided by starting with a fairly wide $N_c = N_c(0)$ and letting it shrink with time. The initial radius of N_c could even be more than half the diameter of the network. During the first 1000 steps or so, when the proper ordering takes place, and $\alpha = \alpha(t)$ is fairly large, the radius of N_c can shrink linearly to, say, one unit; during the fine-adjustment phase, N_c should still contain the nearest neighbors of neuron c.

A Numerical Example: Taxonomy (Hierarchical Clustering) of Abstract Data

Although the more practical applications of self-organizing maps can be found in pattern recognition and modeling of the sensory systems, it may be intriguing to apply this principle to abstract data vectors consisting of hypothetical attributes or characteristiccs. In the example considered here, there are implicitly defined structures in the primary data which the map algorithm is able to reveal. Although this system is a single-level network, it can be shown to be able to produce on it a hierarchical representation of the relations between the primary data.

The most central result in self-organization is that if the input signals have a well-defined probability density function, then the weight vectors of the neurons are trying to imitate it, however complex its form is. It is even possible to perform a kind of numerical taxonomy on this model. As there are no restrictions to the semantic content of the input signals, they can be regarded as any attributes, discrete or continuous valued. In Table 16.1, a total of 32 items, with 5 hypothetical attributes each, were recorded in a data matrix. (This example is completely artificial.) Each of the columns represents one item, and for later inspection it is labeled A through 6, although these labels were not referred to during learning.

The attribute values $(\xi_1, \xi_2, \ldots, \xi_5)$ constitute the pattern vector x, which acts as a set of signal values at the inputs of the network of the type of Figure 16.2. This time the vectors x were picked from Table 16.1 by a random choice, and the state of the network was changed in each representation. Sampling and adaptation were continued iteratively until one could regard the asymptotic state as stationary. Such a "learned" network was then calibrated using the items from Table 16.1 and labeling the units according to the maximum response caused by the different items. Figure 16.5 is such a calibrated map. It is discernible that the "images" of different items are related according to a taxonomic graph where the different branches are visible. Figure 16.6 illustrates, for comparison, what kind of minimal spanning tree would describe the similarity relations of the items of Table 16.1. The following system parameters are engaged in this process.

$\alpha = \alpha(t)$:

During the first 1000 steps, α decreased linearly with time from 0.5 to 0.04 (the initial value could have been closer to unity, say, 0.9). During the subsequent 10,000 steps, α decreased from 0.04 to 0 linearly with time. [Exponential laws for $\alpha = \alpha(t)$ may yield a faster convergence; if the problem is not familiar, however, it is safer and more robust to use the piecewise linear laws.]

$N_c = N_c(t)$:

The lattice was hexagonal, 7 by 10 units, and during the first 1000 steps the radius of N_c decreased from the value 6 (encompassing the majority of cells in the network) to 1 (encompassing neuron c and its six neighbors) linearly with time, thereafter staying at the value 1.

TABLE 16.1   Input Data Matrix

	Item														
Attribute	A	B	C	D	E	F	G	H	I	J	K	L	M	N	O
ξ_1	1	2	3	4	5	3	3	3	3	3	3	3	3	3	3
ξ_2	0	0	0	0	0	1	2	3	4	5	3	3	3	3	3
ξ_3	0	0	0	0	0	0	0	0	0	0	1	2	3	4	5
ξ_4	0	0	0	0	0	0	0	0	0	0	0	0	0	0	0
ξ_5	0	0	0	0	0	0	0	0	0	0	0	0	0	0	0

DISTRIBUTED ASSOCIATIVE MEMORY

A model of autoassociative memory can be derived from the general scheme of Figure 16.1. For that discussion we need not consider details of the input connections; any activity pattern, either an image or activity distribution referring to the sensory maps, may be imposed on the cells in one way or another, and this becomes the information to be stored and recalled.

Assume that the feedback connections of Figure 16.1 are now of the long-range type and time variable and they are distributed all over the network. Modification of their strengths will be approximated by Hebb's law, and this time the forgetting effects are ignored. If the strength of connection between cells i and j is denoted v_{ij}, then

$$dv_{ij}/dt = \alpha'\eta_i\eta_j \qquad (9)$$

where the η_i are components of the output vector y and α' is another parameter.

The state of the network—the set of synaptic interconnections represented by the matrix N—is thus changed, and these changes represent the memory traces stored in the network. This memory can be read associatively only; for instance,

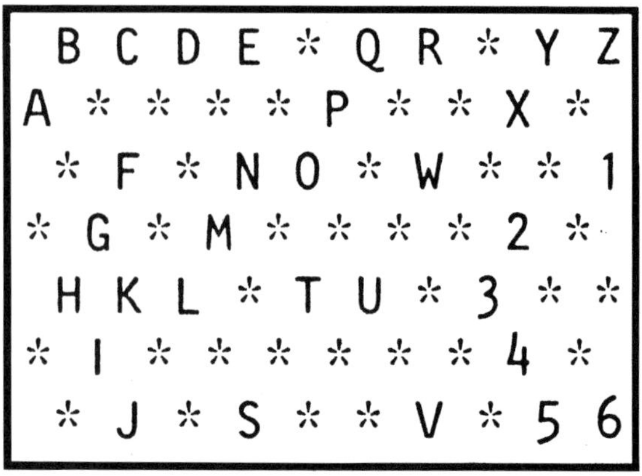

FIGURE 16.5. Mapping of the items of Table 16.1 onto the neural network.

P	Q	R	S	T	U	V	W	X	Y	Z	1	2	3	4	5	6
3	3	3	3	3	3	3	3	3	3	3	3	3	3	3	3	3
3	3	3	3	3	3	3	3	3	3	3	3	3	3	3	3	3
6	7	8	0	3	3	3	6	6	6	6	6	6	6	6	6	6
0	0	0	1	2	3	4	1	2	3	4	2	2	2	2	2	2
0	0	0	0	0	0	0	0	0	0	0	1	2	3	4	5	6

one may start with some partial activation of the network (key), which then spreads into the other parts (recollection). Numerous studies have demonstrated the ability of these networks to recall a previously stored pattern if the initial activation is a part of it. This possibility was pointed out long ago.

For brevity, I am citing only a result that was obtained long ago (Kohonen, 1984; Kohonen et al., 1977). Figure 16.7a represents one sample of 500 different photographic images used as the input patterns. Here each dot corresponds to one cell in the network, and the size of the dot is proportional to its activity value. Figure 16.7b is the key activation, and Figure 16.7c is the recollection that was obtained after spreading of activation into the inactive cells. Notice that the memory traces left by all 500 images were really superimposed on the same network.

DISCUSSION OF SOME EXTENSIONS OF THE MODELS

After the theoretical approaches made above one might expect that comments are possible on certain other phenomena known to occur in the neural realms.

Brain Waves

Many researchers have expressed the wish that the models exhibit certain dynamical phenomena that then could be related to the observed neural signals.

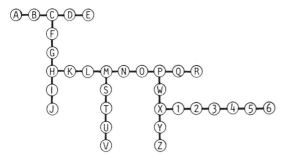

FIGURE 16.6. The minimal spanning tree of the items of Table 16.1.

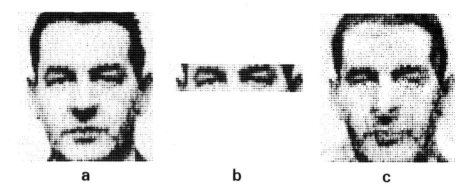

FIGURE 16.7. Demonstration of associative recall in a distributed network: (a) one of the 500 images stored; (b) key pattern used for excitation; (c) recollection. (Adapted from Kohonen, 1984)

The general mechanisms by which oscillations and waves in distributed media are generated are, of course, well understood, but the problem lies in our incomplete knowledge of the neural tissue as a wave-propagating medium. The phase velocities may depend on signal propagation in the excitable membranes, chemical diffusion phenomena, and the like, and the signals may "skip" long distances. It seems unrealistic and unnecessary to describe such phenomena by network models.

Structured Sequences of Signals

Especially in the discussion of memory, one might expect that the production of temporal associations should be described in more detail. It has been shown in the classical theories of automata that structured sequences of system states directly follow from recurrent feedback connections that have a sufficient delay. Detailed modeling is difficult, due to the complexity of brain networks.

Short-Term and Long-Term Memory

It has often been maintained that short-term memory (STM) should be identified with reverberating signal patterns and long-term memory (LTM) with changes in network connectivity. At least the view held of STM ought to be revised; it seems that due to feedback some activity state may persist after simulation, but maintenance of signal patterns in neural lines for any significant period seems impossible. On the other hand, the connections may be altered temporarily, having shorter time constants than with LTM. The strengths and ranges of the STM and LTM connectivities may be different, too. Another problem seems to be more important: How can the memory traces be formed quickly but stay permanent? Obviously very complicated chains of chemical reactions, proceeding automatically after initial triggering, may take place at the synapses.

REFERENCES

Hebb, D. (1949). *Organization of behavior.* New York: Wiley.

Kohonen, T. (1984). *Self-organization and associative memory.* Heidelberg: Springer-Verlag.

Kohonen, T., Lehtiö, P., & Rovamo, J. (1974). Modelling of neural associative memory. *Annales Academiae Scientarium Fennicae* (Series A: V Medica, No. 167).

Kohonen, T., Lehtiö, P., Rovamo, J., Hyvärinen, J., Bry, K., & Vainio, L. (1977). A principle of neural associative memory. *Neuroscience (IBRO), 2,* 1065–1076.

Levy, W., & Burger, B. (1987, June 21–24). *Electrophysiological observations which help describe an associative synaptic modification rule.* Paper presented at the First International Conference on Neural Networks, San Diego.

17

Building Network Learning Algorithms from Hebbian Synapses

TERRENCE J. SEJNOWSKI
GERALD TESAURO

In 1949 Donald Hebb published *The Organization of Behavior,* in which he introduced several hypotheses about the neural substrate of learning and memory, including the Hebb learning rule, or Hebb synapse. We now have solid physiological evidence, verified in several laboratories, that long-term potentiation (LTP) in some parts of the mammalian hippocampus follows the Hebb rule (Brown, Ganong, Kariss, Keenan, & Kelso, 1989; Kelso, Ganong, & Brown, 1986; Levy, Brassel, & Moore, 1983; McNaughton, Douglas, & Goddard, 1978; McNaughton & Morris, 1987; Wigstrom and Gustafsson, 1985). The Hebb rule and variations on it have also served as the starting point for the study of information storage in simplified "neural network" models (Hopfield & Tank, 1986; Kohonen, 1984; Rumelhart & McClelland, 1986; Sejnowski, 1981). Many types of networks have been studied—networks with random connectivity, networks with layers, networks with feedback between layers, and a wide variety of local patterns of connectivity. Even the simplest network model has complexities that are difficult to analyze.

In this chapter we will provide a framework within which the Hebb rule serves as an important link between the implementation level of analysis, the level at which experimental work on neural mechanisms takes place, and the algorithmic level, on which much of the work on learning in network models is being pursued.

LEARNING MECHANISMS, LEARNING RULES, AND LEARNING ALGORITHMS

Long-term potentiation has been found in a variety of preparations. The common denominator is a long-lasting change in synaptic efficacy or spike coupling following afferent stimulation with a high-frequency tetanus. There are probably several different molecular mechanisms underlying LTP in different preparations. For example, LTP in the CA1 region of the rat hippocampus can be blocked with 2-amino-5-phosphonovaleric acid (APV), but the same application of APV does not block LTP from the mossy fibers in the CA3 region of the hippocampus (Chattarji, Stanton, & Sejnowski, 1988). How LTP is implemented in these different regions is a question at the level of the learning mechanism.

The Hebb synapse, in contrast, is a rule rather than a mechanism. That is, many mechanisms can be used to implement a Hebb synapse, as we will show in a later section. A learning rule specifies only the general conditions under which plasticity should occur, such as the temporal and spatial relationships between the presynaptic and postsynaptic signals, but not the locus of plasticity, or even the neuronal geometry. As an extreme example, we show how the Hebb rule can be implemented without synaptic plasticity.

A learning algorithm is more general than a learning rule since an algorithm must also specify how the learning rule is to be used to perform a task, such as storing information or wiring up a neural system. Thus a description of the task to be performed and the type of information involved are essential ingredients of a learning algorithm. Several examples of learning algorithms will be discussed in later sections.

IMPLEMENTATIONS OF THE HEBB RULE

The Hebb Rule

Before considering the various possible ways of implementing the Hebb rule, one should examine what Hebb actually proposed:

> When an axon of cell *A* is near enough to excite cell *B* or repeatedly or persistently takes part in firing it, some growth process or metabolic change takes place in one or both cells such that *A*'s efficiency, as one of the cells firing *B*, is increased. (p. 62)

This statement can be translated into a precise quantitative expression as follows. We consider the situation in which neuron *A*, with average firing rate V_A, projects to neuron *B*, with average firing rate V_B. The synaptic connection from *A* to *B* has a strength value T_{BA}, which determines the degree to which activity in *A* is capable of exciting *B*. (The postsynaptic depolarization of *B* due to *A* is usually taken to be the product of the firing rate V_A times the synaptic strength value T_{BA}.) Now the preceding statement by Hebb states that the strength of the synapse T_{BA} should be modified in some way that is dependent on both activity in *A* and activity in *B*. The most general expression that captures this notion is

$$\Delta T_{BA} = F(V_A, V_B) \tag{1}$$

which states that the change in the synaptic strength at any given time is some as yet unspecified function *F* of both the presynaptic firing rate and the postsynaptic firing rate. Strictly speaking, we should say that $F(V_A, V_B)$ is a functional, since the plasticity may depend on the firing rates at previous times as well as at the current time. Given this general form of the assumed learning rule, it is then necessary to choose a particular form for the function $F(V_A, V_B)$. The most straightforward interpretation of what Hebb said is a simple product:

$$\Delta T_{BA} = \epsilon V_A V_B \qquad (2)$$

where ϵ is a numerical constant usually taken to be small. There are many other choices possible for the function $F(V_A, V_B)$; the choice depends on the particular task at hand. Equation 2 might be appropriate for a simple associative memory task, but for other tasks one would need different forms of the function $F(V_A, V_B)$ in Eq. 1. For example, in classical conditioning, as we shall see in the following section, the precise timing relationships of the presynaptic and postsynaptic signals are important, and the plasticity must then depend on the rate of change of firing, or on the "trace" of the firing rate (i.e., a weighted average over previous times), rather than simply depending on the current instantaneous firing rate. Once the particular form of the learning algorithm is established, the next step is to decide how the algorithm is to be implemented. We shall describe here three possible implementation schemes. This is meant to illustrate the variety of schemes possible.

Three Implementations

The first implementation scheme, seen in Figure 17.1a, is the simplest way to implement the proposed plasticity rule. The circuit consists solely of neurons A and B and a conventional axodendritic or axosomatic synapse from A to B. One postulates that there is some molecular mechanism operating on the postsynaptic side of the synapse which is capable of sensing the rate of firing of both cells and which changes the strength of synaptic transmission from cell B to cell A according to the product of the two firing rates. This is in fact similar to the recently discovered mechanism of associative LTP that has been studied in rat hippocampus (Brown et al., 1989). (Strictly speaking, the plasticity in LTP depends not on the postsynaptic firing rate, but instead on the postsynaptic depolarization. However, in practice these two are usually closely related [Kelso et al., 1986].) Even here, many different molecular mechanisms are possible. For example, even though the induction of plasticity occurs at a postsynaptic site, the long-term structural change may well be presynaptic (Dolphin, Errington, & Bliss, 1982).

A second possible implementation scheme for the Hebb rule is seen in Figure 17.1b. In this circuit there is now a feedback projection from the postsynaptic neuron, which forms an axoaxonic synapse on the projection from A to B. The plasticity mechanism involves presynaptic facilitation: one assumes that the strength of the synapse from A to B is increased in proportion to the product of the presynaptic firing rate times the facilitator firing rate (i.e., the postsynaptic

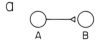

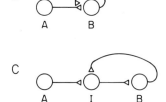

FIGURE 17.1. Three implementations of the Hebb rule for synaptic plasticity. The strength of the coupling between cell A and cell B is strengthened when they are both active at the same time. (a) Postsynaptic site for coincidence detection. (b) Presynaptic site for coincidence detection. (c) Interneuron detects coincidence.

firing rate). This type of mechanism also exists and has been extensively studied in *Aplysia* (Carew, Hawkins, & Kandel, 1983; Kandel et al., 1987). Several authors have pointed out that this circuit is a functionally equivalent way of implementing the Hebb rule (Gelperin, Hopfield, & Tank, 1985; Hawkins & Kandel, 1984; Tesauro, 1986).

A third scheme for implementing the Hebb rule—one that does not specifically require plasticity in individual synapses (Tesauro, 1988)—is seen in Figure 17.1c. In this scheme the modifiable synapse from *A* to *B* is replaced by an interneuron *I* with a modifiable threshold for initiation of action potentials. The Hebb rule is satisfied if the threshold of *I* decreases according to the product of the firing rate in the projection from *A* times the firing rate in the projection from *B*. This is quite similar, although not strictly equivalent, to the literal Hebb rule, because the effect of changing the interneuron threshold is not identical to the effect of changing the strength of a direct synaptic connection. A plasticity mechanism similar to the one proposed here has been studied in *Hermissenda* (Alkon, 1987; Farley & Alkon, 1985).

The three methods for implementing the Hebb rule seen in Figure 17.1 are by no means exhaustive. There is no doubt that nature is more clever than we are at designing mechanisms for plasticity, especially since we are not aware of most evolutionary constraints. These three circuits can be considered equivalent circuits since they effectively perform the same function even though they differ in the way that they accomplish it. There also are many ways that each circuit could be instantiated at the cellular and molecular levels. Despite major differences between them, we can nonetheless say that they all implement the Hebb rule.

Most synapses in cerebral cortex occur on dendrites where complex spatial interactions are possible. For example, the activation of a synapse might depolarize the dendrite sufficiently to serve as the postsynaptic signal for modifying an adjacent synapse. Such cooperativity between synapses is a generalization of the Hebb rule in which a section of dendrite rather than the entire neuron is considered the functional unit (Finkel & Edelman, 1987). Dendritic compartments with voltage-dependent channels have all the properties needed for non-linear processing units (Shepherd et al., 1985).

USES OF THE HEBB RULE

Conditioning

The Hebb rule can be used to form associations between one stimulus and another. Such associations can either be static, in which case the resulting neural circuit functions as an associative memory (Anderson, 1970; Kohonen, 1970; Longuet-Higgins, 1968; Steinbuch, 1961); or they can be temporal, in which case the network learns to predict that one stimulus pattern will be followed at a later time by another. The latter case has been extensively studied in classical conditioning experiments, in which repeated temporally paired presentations of a conditioned stimulus (CS) followed by an unconditioned stimulus (US) cause the animal to respond to the CS in a way that is similar to its response to the US. The animal has learned that the presence of the CS predicts the subsequent presence of the US. A simple neural circuit model of the classical conditioning process that uses the Hebb rule is illustrated in Figure 17.2. This circuit contains three neurons: a sensory neuron for the CS, a sensory neuron for the US, and a motor neuron, R, which generates the unconditioned response. There is a strong, unmodifiable synapse from US to R, so that the presence of the US automatically evokes the response. There is also a modifiable synapse from CS to R, which in the naive untrained animal is initially weak.

One might think that the straightforward application of the literal interpretation of the Hebb rule, as expressed in Eq. 2, would suffice to generate the desired conditioning effects in the circuit of Figure 17.2. However, there are a number of serious problems with this learning algorithm. One of the most serious is the lack of timing sensitivity in Eq. 2. Learning would occur regardless of the order in which the neurons came to be activated. However, in conditioning we know that the temporal order of stimuli is important: if the US follows the CS, then learning occurs, whereas if the US appears before the CS, then no learning occurs. Hence Eq. 2 must be modified in some way to include this timing sen-

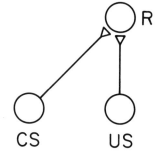

FIGURE 17.2.   Model of classical conditioning using a modified Hebb synapse. The US elicits a response in the postsynaptic cell (R). Coincidence of the response with the CS leads to strengthening of the synapse between CS and R.

sitivity. Another serious problem is a sort of "runaway instability" that occurs when the CS–R synapse is strengthened to the point where activity in the CS neuron by itself causes the R neuron to fire. In that case, Eq. 2 would cause the synapse to be strengthened upon presentation of the CS alone, without being followed by the US. However, in real animals we know that presentation of CS alone causes a learned association to be extinguished, that is, the synaptic strength should decrease, not increase. The basic problem is that algorithm 2 is capable of generating positive learning only, and has no way to generate zero or negative learning.

It is clear then that the literal Hebb rule needs to be modified to produce desired conditioning phenomena (Klopf, 1987; Tesauro, 1986). One of the most popular ways to overcome the problems of the literal Hebb rule is by using algorithms such as the following:

$$\Delta T_{BA} = \epsilon \dot{V}_B \overline{V}_A \tag{3}$$

Here $\overline{V}_A$ represents the stimulus trace of V_A, or the weighted average of V_A over previous times, and $\dot{V}_B$ represents the time derivative of V_B. The stimulus trace provides the required timing sensitivity so that learning occurs only in forward conditioning and not in backward conditioning. The use of the time derivative of the postsynaptic firing rate, rather than the postsynaptic firing rate, is a way of changing the sign of learning and thus avoiding the runaway instability problem. With this algorithm, extinction would occur because upon onset of the CS, no positive learning takes place due to the presynaptic trace, and negative learning takes place upon offset of the CS. Many other variations and elaborations of Eq. 3 behave differently, taking into account other conditioning behaviors such as second-order conditioning and blocking. For details we refer the reader to Gelperin et al. (1985), Gluck and Thompson (1987), Klopf (1987), Sutton (1987), Sutton and Barto (1981), and Tesauro (1986). However, all of these other algorithms are built on the same basic notion of modifying the literal Hebb rule to incorporate a mechanism of timing sensitivity and a mechanism for changing the sign of learning.

Associative Memory

Memory and learning are behavioral phenomena, but there are correlates at many structural levels, from the molecular to the systems levels. Hebb (1949) went beyond the synaptic and cellular levels to speculate about information processing in networks of neurons, or assemblies as he called them, which he considered the fundamental unit of processing in the cerebral cortex. Information from the environment is encoded in an assembly by changing the synaptic strengths at many snapses simultaneously. Even though the Hebb rule is local, in the sense that only local information is needed to make a decision about how to change the strength of the synapse, the global behavior of the network of neurons may be affected. This raises the possibility that new principles might emerge when assemblies of neurons are studied.

Probably the most important and most thoroughly explored use of the Hebb rule is in the formation of associations between one stimulus or pattern of activity and another. The Hebb rule is appealing for this use because it provides a way of forming global associations between macroscopic patterns of activity in assemblies of neurons using only the local information available at individual synapses.

The earliest models of associative memory were based on network models in which the output of a model neuron was assumed to be proportional to a linear sum of its inputs, each weighted by a synaptic strength. Thus

$$V_B = \sum_{A=1}^{N} T_{BA} V_A \qquad (4)$$

where V_B are the firing rates of a group of M output cells, V_A are the firing rates of a group of N input cells, and T_{BA} is the synaptic strength between input cell A and output cell B. Note that A and B are being used here as arbitrary indices to represent one out of a group of cells.

The transformation between patterns of activity on the input vectors to patterns of activity on the output vectors is determined by the synaptic weight matrix, T_{BA}. How should this matrix be chosen if the goal of the network is to associate a particular output vector with a particular input vector? The earliest suggestions were all based on the Hebb rule in Eq. 2 (Anderson, 1970; Kohonen, 1970; Longuet-Higgins, 1968; Steinbuch, 1961). It is easy to verify by direct substitution of Eq. 2 into Eq. 4 that the increment in the output is proportional to the desired vector and the strength of the learning ϵ can be adjusted to scale the outputs to the desired values.

More than one association can be stored in the same matrix, so long as the input vectors are not too similar to one another. This is accomplished by using Eq. 2 for each input–output pair. This model of associative storage is simple and has several attractive features: (1) the learning occurs in only one trial; (2) the information is distributed over many synapses, so that recall is relatively immune to noise or damage; and (3) input patterns similar to stored inputs will give output similar to the stored outputs, a form of generalization. This model also has some strong limitations. First, stored items with input vectors that are similar (i.e., that have a significant overlap) will produce outputs that are mixtures of the stored outputs. However, discriminations must often be made among similar inputs, such as the phonetic distinction between the labial stops in the words "bet" and "pet." Second, the linear model cannot respond contingently to pairs of inputs (i.e., those that have an output that is different from the sum of the individual outputs). Some deficiencies can be remedied by making the learning algorithm and the architecture of the network more complex, as shown in the next section.

The Covariance Rule

Numerous variations have been proposed on the conditions for Hebbian plasticity (Levy, Anderson, & Lehmkuhle, 1984). One problem with any synaptic modification rule that can only increase the strength of a synapse is that the synaptic strength will eventually saturate at its maximum value. Nonspecific decay can reduce the sizes of the weights, but the stored information will also decay and be lost at the same rate. Another approach is to renormalize the total synaptic weight of the entire terminal field from a single neuron to a constant value (von der Malsburg, 1973). Sejnowski (1977a, 1977b) emphasized the need for a learning rule that decreases the strength of a plastic synapse as specifically as the Hebb rule increases it and proposed a covariance learning rule. According to this rule, the change in strength of a plastic synapse should be proportional to the covariance between the presynaptic firing and postsynaptic firing:

$$\Delta T_{BA} = \epsilon \left(V_B - \langle V_B \rangle \right) \left(V_A - \langle V_A \rangle \right) \tag{5}$$

where $\langle V_B \rangle$ is the average firing rates of the output neurons and $\langle V_A \rangle$ is the average firing rates of the input neurons (see also Chauvet, 1986). Thus the strength of the synapse should increase if the firings of the presynaptic and postsynaptic elements are positively correlated, decrease if they are negatively correlated, and remain unchanged if they are uncorrelated. Evidence for long-term depression has been found in the hippocampus (Levy et al., 1983; Stanton, Jester, Chatterji, & Sejnowski, 1988) and in visual cortex during development (Reiter & Stryker, 1987; Fregnac, Shulz, Thorpe, & Bienenstock, 1988).

The covariance rule is a special case of the general form of the Hebb rule in Eq. 1. It does go beyond the simple Hebb rule in Eq. 2; however, it is easy to show that traditional Hebb synapses can be used to implement Eq. 5, which can be rewritten as

$$\Delta T_{BA} = \epsilon \left(\langle V_B V_A \rangle - \langle V_B \rangle \langle V_A \rangle \right) \tag{6}$$

Both terms on the right-hand side have the same form as the simple Hebb synapse in Eq. 2. Thus the covariance learning algorithm can be realized by applying the Hebb rule relative to a "threshold" that varies with the product of the time-averaged presynaptic and postsynaptic activity levels. The effect of the threshold is to ensure that no change in synaptic strength should occur if the average correlation between the presynaptic and postsynaptic activities is at chance level.

Error-Correction Learning

One of the consequences of the linear associative matrix model with Hebbian synapses is that similar input vectors necessarily produce similar output vectors. Error-correction procedures can be used to reduce this interference. The weights are changed to minimize the difference between the actual and correct output vectors:

$$\Delta T_{BA} = \epsilon \, (V_B^{(a)} - V_B^{(c)}) \, V_A \tag{7}$$

where $V_B^{(a)}$ is the actual output produced by the network by the current set of weights and $V_B^{(c)}$ is the correct output vector supplied by the teacher. Unlike the previous learning algorithms, which learn in one shot, error-correction procedures such as this are incremental and require several presentations of the same set of input vectors. It can be shown that the weights will evolve to minimize the average mean square error over the set of input vectors (Kohonen, 1984).

As with the covariance learning algorithm, the error-correction learning algorithm in Eq. 7 can be rewritten in a form that can be implemented with Hebb synapses:

$$\Delta T_{BA} = \epsilon \, (V_B^{(a)} V_A - V_B^{(c)} V_A) \tag{8}$$

Both terms on the right-hand side have the same form as the simple Hebb synapse in Eq. 2. Thus the error-correction procedure can be realized by applying the Hebb rule twice, first to the actual output produced by the network and then to the correct output supplied by a teacher, but with a negative rather than a positive increment. Alternatively, the difference can be computed by another neuron and used to control the Hebbian learning.

Further improvements have also been made to associative matrix models by introducing feedback connections, so that the networks are autoassociative, and by making the processing units nonlinear (Anderson & Mozer, 1981; Hopfield, 1984; Kohonen, 1984; Sejnowski, 1981; Toulouse, Dehaene, & Changeux, 1986). Associative memory models like this have been proposed for the CA3 region of the hippocampus (Lynch & Baudry, 1988; McNaughton & Morris, 1987; Rolls, 1987).

The learning algorithms for associative memory introduced in this section are supervised in the sense that information about the desired output vectors must be supplied along with the input vectors. One way to provide information about the desired output to a group of neurons is to have a separate "teaching" input that "clamps" the output firing rates to the desired values while the input corresponding to the desired output is simultaneously active. The climbing fibers in the cerebellar cortex, which make strong excitatory synapses on individual Purkinje cells, could have such a teaching role, as first suggested by Brindley (1964) and later developed by Albus (1971) and Marr (1969) in models of the cerebellar cortex as an adaptive filter. Evidence for plasticity in the cerebellar cortex has been found by Ito and his co-workers (Ito, 1982). However, evidence for Hebbian plasticity in the cerebellum does not necessarily imply that its function is associative storage, for there are many other possible functions. Evidence for plasticity in the deep cerebellar nuclei has been found as well (Miles & Lisberger, 1981; Thompson, 1986).

Learning Internal Representations

The class of network models of associative memory discussed in the last section has a severe computational limitation in that all the processing units in the network are constrained by either the inputs or the outputs, so that there are no free units that could be used to form new internal features. What features should be used for the input units and output units if the network is deeply buried in the brain? New learning algorithms have been devised for multilayer networks with nonlinear processing units that overcome some of the limitations of single-layer networks (Hinton & Sejnowski, 1983; Rumelhart & McClelland, 1986). In particular, these algorithms use interneurons, or "hidden units," which become sensitive to the features that are appropriate for solving a specified problem and for performing context-sensitive computation. We will review one of these learning algorithms, based on the Boltzmann machine architecture, which can be implemented by Hebb synapses.

The Boltzmann machine is a network of stochastic processing units that solves optimization problems (Hinton & Sejnowski, 1983, 1986). The processing units in a Boltzmann machine have outputs that are binary valued and are updated probabilistically from summed synaptic inputs, which are graded. As a consequence, the state of the units in a Boltzmann machine fluctuate even for a constant input. The amount of fluctuation is controlled by a parameter that is analogous to the temperature of a thermodynamic system. Fluctuations allow the system to escape from local traps into which it would get stuck if there were no noise in the system. All the units in a Boltzmann machine are symmetrically connected: this allows an "energy" to be defined for the network and ensures that the network will relax to an equilibrium state which minimizes the energy (Hopfield, 1982).

The Boltzmann machine has been applied to a number of constraint satisfaction problems in vision, such as figure–ground separation in image analysis (Kienker, Sejnowski, Hinton, & Schumacher, 1986; Sejnowski & Hinton, 1987), and generalizations have been applied to image restoration (Geman & Geman, 1984), binocular depth perception (Divko & Schulten, 1986), and optical flow (Hutchinson, Koch, Luo, & Mead, 1988). These are problems in which many small pieces of evidence must be combined to arrive at the best overall interpretation of sensory inputs (Ballard, Hinton, & Sejnowski, 1983; Hopfield & Tank, 1986).

Boltzmann machines have an interesting learning algorithm that allows "energy landscapes" to be formed within the hidden units between the input and output layers. Learning in a Boltzmann machine has two phases. In the training phase a binary input pattern is imposed on the input group as well as the correct binary output pattern. The system is allowed to relax to equilibrium at a fixed temperature while the inputs and outputs are held fixed. In equilibrium, the average fraction of time a pair of units is on together, the co-occurrence probability, is computed for each connection:

$$P_{BA}^{+} = \langle S_B S_A \rangle \mid_{\text{clamped}} \qquad (9)$$

where S_B is the output value of the Bth unit, which can take on the values 0 or 1 only. In the test phase the same procedure is followed with only the input units clamped, and the average co-occurrence probabilities are again computed:

$$P_{BA}^{-} = \langle S_B S_A \rangle \mid_{\text{free}} \qquad (10)$$

The weights are then updated according to

$$\Delta T_{BA} = \epsilon \, (P_{BA}^{+} - P_{BA}^{-}) \qquad (11)$$

where the parameter ϵ controls the rate of learning. A co-occurrence probability is related to the correlation between the firing or activation of the presynaptic and postsynaptic units and can therefore be implemented by a Hebb synapse. In the second phase, however, the change in the synaptic strengths is anti-Hebbian since it must decrease with increasing correlation. Notice that this procedure is also error-correcting, since no change will be made to the weight if the two probabilities are the same.

The Boltzmann machine demonstrates that the Hebb learning rule can be used to mold the response properties of interneurons within a network and adapt them for the efficient solution of difficult computational problems. The Boltzmann machine also shows that noise can play an effective role in improving performance of a network, and that the presence of noise in the nervous system does not necessarily imply a lack of precision. Other stochastic network models have also been studied (Barto, 1985). Although the Boltzmann machine is not meant to be a realistic brain model, it does serve as an existence proof that difficult computational problems can be solved with relatively simple processing units and biologically plausible learning mechanisms.

Development

The Hebb synapse has also been used by Linsker (1986) to model the formation of receptive fields in the early stages of visual processing. The model is a layered network having limited connectivity between layers, and it uses the covariance generalization of the Hebb rule given in Eq. 5. As the learning proceeds, the units in the lower layers of the network develop on-center and off-center receptive fields that resemble the receptive fields of ganglion cells in the retina, and elongated receptive fields develop in the upper layers of the network that resemble simple receptive fields found in visual cortex. This model demonstrates that some of the properties of sensory neurons could arise spontaneously during development by specifying the general pattern of connectivity and a few parameters to control the synaptic plasticity. One surprising aspect of the model is that regular receptive fields develop even though only spontaneous activity is present at the sensory receptors. Similar models that require patterned inputs have also been proposed (Barrow, 1987; Bienenstock, Cooper, & Munro, 1982; von der Malsburg, 1973).

The visual response properties of neurons in the visual cortex of cats and monkeys are plastic during the first few months of postnatal life and can be permanently modified by visual experience (Hubel & Wiesel, 1962; Sherman & Spear, 1982). Normally, most cortical neurons respond to visual stimuli from either eye. Following visual deprivation of one eye by eyelid suture during the critical period, the ocular preference of neurons in primary visual cortex shifts toward the nondeprived eye. In another type of experiment, a misalignment of the two eyes during the critical period produces neurons that respond to only one eye, and, as a consequence, binocular depth perception is impaired. These and many other experiments have led to testable hypotheses for the mechanisms underlying synaptic plasticity during the critical period (Bear, Cooper, & Ebner, 1987).

Stent (1973) suggested that the effects of monocular deprivation could be explained if the synaptic weight were to decrease when the synapse is inactive and the postsynaptic cell is active. An alternative mechanism that incorporates another Hebbian form of plasticity was proposed by Bienenstock et al. (1982). The Bienenstock–Cooper–Munro algorithm for synaptic modification is a special case of the general Hebb rule in Eq. 1:

$$\Delta T_{BA} = \phi(V_B, \langle V_B \rangle) V_A \qquad (12)$$

where the function $\phi(V_B, \langle V_B \rangle)$ is shown in Figure 17.3. The synapse is strengthened when the average postsynaptic activity exceeds a threshold and is weakened when the activity falls below the threshold level. Furthermore, the threshold varies according to the average postsynaptic activity:

$$\theta = \langle V_B \rangle^2. \qquad (13)$$

Bienenstock et al. (1982) showed that this choice has desirable stability properties and allows neurons to become selectively sensitive to common features in input patterns.

Singer (1987) suggested that the voltage-dependent entry of calcium into spines and the dendrites of postsynaptic cells may trigger the molecular changes required for synaptic modification. This hypothesis is being tested at a molecular level using combined pharmacological and physiological techniques. N-methyl-D-aspartic acid (NMDA) receptor antagonists infused into visual cortex block the shift in ocular dominance normally associated with monocular deprivation (Kleinschmidt, Bear, & Singer, 1986). The NMDA receptor is a candidate mechanism for triggering synaptic modification because it allows calcium to enter a

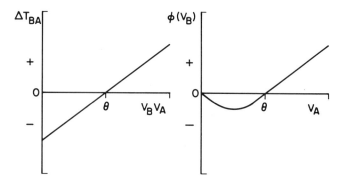

FIGURE 17.3.   (left) Change in coupling strength ΔT_{BA} as a function of the correlation $<V_B V_A>$ between the presynaptic and postsynaptic activity levels, as indicated in Eq. 5. The threshold θ is given by $< V_B >< V_A >$. (right) The postsynaptic factor $\phi(V_B, <V_B>)$ in the Bienenstock–Cooper–Munro learning algorithm in Eq. 1, where the threshold θ is given by $\theta = <V_B>^2$.

cell only if the neurotransmitter binds to the receptor and the postsynaptic membrane is depolarized. In a sense, the NMDA receptor is a "Hebb molecule," since it is activated only when there is a conjunction of presynaptic and postsynaptic activity. The NMDA receptor also is involved in LTP in the hippocampus (Collingridge, Kehl, & McLennan, 1983).

The mechanisms for plasticity in the cerebral cortex during development may be related to the mechanisms that are responsible for synaptic plasticity in the adult. The evidence so far favors the general form of Hebbian plasticity in Eq. 1. However, the details of how this plasticity is regulated at short and long time scales may be quite different during development and in the adult.

CONCLUSIONS

The algorithmic level is a fruitful one for pursuing network models at the present time for two reasons. First, working top-down from functional considerations is difficult, since our intuitions about the functional level in the brain may be wrong or misleading. Knowing more about the computational capabilities of simple neural networks may help us gain a better intuition. Second, working from the bottom up can be treacherous, since we may not yet know the relevant signals in the nervous system that support information processing. The study of learning in model networks can help guide the search for neural mechanisms underlying learning and memory. Thus network models at the algorithmic level are a unifying framework within which to explore neural information processing.

Three principles have emerged from our studies of learning in neural networks. The first is the principle of locality. The Hebb algorithm depends only on information that is present or can be extracted from highly localized regions of space and time. This is of practical importance for any physical system since nonlocal algorithms have a high overhead for the communications needed to bring together the relevant information. In spite of the limitation of locality, networks can nonetheless achieve a global organization during both development and long-term information storage. The second principle is gradient descent. A global energy or cost function can usually be found whenever large-scale network organization emerges from local interactions. That is, global organization is the result of local changes which optimize a function of the entire system (Sejnowski, 1987). This raises the important possibility that such global functions may be exploited in the nervous system and may be discoverable (Sejnowski, 1987). The third is the principle of differences. Given the limited accuracy of signals in neurons, mechanisms that depend on accurate, absolute values are not feasible. Information storage can be made more compact when differences between signals—effectively error signals—are used to make changes at synapses.

Hebb's learning rule has led to a fruitful line of experimental research and a rich set of network models. The Hebb synapse is a building block for many different neural network algorithms. As experiments refine the parameters for Hebbian plasticity in particular brain areas, it should become possible to begin refining network models for those areas. There is still a formidable gap between the complexity of real brain circuits and the simplicity of the current generation of network models. As models and experiments evolve the common bonds linking them are likely to be postulates like the Hebb synapse that serve as algorithmic building blocks.

Acknowledgment

This chapter was prepared with the support of the Mathers Foundation.

REFERENCES

Albus, J. S. (1971). A theory of cerebellar function. *Mathematical Biosciences, 10,* 25–61.

Alkon, D. L. (1987). *Memory traces in the brain.* Oxford: Oxford University Press.

Anderson, J. A. (1970). Two models for memory organization using interacting traces. *Mathematical Biosciences, 8,* 137–160.

Anderson, J. A., & Mozer, M. C. (1981). Categorization and selective neurons. In G. E. Hinton & J. A. Anderson (Eds.), *Parallel models of associative memory.* Hillsdale, N.J.: Erlbaum.

Ballard, D. H., Hinton, G. E., & Sejnowski, T. J. (1983). Parallel visual computation. *Nature, 306,* 21–26.

Barrow, H. G. (1987). Learning receptive fields. In M. Caudill & C. Butler (Eds.), *Proceedings of the First International Conference on Neural Networks* (Vol. 4, pp. 115–121). San Diego: SOS Press.

Barto, A. G. (1985). Learning by statistical cooperation of self-interested neuron-like computing elements. *Human Neurobiology, 4,* 229–256.

Bear, M., Cooper, L. N., & Ebner, F. F. (1987). A physiological basis for a theory of synapse modification. *Science, 237,* 42–48.

Bienenstock, E. L., Cooper, L. N., & Munro, P. W. (1982). Theory for the development of neuron selectivity: Orientation specificity and binocular interaction in visual cortex. *Journal of Neuroscience, 2,* 32–48.

Brindley, G. S. (1964). The use made by the cerebellum of the information that it receives from sense organs. *International Brain Research Organization Bulletin, 3,* 80.

Brown, T. H., Ganong, A. H., Kariss, E. W., Keenan, C. L., & Kelso, S. R. (1989). Long-term potentiation in two synaptic systems of the hippocampal brain slice. In J. H. Byrne & W. O. Berry (Eds.), *Neural models of plasticity.* Orlando, Fla.: Academic Press.

Carew, T. J., Hawkins, R. D., & Kandel, E. R. (1983). Differential classical conditioning of a defensive withdrawal reflex in *Aplysia californica. Science, 219,* 397–400.

Chattarji, S., Stanton, P., & Sejnowski, T. J. (1988). Commissural, but not mossy fiber, synapses exhibit both associative long-term potentiation (LTP) and depression (LTD) in the CA3 region of the hippocampus. *Society for Neuroscience Abstracts, 14,* 567.

Chauvet, G. (1986). Habituation rules for a theory of the cerebellar cortex. *Biological Cybernetics, 55,* 201–209.

Churchland, P. S., & Sejnowski, T. J. (1988). Neural representations and neural computations. In L. Nadel (Ed.), *Neural connections and mental computation* (pp. 15–48). Cambridge, Mass.: MIT Press.

Collingridge, G. L., Kehl, S. L., & McLennan, H. (1983). *Journal of Physiology (London), 334,* 33.

DiPrisco, G. V. (1984). Hebb synaptic plasticity. *Progress in Neurobiology, 89,* 98–102.

Divko, R., & Schulten, K. (1986). Stochastic spin models for pattern recognition. In J. S. Denker (Ed.), *AIP Conference Proceedings 151: Neural Networks for Computing* (pp. 129–134). New York: AIP.

Dolphin, A. C., Errington, M. L., & Bliss, T. V. P. (1982). *Nature, 297,* 496.

Farley, J., & Alkon, D. L. (1985). Cellular mechanisms of learning, memory and information storage. *Annual Review of Psychology, 36,* 419–494.

Finkel, L. H., & Edelman, G. M. (1987). Population rules for synapses in networks. In G. M. Edelman, W. E. Gall, & W. M. Cowan (Eds.), *Synaptic function.* (pp. 711–757). New York: Wiley.

Fregnac, Y., & Imbert, M. (1984). Development of neuronal selectivity in the primary visual cortex of the cat. *Physiology Review, 64,* 325.

Fregnac, Y., Shulz, D., Thorpe, S., & Bienenstock, E. (1988). A cellular analogue of visual cortical plasticity. *Nature, 333,* 367–370.

Gelperin, A. (1986). Complex associative learning in small neural networks. *Trends in Neurosciences, 9,* 323–328.

Gelperin, A., Hopfield, J. J., & Tank, D. W. (1985). The logic of Limax learning. In A. Selverston (Ed.), *Model neural networks and behavior* (pp. 237–261). New York: Plenum.

Geman, S., & Geman, D. (1984). Stochastic relaxation, Gibbs distribution and the Bayesian restoration of images. *IEEE Transactions on Pattern Analysis and Machine Intelligence, 3,* 79–92.

Gluck, M. A., & Thompson, R. F. (1987). Modeling the neural substrates of associative learning and memory: A computational approach. *Psychological Review, 94,* 176–191.

Hawkins, R. D., & Kandel, E. R. (1984). Is there a cell-biological alphabet for simple forms of learning? *Psychological Review, 91,* 375–391.

Hebb, D. O. (1949). *Organization of behavior.* New York: Wiley.

Hinton, G. E., & Sejnowski, T. J. (1983). Optimal perceptual inference. In *Proceedings of the IEEE Computer Society Conference on Computer Vision and Pattern Recognition* (pp. 448–453). Silver Spring, Md.: IEEE Computer Society Press.

Hinton, G. E., & Sejnowski, T. J. (1986). Learning and relearning in Boltzmann machines. In D. Rumelhart & J. McClelland (Eds.), *Parallel distributed processing: Explorations in the microstructure of cognition: Psychological and biological models* (pp. 282–317). Cambridge, Mass.: MIT Press.

Hopfield, J. J. (1982). Neural networks and physical systems with emergent collective computational abilities. *Proceedings of the National Academy of Sciences USA, 79,* 2554–2558.

Hopfield, J. J. (1984). Neurons with graded response have collective computation abilities. *Proceedings of the National Academy of Sciences USA, 81,* 3088–3092.

Hopfield, J. J., & Tank, D. W. (1986). Computing with neural circuits: A model. *Science, 233,* 625–633.

Hubel, D. H., & Wiesel, T. N. (1962). Receptive fields, binocular interactions, and functional architecture in the cat's visual cortex. *Journal of Physiology, 160,* 106–154.

Hutchinson, J., Koch, C., Luo, J., & Mead, C. (1988). *IEEE Computer, 21*(3), 52–64.

Ito, M. (1982). Cerebellar control of the vestibulo-ocular reflex—around the flocculus hypothesis. *Annual Review of Neuroscience, 5,* 275–296.

Ito, M. (1984). *The cerebellum and neural control.* New York: Raven.

Kandel, E. R., Klein, M., Hochner, B., Shuster, M., Siegelbaum, S. A., Hawkins, R. D., Glanzman, D. L., & Castellucci, V. F. (1987). Synaptic modulation and learning: New insights into synaptic transmission from the study of behavior. In G. M. Edelman, W. E. Gall, & W. M. Cowan (Eds.), *Synaptic function* (pp. 471–518). New York: Wiley.

Kelso, S. R., & Brown, T. H. (1986). Differential conditioning of associative synaptic enhancement in hippocampal brain slices. *Science, 232,* 85–87.

Kelso, S. R., Ganong, A. H., & Brown, T. H. (1986). Hebbian synapses in hippocampus. *Proceedings of the National Academy of Sciences USA, 83,* 5326–5330.

Kienker, P. K., Sejnowski, T. J., Hinton, G. E., & Schumacher, L. E. (1986). Separating figure from ground with a parallel network. *Perception, 15,* 197–216.

Kleinschmidt, A., Bear, M. F., & Singer, W. (1986). *Neuroscience Letters, 26* (Suppl.), S58.

Klopf, A. H. (1987). *A neuronal model of classical conditioning.* (Technical Report AFWAL-TR-87-1139). Dayton, Ohio: Wright-Patterson Air Force Base Aeronautical Laboratories.

Kohonen, T. (1970). Correlation matrix memories. *IEEE Transactions on Computers, C-21,* 353–359.

Kohonen, T. (1984). *Self-organization and associative memory.* New York: Springer-Verlag.

Komatsu, Y., Fujii, K., Maeda, J., Sakaguchi, H., & Toyama, K. (1988). Long-term potentiation of synaptic transmission in kitten visual cortex. *Journal of Neurophysiology, 59,* 124–141.

Levy, W. B., Anderson, J. A., & Lehmkuhle, W. (1984). *Synaptic change in the nervous system.* Hillsdale, N.J.: Erlbaum.

Levy, W. B., Brassel, S. E., & Moore, S. D. (1983). Partial quantification of the associative synaptic learning rule of the dentate gyrus. *Neuroscience, 8,* 799–808.

Linsker, R. (1986). From basic network principles to neural architecture: Emergence of orientation columns. *Proceedings of the National Academy of Sciences USA, 83,* 8779–8783.

Longuet-Higgins, H. C. (1968). Holographic model of temporal recall. *Nature, 217,* 104–107.

Lynch, G. & Baudry, M. (1988). Structure–function relationships in the organization of memory. In M. S. Gazzaniga (Ed.), *Perspectives in memory research and training* (pp. 23–92). Cambridge, Mass.: MIT Press.

Marr, D. (1969). A theory of cerebellar cortex. *Journal of Physiology, 202,* 437–470.

Marr, D. (1982). *Vision.* San Francisco: Freeman.

McNaughton, B. L., Douglas, R. M., & Goddard, G. V. (1978). Synaptic enhancement in fascia dentata: Cooperativity among coactive afferents. *Brain Research, 157,* 277.

McNaughton, B. L., & Morris, R. G. (1987). Hippocampal synaptic enhancement and information storage within a distributed memory system. *Trends in Neurosciences, 10,* 408–415.

Miles, F. A., & Lisberger, S. G. (1981). Plasticity in the vestibulo-ocular reflex: A new hypothesis. *Annual Review of Neuroscience, 4,* 273–299.

Moore, J. W., Desmond, J. E., Berthier, N. E., Blazis, D. E. J., Sutton, R. S., & Barto, A. G.

(1986). Simulation of the classically conditioned nicitating membrane response by a neuron-like adaptive element: Response topography, neuronal firing, and interstimulus intervals. *Behavioral Brain Research, 21,* 143–154.

Mpitsos, G. J., & Cohna, C. S. (1986). Discriminative behavior and Pavlovian conditioning in the mollusc. *Journal of Neurobiology, 17,* 469–486.

Reiter, H. O., & Stryker, M. P. (1987). A novel expression of plasticity in kitten visual cortex in the absence of postsynaptic activity. *Society for Neuroscience Abstracts, 13,* 1241.

Rolls, E. T. (1987). Information representation, processing and storage in the brain: Analysis at the single neuron level. In J.-P. Changeux & M. Konishi (Eds.), *Neural and molecular mechanisms of learning* (pp. 503–540). Berlin: Springer-Verlag.

Rumelhart, D. E., & McClelland, J. L. (1986). *Parallel distributed processing: Explorations in the microstructure of cognition: Vol. 1. Foundations.* Cambridge, Mass.: MIT Press.

Sahley, C., Rudy, J. W., & Gelperin, A. (1981). An analysis of associative learning in a terrestrial mollusc: Higher-order conditioning, blocking, and a transient US pre-exposure effect. *Journal of Comparative Physiology, 144,* 1–8.

Sahley, C. L., Rudy, J. W., & Gelperin, A. (1984). Associative learning in a mollusc: A comparative analysis. In D. Alkon & J. Farley (Eds.), *Primary neural substrates of learning and behavioral change* (pp. 243–258). New York: Cambridge University Press.

Sejnowski, T. J. (1977a). Statistical constraints on synaptic plasticity. *Journal of Mathematical Biology, 69,* 385–389.

Sejnowski, T. J. (1977b). Storing covariance with nonlinearly interacting neurons. *Journal of Mathematical Biology, 4,* 303–321.

Sejnowski, T. J. (1981). Skeleton filters in the brain. In G. E. Hinton & J. A. Anderson (Eds.), *Parallel models of associative memory* (pp. 189–212). Hillsdale, N.J.: Erlbaum.

Sejnowski, T. J. (1987). Computational models and the development of topographic projections. *Trends in Neurosciences, 10,* 304–305.

Sejnowski, T. J., & Hinton, G. E. (1987). Separating figure from ground with a Boltzmann machine. In M. A. Arbib & A. R. Hanson (Eds.), *Vision, brain and cooperative computation* (pp. 703–724). Cambridge, Mass.: MIT Press.

Sejnowski, T. J., & Tesauro, G. (1989). The Hebb rule for synaptic plasticity: Algorithms and implementations. In J. N. Byrne & W. O. Berry (Eds.), *Neural model of plasticity* (pp. 94–103). Orlando, Fla.: Academic Press.

Shepherd, G. M., Brayton, R. K., Miller, J. P., Segev, I., Rinzel, J., & Rall, W. (1985). Signal enhancement in distal cortical dendrites by means of interactions between active dendritic spines. *Proceedings of the National Academy of Sciences USA, 82,* 2192–2195.

Sherman, S. M., & Spear, P. D. (1982). Organization of visual pathways in normal and deprived cats. *Physiological Reviews, 62,* 738.

Singer, W. (1987). Activity-dependent self-organization of synaptic connections as a substrate of learning. In J. P. Changeux & M. Konishi (Eds.), *The neural and molecular bases of learning* (pp. 301–336). New York: Wiley.

Stanton, P., Jester, J., Chattarji, S., & Sejnowski, T. J. (1988). Associative long-term depression (LTD) or potentiation (LTP) is produced in the hippocampus dependent upon the phase of rhythmically active inputs. *Society for Neuroscience Abstracts, 14,* 19.

Steinbuch, K. (1961). Die Lernmatrix. *Kybernetik, 1,* 36–45.

Stent, G. W. (1973). A physiological mechanism for Hebb's postulate of learning. *Proceedings of the National Academy of Sciences USA, 70,* 997–1001.

Sutton, R. S. (1987). *A temporal-difference model of classical conditioning.* (Technical Report TR87-509.2). Waltham, Mass.: GTE Labs.

Sutton, R. S., & Barto, A. G. (1981). Toward a modern theory of adaptive networks: Expectation and prediction. *Psychological Review, 88,* 135–170.

Tesauro, G. (1986). Simple neural models of classical conditioning. *Biological Cybernetics, 55,* 187–200.

Tesauro, G. (1988). A plausible neural circuit for classical conditioning without synaptic plasticity. *Proceedings of the National Academy of Sciences USA, 85,* 2830–2833.

Thompson, R. F. (1986). The neurobiology of learning and memory. *Science, 233,* 941–947.

Toulouse, G., Dehaene, S., & Changeux, J. P. (1986). Spin glass model of learning by selection. *Proceedings of the National Academy of Sciences USA, 83,* 1695–1698.

von der Malsburg, C. (1973). Self-organization of orientation sensitive cells in striate cortex. *Kybernetik, 14,* 85.

Wigstrom, H., & Gustafsson, B. (1985). On long-lasting potentiation in the hippocampus: A proposed mechanism for its dependence on coincident pre- and postsynaptic activity. *Acta Physiologica Scandinavica, 123,* 519.

Wilshaw, D. (1981). Holography, associative memory, and inductive generalization. In G. E. Hinton & J. A. Anderson (Eds.), *Parallel models of associative memory* (pp. 83–104). Hillsdale, N.J.: Erlbaum.

Woody, C. D. (1982). *Memory, learning and higher function.* Berlin: Springer-Verlag.

18

A Neural Architecture
for the Representation of Scenes

CHRISTOPH VON DER MALSBURG

Learning and memory deal with the process by which knowledge and skills are absorbed and stored in the brain. To understand them it is important to have precise ideas about the stuff that is being stored: What is its nature? How is it organized? How is it implemented in neural hardware? The neuroscience of learning and memory is at present conditioned by a set of concepts based on specific answers to these questions. In this chapter I will raise a number of issues that are not solved in this framework. These issues have come up during attempts at model reconstructions of elementary capabilities of the brain, such as pattern recognition, perceptual segmentation, and scene representation. Backengineering is an important window to the brain. It is true that if a given functional problem had a million technical solutions, the construction of any one of them would say nothing about nature's solution. However, there is good reason to believe that relevant functional problems have very few solutions, and any one of them will suggest important constraints to the neuroscience of brain function. Backengineering is a fruitful exercise because it necessitates whole-system solutions. This puts it in contrast to many studies that limit their view to small subtasks and subsystems, thus leaving out essential aspects. This chapter continues a series of conceptual discussions (von der Malsburg, 1981, 1987b; von der Malsburg & Bienenstock, 1986). More technical accounts of the approach advocated here are contained in Bienenstock and von der Malsburg (1987), von der Malsburg (1985, 1988), von der Malsburg and Schneider (1986), von der Malsburg and Bienenstock (1987) and Werman (1987).

THE ISSUE OF ARCHITECTURE

In computer science one often speaks of the architecture of a system. The term refers to a conceptual level of structure which abstracts from details of implementation and from consideration of particular applications. It has been said that the brain is just an incoherent collection of simple tricks, each one to be understood on its own. If that was true, nothing could be discussed on a general abstract level and there would be no functional architecture to the brain.

This view is conceivable, but is it likely to be realistic? How could such unprincipled structure have come about in the brain? The obvious answer is that evolution created it through simple trial and error. If there really were no general design principles, this would be a very inefficient process. A generous estimate limits genetic information that can have accumulated over the course of evolution to a few billion bits (von der Malsburg & Singer, 1988). This is in line with the amount of information in our genes. Since about 33 bits are required to designate one out of the 10^{10} cells in our cerebral cortex, the specification of its 10^{14} synapses needs slightly more than 33×10^{14} bits (not speaking about the rest of the brain and nervous system). Evolution therefore must have made use of regularities and strategies, otherwise it could not have developed the brain (von der Malsburg, 1987a). These strategies and regularities certainly constitute an architecture.

The point just made can be illustrated by the analogy to computer programs. Each little algorithm in a software system could be a realization of an independent little trick. There is no inherent necessity to conform to any abstract style or architecture. But that is not what you find in actual programs. A very important aspect of the recent history of computer science is the development of high-level computer languages, programming styles, verification procedures, and data structures. This was important to speed up "evolution." Developing or debugging an architecturally unstructured sequence of machine instructions would simply be prohibitively slow. The same reason must have forced evolution to develop an architecture.

More specifically, the view has been expressed that the brain had no representation of its environment; that is, there was no coherent system by which a one-to-one correspondence could (in principle) be established between stiuations in the environment and states of the brain. In terms of an analogy, a car is designed to deal with road situations but it would be very difficult or impossible to find any kind of "representation" of road situations in the structure or dynamical state of the car. It is much better understood in terms of a collection of devices and mechanisms to solve individual problems one at a time. Analogously, the brain could be just a collection of reflexes and mechanisms designed to deal with individual problems and situations.

The issue of correspondence between mind and reality is a very important and a very old subject of philosophy. We can, of course, have no knowledge of reality in any direct sense *(Ding an sich)*. When we speak of "reality" we refer to a mental construction that is objective in the sense that it is not subject to individual arbitrary choices and that we can communicate and agree about it. It would therefore be absurd to claim we had no mental representation of reality. In a dualist point of view this statement about mind still leaves open the issue of existence of a representation in the brain. To avoid a lengthy philosophical discussion let me leave this line of argument to the reader.

There is a further argument in favor of the existence of a representation of our environment in the brain, again based on development, this time on the time scale of individual learning and memory. When we are thrown into a new and unfamiliar environment we repeatedly run into situations to which we cannot react in appropriate ways. After a while, however, we acquire experience and learn to deal flexibly with every new situation. This is possible only on the basis of a perceptive system able to make all distinctions necessary for appropriate decisions, although many of these decisions had never been met before. Our level of success in dealing with new situations in familiar environments indicates that the raster of distinctions that can be made by our perceptive system is complete in a certain sense. This raster of distinctions is a perception of the environment and may certainly be called a representation of it.

Proceeding on the assumption that there is indeed an abstract and coherent architecture to the brain, let me briefly discuss the two aspects of neural architecture, network topology and dynamics. Network dynamics deals with the nature of signals and the mechanisms by which they are processed in neurons. It also deals with the way in which processing mechanisms are plastically changed and organized. Network topology speaks about the connectivity diagram of brain networks, their subdivision into areas, the fiber projections between areas, and the internal structure of connections within them. The term brain architecture is often seen as synonymous with network topology. On the other hand, neural dynamics is far from being clear in its details and deserves more attention. My concern here is mainly with neural dynamics, although I am aware of the importance of more intensive work on network topology.

THE PROBLEM OF SCENE REPRESENTATION

Associative memory (Anderson, 1970; Cooper, 1974; Hopfield, 1982; Kohonen 1977; Palm, 1980; Steinbuch, 1961; Willshaw, Buneman, & Longuet-Higgins, 1969) crystallizes a set of answers to many issues of brain architecture. It suggests a data structure that can be decomposed into elementary symbols or propositions. Each element corresponds to a neuron or to a small set of neurons. Dynamics takes the form of an exchange of excitation and inhibition such that activity stabilizes in certain stationary states. New stationary states can be stored as memory traces with the help of Hebbian plasticity. Associative memory suggests a network topology in which the brain is cut into subsystems, each of which has complete connectivity (or something like a sparse random subset of the complete network), with sparse and regular connections between subsystems.

Memory traces can be dynamically reconstructed from partial information. Thus incomplete sensory information regarding a familiar object can be completed by the addition of missing elements and by the addition of abstract descriptors and names; or a sensory stimulus can be completed by the dynamic reconstruction of a response which was once learned to be associated to the stimulus. With these properties associative memory is a candidate concept for brain architecture.

Is this the complete answer to the question of brain function? One big unsolved problem with associative memory is appropriate generalization from one situation in which something has been learned to other, different, situations in which the knowledge is applied. The main problem here is that situations never recur identically in natural environments, and that generalization is an absolute necessity for an animal to survive. The only type of generalization inherent in associative memory is over Hamming distance, that is, between states which have a large cell-wise overlap with each other.

The issue of generalization cannot be discussed without specifying the nature of the general task of the nervous system. This is to control an organism in a temporally changing scene in order to achieve goals and avoid disaster. The central entity for the nervous system is thus a *generalized scene*. Its internal representation, its creation from perceptual data and stored knowledge, as well as its manipulation and transformation are the central issues of brain architecture. The generalized scene comprises the scene in the more narrow sense which surrounds the organism: descriptions of objects, their parts, their relationships, and their state of movement, including the organism itself. This will mostly be built up by visual image interpretation helped by stored knowledge. Beyond that, the scene describes objects in terms of interpretation, role, significance, material, and the like; it represents action plans, including those of other agents within the scene. The generalized scene is not limited to static situations, dealing also with temporal processes. Finally, motor patterns concerning manipulation, navigation, and communication are to be created as part of the generalized scene.

The term *scene* implies static structure. This needs comment. A scene has to be organized by a temporal process in the nervous system. This process cannot be regulated by specific procedures for specific scenes. Flexibility calls for a very general mechanism of organization. Associative memory, and indeed all known systems displaying self-organization, are based on mechanisms of relaxation toward stationary states. If the generalized scene is to comprise temporal processes such as motor patterns, then there seems to be a problem: How can such patterns be created as stationary states? The solution very likely lies in the possibility of representing temporal processes in a nontemporal way. Any graphical representation with time as abscissa is an example of a nontemporal representation of a temporal process. A neural implementation of such representation is represented by the holophone (Longuet-Higgins 1967). After a motor pattern has been created in a stationary representation it can be "read off" by a standard mechanism which transforms it into the temporal domain.

THE GENERALIZATION PROBLEM

The usual basis for generalization is abstraction, by which a situation is freed from its particular context and is thus made available for many contexts. This can be done by an incomplete description of a situation in a way that reduces it to a useful principle that can be frequently applied. An abstract situation or scheme is applied by attaching it to a new scene. Thus generalization involves three difficult steps:

1. Useful abstractions must be discovered. Not any part of one scene is applicable to others. One important step to abstraction is the decomposition of a scene into subsituations that are coherent in some sense.
2. When a useful abstraction or principle has been formed its applicability to a new scene must be discovered. This step necessitates a concept of structural relatedness, possibly based on partial overlap or on some kind of isomorphy.
3. There has to be a way to attach an abstract descriptor to a new situation and thereby modify its processing.

Opportunities to generalize are based on the existence of regularities and symmetries. In a biological context an important source of regularity is the genetical reproduction of structures. Another important practical example is generalization on the basis of perceptual invariance. A single object in the external world can create a large variety of stimulus patterns on sensory surfaces, depending on incidental variables. For instance, the retinal image created by light reflected by an object depends in its position, size, shape, color, and intensity distribution on eye position, object distance and orientation, and on illumination. It is important for an organism to have an internal representation of an object which is independent of incidental variables and on the basis of which it can generalize from one retinal image to others of the same object.

The ability to generalize is an important criterion in the discussion of neural architectures. The three steps necessary for generalization are realized in associative memory at best in a very rudimentary form. The reason for its limitations is its inadequate structure concept, which is based on overlap, or Euclidean or Hamming distance, between two states. It has been shown (Cooper, 1974; Kohonen, 1977) that associative memory can be made to abstract a prototype from a set of patterns which have large overlap with each other. Thus a noise-free prototype can be abstracted from a sequence of noisy exemplars. Applicability of a memory trace to an input pattern is discovered on the basis of sufficient overlap between the two. Application of this "abstract descriptor" is done by replacing the input pattern by the stored one. This mechanism of generalization has serious weaknesses. The first is that situations are treated in a monolithic fashion. Segmentation of a situation into subsituations is not possible in a flexible way (it has to be imposed by a rigid connection pattern between subsystems). Thus the recurrence of a subpattern in different situations cannot be put to profit. Second, a subpattern b can be applied to an input pattern a only if b has been previously associated and attached to a by synaptic plasticity. The appearance of a then leads to the coactivation of b. There is no concept of structural similarity that could lead to the *discovery* within the system of a relationship between a and b such that they can be associated spontaneously. Finally, the principle by which descriptors are attached to other subpatterns, simple coactivation, is very poorly structured. If, for instance, a descriptor symbol b is to be attached to symbol a and a descriptor b' to symbol a' at the same time, an ambiguity arises if all four symbols are simply coactivated because an attachment $b \leftrightarrow a'$ and $b' \leftrightarrow a$ would lead to the same neural state. This is the syntax problem which is the main subject of this chapter.

The poor generalization properties of associative memory are considerably improved in layered systems (Ackley, Hinton, & Sejnowksi, 1985; Fukushima, 1980; Marko & Giebel, 1970; Rosenblatt, 1961; more references are found in Rumelhart & McClelland, 1986). The central concept here is feature detectors (or association units or hidden units). These are enabled to detect subpatterns in an input stimulus by appropriate connections restricted to those neurons on which the subpatterns are defined. A feature dector generalizes over all input patterns which share the required subpattern. Layered structures have much more power to generalize than associative memory and are especially not limited to small Hamming distance between input patterns. The basis of this higher power to generalize is a restriction of connectivity. Whereas in associative memory a neuron receives connections from all other neurons with which it is coactive in some memory state (although for reasons of economy only a sample thereof is realized), connections in layered structures are restricted to those between layers (which is, of course, the essence of layering) and, further, to small subsets of all connections between layers.

Steps 2 and 3 of our generalization scheme are easily accomplished in layered structures: The applicability of abstractions is discovered with the activation of association units. Activation of an association unit in turn activates the correct output units to which it has been connected. The first step, however—discovery of opportunities to abstract and generalize and implementation of appropriate connections with input and output layers of the sysem—is difficult. The difficulty has to do precisely with the important restriction of interlayer connections. Let us consider an individual excitatory connection between two neurons α and β as an elementary rule of the kind "If α is on, then β also should be on." The problem of finding the right connections is equivalent to finding the right elementary rules. For associative memory this is simple. During storage of a state the activity of all neurons is controlled from outside, and if neurons α and β are simultaneously active in a state to be memorized, then α and β are to be connected with each other. In a layered structure in which activity in input and output layers is controlled from outside an appropriate subset of hidden units is to be activated and then appropriate connections are to be introduced or strengthened. The previous idea of strengthening all connections between coactive neurons in different layers introduces too many connections. Instead, all those connections that fit only a particular situation and do not generalize should be left out.

A solution to this problem which is implicit in many of the neural systems that have been proposed (see, for instance, Ackley et al., 1985; Rosenblatt, 1961; more references in Rumelhart & McClelland, 1986) is based on statistical properties of large sets of situations. A starting configuration of connections is given. This may be random or it may already implement some general property of the problem at hand, such as locality of connections. Then a sequence of situations is presented by the activation of input neurons. In each situation hidden units and output units settle into activity states on the basis of current connections. Connections are changed in small increments according to some rule which has the important property of stabilizing the system in a state of satisfactory reaction and of modifying it in states of unsatisfactory reaction (where the satisfactory/unsatisfactory decision is taken by some external teacher who knows correct responses). The final connectivity pattern is shaped by statistical properties of the set of applied stiuations. Those subpatterns on input and output layers are finally represented by hidden units which have consistently appeared in many successful situations. If, for instance, mirror symmetry about a given axis is to be detected in an input plane, then pairs of symmetrically lying pixels come to be represented (Sejnowski, Kienker, & Hinton, 1986).

A problem with this method is that it may necessitate extreme numbers of training situations (dozens of thousands of input patterns were necessary to train the system just cited). This will be particularly worrisome in numerically large systems and especially with problems in which generalization necessitates detection of large subpatterns. In contrast, there are many types of phenomena for which the structure of a problem and potent generalizations can be deduced from very few exemplars. This is possible only if a system can detect significant subpatterns in individual situations without having recourse to the statistics of many situations. In the example in which the symmetry of pixel patterns is to be classified this is possible by the detection of structural relationships between symmetrically lying parts of a single pattern.

The detection and processing of structural relationships and of significant patterns *before* they are represented by association units, such that they can help in the establishment of such units, is not possible in the neural architecture implicit in associative memory and in the layered structures discussed. A modification of neural architecture that permits the processing of this type of syntactical information is introduced below.

SYMBOL SYSTEMS WITH SYNTAX

According to the *Concise Oxford Dictionary,* syntax is "the grammatical arrangement of words in speech or writing to show their connection and relation; set of rules governing this arrangement." Syntax is an important and integral aspect of all known symbol systems. This will be illustrated shortly. Neural networks, as discussed thus far, are a notable example.

Any symbol system consists of elementary symbols, which can be combined into more complex composite symbols. The elmentary symbols of written language are letters and other characters. These are combined into words, phrases, sentences, paragraphs, chapters, and books. Since text ultimately refers to the temporal process of spoken language, the syntactical arrangement of subsymbols into higher symbols is a linear chain. The whole information content of a long textual communication is contained in the syntactical arrangement of characters. In mathematics complex formulas are composed by combining elementary characters and other symbols. It is possible to replace a whole formula like $(2a\int_0^\infty e^{-a^2x^2}dx)^2$ by another elementary symbol, say π, but it is clear that new abbreviations cannot replace syntactically structured composite symbols altogether. The processing of syntactical structures is the whole subject of algebra! The introduction of new abbreviations has to be preceded by the recognition of significant constellations of symbols. For this reason alone processing of unabbreviated syntactical arrays of symbols must be possible.

Compare this to a neural network. A complex symbol in a network is an activity pattern. This can be decomposed into elementary symbols, active neurons. An unstructured list of the neurons that are active in a state is all the information there is. (With analog signals a vector of numbers is required.) The arrangement of entries in the list is immaterial since there are no dynamical variables that could code different arrangements. The structure of connections between neurons is important for the establishment of activity states but it cannot be read off signals. Consequently, neural networks of the kind discussed so far have only one composition rule by which a single complex symbol can be formed at a time: by the simultaneous activation of a set of neurons.

Let me illustrate this point by the contrast to another symbol system, data structures in computer science. An important general data structure consists of hierarchical lists. Take the three lists, $A = (a\ b\ c\ d)$, $B = [(a\ b)\ (c\ d)]$, and $C = [(a\ d)\ (c\ b)]$. Although they comprise the same elementary symbols, these lists are discriminable objects and the distinction between them is important. Only A is natural to the neural architecture discussed so far, the distinction between A, B, and C being impossible. This point was raised a long time ago. Rosenblatt (1961, p. 478) discussed the following situation. A layered structure, a "perceptron," has been trained to respond (with four output units) to squares and triangles in all positions on a retina. Unit $r_\triangle$ responds to a triangle, $r_\square$ responds to a square, r_{top} responds to a stimulus in the top half of the retina, and r_{bot} responds to a stimulus in the bottom half. What if there is a triangle in the top half and square in the bottom half of retina? All four units go on, corresponding to the list $(r_\triangle\ r_{\text{top}}\ r_\square\ r_{\text{bot}})$. This state does not discriminate the situation from another one in which the positions of square and triangle are interchanged. A list $[(r_\triangle\ r_{\text{top}})\ (r_\square\ r_{\text{bot}})]$ would describe the situation correctly, the other situation being described by $[(r_\triangle\ r_{\text{bot}})\ (r_\square\ r_{\text{top}})]$. Rosenblatt proposed solving the problem with the help of selective attention. He added back-coupling to his system, which introduced an instability such that the system either activated only units $(r_\triangle\ r_{\text{top}})$ or only units $(r_\square\ r_{\text{bot}})$, depending on chance or on influences from other modalities.

A very similar problem was experimentally investigated by Treisman and Gelade (1980). A visual situation is presented tachistoscopically in which there are colored letters together with distractor digits. After a short presentation time (typically 120 msec) the display is masked by visual noise. The surprising result is that subjects make many conjunction errors, mistaking, for instance, a red O and a green X for a red X and/or a green O. This happens in every two or three trials. No such errors occur, of course, if the pattern is displayed sufficiently long. The interpretation seems straightforward. There are four types of neurons, responding to red (r_{red}), green (r_{grn}), letter X (r_X), and letter O (r_O). After a short presentation active neurons are described by the list $A = (r_X\ r_{red}\ r_O\ r_{grn})$. Syntactical information is missing. The system knows that there has to be syntactical binding between letters and colors and proceeds by guessing one of the possibilities, say $B = [(r_X\ r_{grn})\ (r_O\ r_{red})]$. Theoretically, the problem could be mended by the introduction of new types of neurons, encoding conjunctions $(r_X\ r_{red})$, $(r_O\ r_{grn})$, and so on. The experiment shows that either these units do not exist or they can be activated only indirectly with great delay. Treisman and Gelade propose attention to solve the problem. Given enough time, the visual system concentrates attention sequentially on one letter after another, thereby coactivating all feature units that correspond to one letter. The rest of the brain then can read off syntactical relations from the temporal conjunctions thus created.

Another important type of experiment in which syntactical relationships play a central role is described by Julesz (1984). This work deals with the perception of fields formed out of small figural elements, called textons. Segregation of figure from ground is found to be effortless and rapid if figure and ground differ in their mix of texton types. Segregation is tedious and slow if figure and ground differ only in local syntactical bindings of the same texton elements. One may again conclude that syntax is processed in the temporal domain, with the help of a sequence of local fixations of attention.

NEURAL REPRESENTATION OF SYNTAX

Is there a coherent and general way in which syntax can be represented in neural architecture? The problem has always been camouflaged by the fact that any rigid predetermined set of syntactical relations can be represented by neurons again, as in our previous example by a neuron $r_{X_{red}}$ encoding the binding $(r_X\ r_{red})$ of neurons r_X and r_{red}. The point made here, however, is that for learning it is important to process syntactical information which is not yet represented by neurons, in order to detect syntactical combinations that are worth being represented by new neurons. Even in a static, nonlearning system it may be advantageous to have the possibility to represent and process syntax which is not represented by neurons, either because the required number of neurons would be prohibitive or, more importantly, because those neurons would be too special to be a basis for generalization. The psychophysical work cited (Julesz, 1984; Treisman & Gelade, 1980) is an illustration of this.

To pose the syntax problem clearly let us speak of a neural system that has a fixed connectivity structure and in which, consequently, each neuron can be interpreted as a symbol with fixed meaning. Let us refer to all of them as elementary symbols, although their majority actually codes for combinations of others. We are now interested in an architecture that is able to represent and process syntactical structure on these elementary symbols in a flexible way.

The mathematical structure of syntax is not clear. Let there be N elementary symbols. A simple version of syntax assigns a single variable to each pair of elementary symbols. There would then be N^2 such variables, and the complete structure would be a graph with elementary symbols as nodes and syntax variables as links. A graph assigns a syntax variable to each pair of nodes. More complex systems would assign variables to larger sets of nodes, say tripletts or quadrupletts. A system assigning variables to sets of not more than n neurons is said to be "of order n."

A conceptually simple way of representing syntax is the introduction of a two-class system of neurons. Class 1 neurons act as elementary symbols, class 2 neurons encode syntax variables. In the simplest case, a system of order 2 representing graphs on N nodes or class 1 neurons could be constructed with the help of N^2 class 2 neurons. Such systems have been described in the literature (Hopfield & Tank, 1986; Kree & Zippelius, 1988; McClelland, 1985; Phillips, Hancock, Willson, & Smith, 1988; Sejnowski, 1981). It is important also to process higher order relations. The direct method of representing them in a complete way by neurons is not practical. The number of neurons required would be prohibitive. It is conceivable, however, that a combinatorial code can be found in which sets of class 2 neurons represent higher order relations.

REPRESENTATION OF SYNTAX BY SIGNAL CORRELATIONS

A much more parsimonious and extremely flexible representation of syntax can be based on temporal correlations between neural signals (von der Malsburg, 1981, 1985, 1987; von der Malsburg & Bienenstock, 1986, 1987). Only node neurons and their connections are required for the system. Minor alterations to conventional neural architecture are necessary. If s_i denotes the membrane potential of neuron i, σ_i its axonal signal, and W_{ij} the synaptic weight connecting neuron j to neuron i, then neural signal dynamics is usually written as

$$\dot{s}_i = -\alpha s_i + \sum_j W_{ij}\sigma_j - \beta \sum_j \sigma_j + \rho_i \qquad (1)$$

where α and β are parameters. Neurophysiology has in this formulation been simplified in several respects in order to show essentials. Inputs to the system may be formally subsumed under the second term. A rudimentary inhibitory system is modeled by the third term, the idea being that inhibition is a service system to keep the sum of all signals in the system at about a constant level. Noise may originate in a number of places—in the statistical process of spike generation, as a consequence of the complexities of synaptic transmission, or within the membrane—and it is symbolically represented here by an additive term ρ_i. The axonal signal is derived from the membrane potential by some functional

$$\sigma_j = \varphi(s_j, \sigma_j) \qquad (2)$$

which models a threshold function, refractory time, and may also have stochastic aspects to it. The form of Eqs. 1 and 2 is completely conventional. However, whereas these equations are normally implemented to tend to stationary signal levels (as long as input signals are constant), I propose here to set noise level and parameters to create stochastic fluctuations in signal levels. Due to structured input signals and to excitatory and inhibitory connections between neurons, fluctuations in the signals of different neurons are correlated with each other. Syntactical binding between neurons is simply expressed by a correlation between their signals (Fig. 18.1). There is no limit to the syntactical order that can be represetned. There are, however, limits to the amount of syntactical information which can be expressed in a given time interval, due to limited temporal resolution of neural signals.

When coming to the issue of dynamical processing of syntax a more radical deviation from conventional network dynamics is required. To this end the single synaptic weight variable W_{ij} is replaced by two variables, T_{ij} and W_{ij}. According to Eq. 1, variable W_{ij} is the efficiency with which synapse ij transmits signal σ_j to cell i. This variable is allowed to change on a fast time scale (see below). The quantity $T_{ij} \geq 0$, on the other hand, is a constant (although it may slowly change due to synaptic plasticity) and determines the range over which W_{ij} is allowed to change:

$$0 \leq W_{ij} \leq T_{ij} \qquad (3)$$

Synapses that do not exist, $T_{ij} = 0$, cannot be switched on. Dynamic synaptic weights are regulated by a functional

$$\Delta W_{ij} = f(\sigma_j, s_i, W_{ij}, T_{ij}) \qquad (4)$$

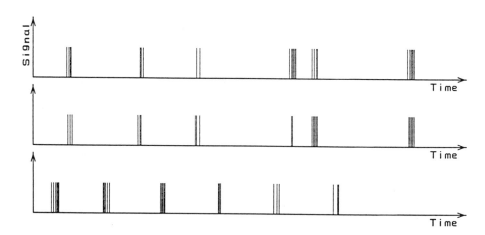

FIGURE 18.1.   Syntactical binding in the temporal domain. The signals of three cells are shown. Each vertical line represents an action potential. The upper two cells are syntactically bound to each other, their spikes being correlated in time with a certain temporal resolution. The lower two cells avoid firing simultaneously and are not bound to each other.

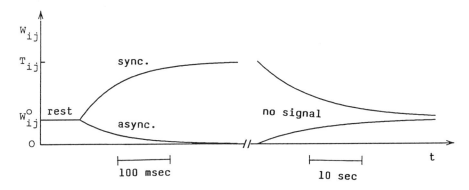

FIGURE 18.2. Dynamic control of the synaptic weight W_{ij} between cells j and i. If there are no signals in cells i and j, the dynamic weight has the resting value W^o_{ij}. Under the control of synchronous signals σ_i and σ_j (upper pair in Fig. 18.1), W_{ij} can be increased within fractions of a second to the upper limit, T_{ij} (upper branch in left half of figure). If signals σ_i and σ_j are asynchronous (lower pair in Figure 18.1), W_{ij} can be lowered to 0 (lower branch). When the signal σ_i in the postsynaptic neuron ceases W_{ij} decays with the time constant of short-term memory to the resting value (right part of figure).

which is somewhat analogous to Hebbian plasticity, though on a faster time scale: coincidences between incoming signal σ_j and strong depolarization of membrane potential s_i increase W_{ij}, at most up to the limit T_{ij}, whereas a signal σ_j hitting an undepolarized or hyperpolarized cell i decreases W_{ij}. Time constants for these actively controlled changes are fractions of a second. When there is no incoming signal the synapse slowly decays to a resting value intermediate between 0 and T_{ij} (Fig. 18.2).

Synaptic plasticity—change in the "permanent" synaptic parameter T_{ij}—is controlled by the dynamic weight W_{ij}:

$$\Delta T_{ij} = F(W_{ij}), \qquad > 0 \text{ for } W_{ij} \approx T_{ij} \qquad (5)$$

The function $F(W_{ij})$ is shaped according to the idea that a connection is allowed to grow only if the two neurons involved have something to do with each other, that is, are syntactically bound to each other, which in turn is expressed by signal correlations and a maximally activated dynamic weight W_{ij}. As far as learning and memory are concerned, this is the point of the exercise: to limit synaptic plasticity to those pairs of neurons which are syntactically bound to each other in a given situation, although many more neurons are active in that situation.

DYNAMICS OF SYNTACTICAL STRUCTURES

The formulation given here is meant to be sketchy and leaves out many details that would have to be specified in a simulation. Various concrete versions have been tried, each one optimizing its own set of goals (Bienenstock & von der Malsburg, 1987; von der Malsburg, 1985, 1988; von der Malsburg & Bienenstock, 1987; von der Malsburg & Schneider, 1986). Important aspects, however, are common to all of them. Very few or no arbitrary choices have been made in Eq. 1 to 5, yet they favor syntactical patterns of very specific structure. The momentary set $\{W_{ij}\}$ of synaptic weights together with an ensemble of input signals determines the statistical structure of signals according to Eqs. 1 and 2. These signals contain certain correlations which are shaped by correlations in the input signals and by cooperating sets of active connections. These correlations in turn act back on the connectivity structure according to Eq. 4. If input signals are sufficiently stationary in their statistical properties, this feedback loop between the connectivity state and internal signal statistics continues to change the dynamic state of the system until stationarity is reached in terms of connectivity and signal statistics, that is, in terms of syntactical structure.

What is the structure of connectivity patterns which are favored by this dynamical process? The graph of active connections in a connection patterns is sparse in the present formulation due to the β term in Eq. 1 which limits activity to fairly small sets of active neurons in each time slice. (A tendency to form sparse connection patterns is one of the very few "arbitrary" choices to be implemented in the system. Without this tendency the system would tend to the uninteresting and featureless total connectivity state.) The sparse graph of a connectivity pattern can locally be characterized by cooperative combinations of active connections: combinations that are effective in creating strong correlations. A favorable local constellation of connections is, for instance, a small set of neurons with complete connectivity (the set has to be small due to the sparseness constraint). Another favorable constellation is a set of short alternative pathways of equal delay between two cells a and b: if a fires, a wave of activity is transported over the several pathways to b where, accordingly, all participating synapses experience a favorable event.

If the dynamical aspect of brain architecture is described realistically here, there is an *a priori* structure imposed on all dynamic states of the brain. This limits activity to a certain universe of syntactical structures or connectivity-and-correlation patterns. There is thus a potent structure concept, as was asked for earlier. Global characterization of these connectivity patterns is an important unsolved problem. It has already been shown, however, that some very useful properties are implicit in the system. Two-dimensional topological graphs, which are ideal for representing and storing visual images, belong to the favored universe (von der Malsburg & Bienenstock, 1987). If there are two isomorphic connectivity patterns in different parts of the network, connectivity dynamics is able to discover this fact and activate a connectivity pattern which maps the two networks to each other in terms of the isomorphism (Bienenstock & von der Malsburg, 1987; von der Malsburg, 1988; von der Malsburg & Bienenstock, 1986). This can be conveniently used for position-invariant image recognition (Bienenstock & von der Malsburg, 1986; von der Malsburg, 1981, 1988). Many different connectivity patterns on the same set of neurons can be stored and retrieved (von der Malsburg, 1985; von der Malsburg & Bienenstock, 1987). Finally, separation of figure from ground has been demonstrated (von der Malsburg & Schneider, 1986).

THE GENERALIZED SCENE IN NEURAL ARCHITECTURE

The dynamical architecture described here is not an easy blueprint for the solution of all brain problems. The other aspect to architecture, permanent connectivity structure $\{T_{ij}\}$, is a much more voluminous issue. However, many problems that have proved to be difficult in conventional architecture may be much more easily solved in an architecture able to process syntactical structure.

One of the great problems awaiting solution is representation of the generalized scene in neural architecture. The difficulty arises from a number of aspects. One is the necessity to represent many components coexisting in a scene. A rigid representation of a visual scene, like a photograph, is not a basis for generalization and thus is not acceptable. The main reason is that accidental aspects, like the relative positions of objects, and essential aspects, like geometrical relationships within an object, are mixed with each other. In addition, a pictorial representation cannot accommodate abstract aspects of generalized scenes. The situation cries for a symbol system with syntax. Let me try to indicate the style of representation that would be possible.

Let us first talk about the representation of a single object. In a syntactical system designators can be attached to it which specify various aspects of functional importance. There may be a great variety of designators. Some may specify the position of the object in various frames of reference, for example, in world coordinates, in body coordinates, or in visual coordinates. Another kind of designator may specify geometrical relations of the object to others. Designators may attach to an object type information, names, or material. Also important is the attachment of designators of functional role: Is it edible? Is it dangerous? Is it agreeable or disagreeable? Is it the target of my intended movement? Does it play a causal role in some process? For a linguistic object grammatical role has to be attached. The alternative to the attachment of a designator in a system without syntax would be the creation of a new symbol whenever some specification is to be added.

If there was only one object in the whole scene, attachment of designators would be possible by simply activating the corresponding symbols. In realistic scenes, however, there have to be many objects at the same time. In a grammatical sentence with two nouns it is, for instance, necessary to attach the role of subject to one and the role of object to the other. Simple simultaneous activity in the symbols involved would lead to conjunction ambiguity, as illustrated above. If there is a flexible syntax system, however, complicated networks of objects and designators can be created. The designators themselves can be further specified by more designators. Also what is perceived as a single object may be represented by a network of descriptors and relationships (Bienenstock & von der Malsburg, 1987), so that the object cannot be identified with any elementary symbol. A single object is then represented as a scene.

The great distinction between cultural communication symbols and symbols in the brain lies in the way they are used. Communication signals are passive until they are interpreted by a receiver. Brain symbols form a dynamical system in themselves. The whole significance of one symbol lies in its ability to create another symbol in the next moment, in another part of the brain or in the same. An object represented by a network of cross-referencing designators acts as boundary condition for other pattern formation processes in which more connection patterns are formed. It is claimed here that a fixed neural architecture constructed along lines similar to those discussed around Eq. 1 to 4 suffices to act as the "set of rules governing this arrangement," as required by our dictionary definition. These general metagrammatical rules are to be specified to the needs of particular types of scenes and objects with the help of specific restrictions to connectivity imposed by the "permanent" parameters T_{ij}, which in turn can be modified by plasticity of the type in Eq. 5. A constellation like "there is an apple; it is an edible object; it is within the reach of my hand; it is my property," together with the symbol "I am hungry," is able to induce another complex symbol, "I have the intention to grasp; the object of the grasp is an edible object; this object is the apple; the apple has such and such body-frame coordinates," together with motor descriptions of appropriate movements of my arm and hand.

The claim I am making here will have to be validated in the course of a long reasearch program. Just now it is not much more than a vision and a scientific program. At best I may be able to convince a few specialists who are aware of the difficulties and problems involved in modeling even the most elementary capabilites of our brain. Only the very first simple steps of the program (von der Malsburg, 1981) have been demonstrated so far, as cited above. Experimental demonstration of some aspects of the dynamical architecture formulated in Eqs. 1 to 5 would be useful. Possible experiments have been described (von der Malsburg, 1987). The crucial test will, however, be technical demonstrations. If these are successful, their authority will influence our neurobiological thinking.

REFERENCES

Ackley, D. H., Hinton, G. E., & Sejnowski, T. J. (1985). A learning algorithm for Boltzmann machines. *Cognitive Science, 9,* 147–169.

Anderson, J. A. (1970). Two models for memory organization using interacting traces. *Mathematical Biosciences, 8,* 137–160.

Bienenstock, E., & von der Malsburg, C. (1987). A neural network for invariant pattern recognition. *Europhysics Letters, 4*(1), 121–126.

Cooper, L. N. (1974). A possible organization of animal memory and learning. In B. Lundquist & S. Lundquist (Eds.), *Proceedings of the Nobel Symposium on Collective Properties of Physical Systems* (pp. 252–264). New York: Academic Press.

Fukushima, K. (1980). Neocognitron: A self-organizing neural network model for a mechanism of pattern recognition unaffected by shift in position. *Biological Cybernetics, 36,* 193–202.

Hopfield, J. J. (1982). Neural networks and physical systems with emergent collective computational abilities. *Proceedings of the National Academy of Sciences USA, 79,* 2554–2558.

Hopfield, J. J., & Tank, D. W. (1986). Collective computation with continous variables. In E. Bienenstock, F. Fogelman Soulié, & G. Weisbuch (Eds.), *Disordered systems and biological organization* (NATO ASI Series, Vol F20, pp. 155–170). Berlin: Springer-Verlag.

Julesz, B. (1984, February). A brief outline of the texton theory of human vision. *Trends in Neurosciences,* 41–45.

Kohonen, T. (1977). *Associative memory.* Berlin: Springer-Verlag.

Kree, R., & Zippelius, A (1988). Recognition of topological features of graphs and images in neural networks. *Journal of Physics, A21,* L813.

Longuet-Higgins, H.-C. (1967). Holographic model of temporal recall. *Nature, 217,* 104.

Marko, H., & Giebel, H. (1970). Recognition of handwritten characters with a system of homogeneous layers. *Nachrichtentechnische Zeitschrift, 9,* 455–459.

McClelland, J. L. (1985). Putting knowledge in its place: A scheme for programming parallel processing structures on the fly. *Cognitive Science, 9,* 113–146.

Palm, G. (1980). On associative memory. *Biological Cybernetics, 36,* 19–31.

Phillips, W. A., Hancock, P. J. B., Willson, N. J., & Smith, L. S. (1988). On the acquisition of object concepts from sensory data. In R. Eckmiller & C. von der Malsburg (Eds.), *Neural computers* (NATO ASI Series: Computer Systems Sciences, Vol. 41). Berlin: Springer-Verlag.

Rosenblatt, F. (1961). *Principles of neurodynamics: Perceptrons and the theory of brain mechanisms.* Washington, D.C.: Spartan Books.

Rumelhart, D. E., & McClelland, J. L. (Eds.). (1986). Parallel distributed processing (Vol. 1). Cambridge, Mass.: MIT Press.

Sejnowski, T. J. (1981). Skeleton filters in the brian. In G. E. Hinton & J. A. Anderson (Eds.), *Parallel models of associative memory* (pp. 190–212). Hillsdale, N.J.: Erlbaum.

Sejnowski, T. J., Kienker, P. K., & Hinton, G. E. (1986). Learning symmetry groups with hidden units: Beyond the perceptron. *Physica, 22D,* 260–275.

Steinbuch, K. (1961). Die Lernmatrix. *Kybernetik, 1,* 1-36.

Treisman, A. M., & Gelade, G. (1980). A feature-integration theory of attention. *Cognitive Psychology, 12,* 97–136.

von der Malsburg, C. (1981). *The correlation theory of brain function* (Internal Report 81-2). MPI Biophysical Chemistry, P.O. Box 2841, 3400 Göttingen, West Germany.

von der Malsburg, C. (1985). Nervous structures with dynamical links. *Berichte Bunsengesellschaft fuer Physikalische, Chemie, 89,* 703–710.

von der Malsburg, C. (1987a). Ist die Evolution blind? In B.-O. Küppers (Ed.), *Ordnung aus dem Chaos.* Munich: Piper.

von der Malsburg, C. (1987b). Synaptic plasticity as basis of brain organization. In J.-P. Changeux & M. Konishi (Eds.), *The neural and molecular bases of learning, Dahlem Konferenzen* (pp. 411–431). Chichester: Wiley.

von der Malsburg, C. (1988). Pattern recognition by labeled graph matching. *Neural Networks, 1,* 141–148.

von der Malsburg, C., & Bienenstock, E. (1986). Statistical coding and short-term synaptic plasticity: A scheme for knowledge representation in the brain. In E. Bienenstock, F. Fogelman, & G. Weisbuch (Eds.), *Disordered systems and biological organization* (NATO ASI Series, Vol. F20, pp. 247–272). Berlin: Springer-Verlag.

von der Malsburg, C. & Bienenstock, E. (1987). A neural network for the retrieval of superimposed connection patterns. *Europhysics Letters, 3*(11), 1243–1249.

von der Malsburg, C., & Schneider, W. (1986). A neural cocktail-party processor. *Biological Cybernetics, 54,* 29–40.

von der Malsburg, C., & Singer, W. (1988). Principles of cortical network organization. In P. Rakic & W. Singer (Eds.), *Neurobiology of neocortex* (pp. 69–99). Chichester: Wiley.

Werman, M. (1987). *The capacity of k-gridgraphs as associative memory* (Reports in Pattern Analysis No. 146). Providence, R.I.: Brown Unversity, Division of Applied Mathematics.

Willshaw, D. J., Buneman, O. P., & Longuet-Higgins, H.-C. (1969). Non-holographic associative memory. *Nature, 222,* 960–962.

COMMENTARIES AND
ALTERNATIVE PERSPECTIVES

19

Representations: Who Needs Them?

WALTER J. FREEMAN
CHRISTINE A. SKARDA

Biologists by tradition have seldom used the term *representation* to describe their findings. Instead they have relied on phrases such as "receptor field" on the sensory side and "command" or "corollary discharge" on the motor side when discussing neural control of sensation and motion in goal-directed behavior. Such words connote dynamic process rather than symbolic content. One might suppose that this neglect of a now common word reflects diffidence about discussing so-called higher functions of the brain, owing to a humbling lack of understanding of the brain's complexity. Inspection of biology textbooks belies this view. Biologists have shown no lack of hubris in pontificating about the properties of the brain supporting mental functions. On the contrary, they have always taken pride in being uniquely qualified to explain brain function to anyone willing to listen.

A turning point came in the 1940s with the popularization of digital and analog computers as "giant brains" and with the adoption of the Turing machine as a model for explanation. In this conception, which is lucidly illustrated by von der Malsburg (Chapter 18, this volume), the human ability to understand the world is likened to the procedure of incorporating information on a tape into a machine by means of symbols. Cognitive operations are interpreted as the manipulation of these symbols according to certain semantic rules. At present we are all so accustomed to this metaphor that it seems self-evident (Goldman-Rakic, 1987). The brain's job is to incorporate features of the outside world and make internal syntactical representations of these data, which together constitute a world model that serves to control motor output. Any other account appears to be "noncognitive" (Earle, 1987) and counterintuitive. In short, to question this commonsense notion seems quixotic, sophistic, and arbitrary.

We propose, however, that physiologists avoid this way of thinking for two reasons. One is that no one now understands how brains work, but the use of the term representation and its attached concepts tends to obscure this fact. The term gives us the illusion that we understand something that we do not. We suggest that the idea of representation is seductive and ennervating, promising good deals but delivering nothing new. When researchers refrain from using the term, knowledge of brain function is not significantly affected. We conclude that use of the term is unnecessary to describe brain dynamics.

The second reason is that the use of the metaphor points us in a direction that carries physiological research away from more profitable lines of inquiry. We have found that thinking of brain function in terms of representation seriously impedes progress toward genuine understanding.

An example is taken from our studies of the behavioral correlates of the electroencephalograms (EEGs) of the olfactory system under conditioning (Freeman & Skarda, 1985). The EEGs of the olfactory bulb and cortex show a brief oscillatory burst of potential that accompanies each inhalation. This can be likened to a burst of energy carried by a wave of neural activity at a common frequency. Each burst exists over the entire bulb or cortex with a spatial pattern of amplitude that varies from one burst to the next. We have shown that a stereotypical pattern recurs whenever a particular odorant is presented that the animal has been trained to respond to.

For more than 10 years we tried to say that each spatial pattern was like a snapshot, that each burst served to represent the odorant with which we correlated it, and that the pattern was like a search image that served to symbolize the presence or absence of the odorant that the system was looking for. But such interpretations were misleading. They encouraged us to view neural activity as a function of the features and causal impact of stimuli on the organism and to look for a reflection of the environment within by correlating features of the stimuli with neural activity. This was a mistake. After years of sifting through our data, we identified the problem: it was the concept of representation.

Our research has now revealed the flaws in such interpretations of brain function. Neural activity patterns in the olfactory bulb cannot be equated with internal representations of particular odorants to the brain for several reasons. First, simply presenting an odorant to the system does not lead to any odor-specific activity patterns being formed. Only in motivated animals, that is, only when the odorant is reinforced leading to a behavioral change, do these stereotypical patterns of neural activity take shape. Second, odor-specific activity patterns are dependent on the behavioral response; when we change the reinforcement contingency of a CS we change the patterned activity. Third, patterned neural activity is context dependent: the introduction of a new reinforced odorant to the animal's repertoire leads to changes in the patterns associated with all previously learned odorants. Taken together these facts teach us that we who have looked at activity patterns as internal representations of events have misinterpreted the data. Our findings indicate that patterned neural activity correlates best with reliable forms of interaction in a context that is behaviorally and environmentally co-defined by what Steven Rose (1976) calls a dialectic. There is nothing intrinsically representational about this dynamic process until the observer intrudes. It is the experimenter who infers what the observed activity patterns represent to or in a subject, in order to explain his results to himself (Werner, 1988a, 1988b).

The impact of this insight on our research has been significant. Once we stopped looking at neural activity patterns as representations of odorants, we began to ask a new set of questions. Instead of focusing on pattern invariance and storage capacity, we began to ask how these patterns could be generated in the first place from less ordered initial conditions. What are the temporal dynamics of their development and evolution? What are their effects on the neurons to which they transmit? What kinds of structural changes in brains do they require and do they lead to? What neuromodulators do these pattern changes require? What principles of neural operations do these dynamical processes exemplify and instantiate? In short, we began to focus less on the outside world that is being put into the brain and more on what brains are doing.

Our efforts to answer these questions led us to develop mathematical, statistical, and electronic models that describe and explain the neural dynamics of pattern generation. These models have, in turn, caused radical changes in our views of how brains operate. In particular, we now see brains as physicochemical systems that largely organize themselves, rather than reacting to and determined by input. As Carew and co-workers (Chapter 2, this volume) showed, each brain has a history that begins with simple structures and that evolves through innumerable stages and phases of growth and development to increasing order and complexity. The patterns are formed from within and not imposed from outside, as is commonly supposed to occur in brains under sensory stimulation. We have found that an essential condition for these patterns to appear is the prior existence of unpatterned energy distributions which appear to be noise, but which in reality are chaos. New forms of order require that old forms of order collapse back into this chaotic state before they can appear. Therefore, in the EEG we see each burst appearing from chaotic basal activity and collapsing back into chaos, thereby clearing the way for the next burst of patterned activity (Skarda & Freeman, 1987).

These findings challenge two widely held assumptions concerning brain dynamics. First, conventional theory holds that full information is delivered into the system and that thereafter it is degraded by noise. This property is analogized to entropy. However, chaotic systems like the brain are open and, by virtue of energy throughput, operate far from equilibrium. They internally create new information and can be described as negentropic (Tsuda & Shimizu, 1985). The brain has immunity from the first and second laws of thermodynamics because its assured blood supply brings it more energy than it can use and carries off waste heat and entropy. As a result the formalisms of information theory that underlie the representation-based computational metaphor of brain dynamics do not apply to the neural networks of biological systems, because these formalisms make no sense in systems with positive information flow.

Second, the conventional description of signals embedded in noise is inappropriate. The same neural system that generates bursts (signals) also generates the background state of chaotic activity (often thought to be noise). When the system switches (bifurcates) from chaos to burst activity, the chaotic activity stops and the signal starts. Chaos operates up to the moment of bifurcation. It plays no role of "annealing" thereafter because response selection has already taken place, convergence is assured, and there is no role for "noise." The metaphor of the "signal to noise ratio" is inappropriate for brain function, yet it is essential for representation in man-made systems.

These considerations are well illustrated by the preceding four chapters. Of these the report by Cooper, Bear, Ebner, and Scofield (Chapter 15) deals most directly with neurophysiological data, and they alone make no reference to representations. Their model describes the dynamics of modifiable synapses over the time scale of learning. It does not address the dynamic of stimulus-induced neural activity on the time scale of responding. It attempts to explain the dynamics in terms of membrane conductances and calcium fluxes and not the semantic content of the input. The strength of their model lies in the identification of global variables as important for consideration; the main weakness is their decision to "delay consideration of the global variables by assuming that they act to render cortical synapses modifiable or nonmodifiable by experience."

Their chapter emphasizes the great value of the "mean field" state variable for the analysis and understanding of physical systems composed of ensembles. They elect not to consider the basis for defining and using such variables in their work with neural networks, thereby depriving themselves and their readers of access to the existing literature, including well-reasoned approaches to brain systems from the classical standpoints of statistical mechanics (Amari, 1974; Wilson & Cowan, 1972) and of nonequilibrium thermodynamics from the school of Prigogine (Babloyantz & Kaczmarek, 1981; Freeman, 1975). Both approaches emphasize the importance of mutually excitatory (positive) feedback within laminar distributions of nerve cells by their recurrent collateral axons and the renewal process in cell firing, leading to the emergence of macroscopic state variables to represent the activity of local neighborhoods, that is, axonal pulse density and dendritic current density functions that are continuous in both time and the spatial dimensions of cerebral cortex. These activity states are readily observed in many parts of brains by use of electrodes, magnetic probes, and optical dyes and by computer-implemented spatial filtering, summing, and enhancement of the raw data for visual display (Freeman, 1987). By means of these and related well-documented procedures these investigators and others can test their models directly with respect to brain dynamics.

Chapter 18 by von der Malsburg and part of Chapter 17 by Sejnowski and Tesauro are at the opposite pole and take representation for granted. They are also explicitly about machines and not about brains. "Representations" that are selected and defined by the observer serve as the goals or end points of the evolution of the machines. Sejnowski and Tesauro present elements on both sides. The description of Gerald Westheimer's dynamics of spatial attractors, which in some ways recalls Wolfgang Kohler's field theories, is accounted for by the dynamics of mutually excitatory feedback. This is physiology (Freeman, 1975). When he asks "Who reads the population code?" he gives engineering answers: "find all possible depths and find which matches the closest with minimal error." The algorithms of backpropagation and error correction by the observer-instilled "teacher" and "correct answer" are machine processes that do not exist in biological brains. "NETtalk" can transduce optical characters to sounds that are recognizable by human observers, so it is a machine that can be shaped to read to the blind, but one cannot say that the machine has learned to read in the sense that a schoolchild has.

Kohonen (Chapter 16) most clearly addresses the nature of internal representations as they are needed and used by engineers and machines. Each representation has characteristics and attributes that are to be stored, matched, and retrieved by processes ultimately deriving from mappings. Our physiological data show that episodic storage of odor trials does not happen, that "retrieval" is not recovery but re-creation, always with differences, and that stimulus-bound patterns cannot coexist with re-created patterns to support matching procedures. We agree with Kohonen's statement that we are faced with semantic difficulties, and we conclude that they stem from deep incompatibilities between the dynamics respectively of biological and present-day artificial intelligence. The key words to look for are "best matching" and "error detection," because these refer to machine cognition and not neural cognition.

These considerations give an answer to our question about representations. Who needs them? Functionalist philosophers, computer scientists, and cognitive psychologists need them, often desperately, but physiologists do not, and those who wish to find and use biological brain algorithms should also avoid them. They are unnecessary for describing and understanding brain dynamics. They mislead by contributing the illusion that they add anything significant to our understanding of the brain. They impede further advances toward our goal of understanding brain function, because they deflect us from the hard problems of determining what neurons do and seduce us into concentrating instead on the relatively easy problems of determining what our computers can or might do. In a word, representations are better left outside the laboratory when physiologists attempt to study the brain. Physiologists should welcome the ideas, concepts, and technologies brought to them by brain theorists and connectionists, but they should be aware that representation is like a dose of lithium chloride; it tastes good going down but it doesn't digest very well (Bureš, Chapter 1, this volume).

REFERENCES

Amari, S. (1974). A method of statistical neurodynamics. *Kybernetik, 14,* 201–215.

Amari, S. (1987). *Statistical neurodynamics of associative memory.* (Tech. Rep. METR87-8). Tokyo: University of Tokyo, Department of Mathematics, Engineering, and Instrument Physics.

Babloyantz, A., & Kaczmarek, L. (1981). Self-organization in biological systems with multiple cellular contacts. *Bulletin of Mathematical Biology, 41,* 193–201.

Earle, D. C. (1987). On the differences between cognitive and noncognitive systems. *Brain and Behavioral Science, 10,* 177–178.

Freeman, W. J. (1975). *Mass action in the nervous system.* New York: Academic Press.

Freeman, W. J. (1987). Analytic techniques used in the search for the physiological basis of the EEG. In A. S. Gevins & A. Rémond (Eds.), *EEG Handbook* (pp. 583–664). Amsterdam: Elsevier.

Freeman, W. J., & Skarda, C. A. (1985). Spatial EEG patterns, nonlinear dynamics and perception: The neo-Sherringtonian view. *Brain Research, 10,* 147–175.

Goldman-Rakic, P. (1987). Circuitry of primate prefrontal cortex and the regulation of behavior by representational memory. In F. Plum (Ed.), *Handbook of physiology: Sec. 1. The nervous system* (pp. 373–417). Bethesda Md.: American Physiological Society.

Gray, C. M., Freeman, W. J., & Skinner, J. E. (1986). Chemical dependencies of learning in the rabbit olfactory bulb: Acquisition of the transient spatial pattern change depends on norepinephrine. *Behavioral Neuroscience, 100,* 585–596.

Rose, S. P. R. (1976). *The conscious brain.* New York: Vintage Books.

Skarda, C. A., & Freeman, W. J. (1987). Brain makes chaos to make sense of the world. *Brain and Behavioral Science, 10,* 161–195.

Tsuda, I., & Shimizu, H. (1985). Self-organization of the dynamical channel. In H. Haken (Ed.), *Complex systems: Operational approaches in neurobiology, physics and computers* (pp. 240–251). Berlin: Springer-Verlag.

Werner, G. (1988a). Five decades on the path to naturalizing epistemology. In J. S. Lund (Ed.), *Sensory processing in the mammalian brain* (pp. 345–359). New York: Oxford University Press.

Werner, G. (1988b). The many faces of neuroreductionism. In E. Basar (Ed.), *Dynamics of sensory and cognitive processing by the brain* (pp. 241–257). Berlin: Springer-Verlag.

Wilson, H. R., & Cowan, J. D. (1972). Excitatory and inhibitory interactions in biological populations of model neurons. *Biophysics Journal, 12,* 1–24.

20

Interactions Within Neuronal Assemblies: Theory and Experiment

GEORGE L. GERSTEIN

Models of neuronal networks have been with us since the mid-fifties, starting with the work of Rochester (Rochester, Holland, Haibt, & Duda, 1956) and of Farley (1964; Farley & Clarke, 1961) and their associates. After years of steady growth, the field has become extremely active, as exemplified by the chapters by Cooper and co-workers, Kohonen, von der Malsburg, and Sejnowski and Tesauro in this volume. In contrast, direct experimental access to real neuronal networks in the brain has been possible only since the early eighties. It is the purpose of this chapter to juxtapose some of the ideas and assumptions made in modeling networks to recent experimental results on real neurons.

Neuronal network models typically consist of many nodal elements that have simplified properties intended to mimic some aspects of real neurons. The minimum set of properties for a nodal element specifies the (linear or nonlinear) way its inputs will be combined and defines the conditions (possibly nonlinear) under which an output will occur. The extent to which further properties are incorporated into the nodal elements depends on the purpose of the modeling. It is possible to have nodal elements that mimic large dendritic trees with the attendant spatiotemporal summation of inputs. However, for many purposes it is appropriate to simplify to nodal elements which are, in effect, like "point neurons" without spatial extent.

Connections between nodes in a network model mimic axons and synapses. The important parameters are delay (conduction) time and connection strength or influence. For a network model with N nodes, connections between nodes can be specified by an $N \times N$ matrix. An element of this matrix, say W_{ij}, would represent the influence of node j on node i. Excitatory or inhibitory influence can be represented by the sign of the W_{ij}; its magnitude can reflect the strength of the influence. A value of zero indicates no connection (influence) between the specified nodes.

Many of the studies involving neural network models have examined mechanisms that could be responsible for learning and memory in biological systems.

In principle the necessary modulations of a network model could be accomplished by an evolution of nodal characteristics. It has been more usual, however, to locate the necessary modulations in the connection strengths between the nodal elements. The rules used for such modulations are often based on Hebb's (1949) proposal that the strength (or efficacy) of a synapse will be increased by a small amount every time that the presynaptic and postsynaptic neurons fire in close temporal sequence. Other rules for synaptic modification have been studied and are reviewed by Palm (in press).

An underlying assumption of most of the rules for change of synaptic weight is that such changes take place very slowly, on a time scale appropriate to our conception of learning as a slow process that requires many repetitions of the appropriate input. Thus modelers have taken the W_{ij} matrix of connectivity to be almost a constant, with only a slow evolution of its values during the "training" phases of an experiment. It is precisely this assumption that is challenged by recent experimental results on real neuronal assemblies. It turns out, as I shall show, that the "effective connectivity" between neurons, which corresponds to the modeler's W_{ij}, is dynamic on several time scales and is hardly to be described as a slowly evolving constant.

EXPERIMENTAL AND ANALYTIC TOOLS

The central requirement for experimental observation of neuronal assembly properties is simultaneous recording of the activity of as many individual neurons as technically possible. This class of experiment allows a much greater degree of inference than sequential traditional single neuron observations: instead of being able to examine only the relations between activity of a single neuron and the occurrence of external events (stimulus, movement, etc.), we may now examine the interrelationship of the activities of two (or more) neurons. The technical requirements of this type of multineuron experiment are very demanding, so that relatively few laboratories have built up the necessary instrumentation. For a review of some of the ways that multineuron experiments involve a nonlinear increase indifficulty over the single-neuron experiment, see Gerstein, Bloom, Espinosa, Evanczuk, and Turner (1983) and Kruger (1983).

Current technology allows the simultaneous extracellular observation of up to 30 neurons, although half that amount is a more frequently attained goal. Such numbers are preposterously small on the scale of functional neuron groupings like visual cortical columns, which may involve many thousand neurons. Thus current technology for multineuron experiments leaves us with a difficult sampling problem.

The usual way to assess interrelationships among the observed neurons is to measure the temporal correlation of their firing activity. The use of cross-correlation for two or three neurons is clearly reviewed by Glaser and Ruchkin (1976), who also give many useful references to the original literature. Basically, for two neurons, the cross-correlogram estimates the amount of near-coincident firing and determines whether there is a favored order and delay between spikes in the two trains. Such favored compound events can in principle serve directly as carriers of information, since convergent, near-coincident activity of two synapses is much more effective than activation of either synapse alone.

In addition, however, we may estimate the amount of near-coincident firing that would be expected for two neurons exhibiting the observed individual firing rates (and their possible modulations by stimulus). By subtracting this estimate from the original directly observed correlation, we may estimate the amount of "excess" firing correlation in comparison to the model of two independent neurons. This excess can be interpreted as an "effective connectivity" between the two neurons. Such effective connectivity is not directly related to the actual anatomical connectivity that may exist between the two neurons, although it may be its currently active subset in some cases. Generally the effective connectivity is simply a shorthand for the interconnections of the simplest two neuron model that would replicate the experimentally observed cross-correlograms. In this respect it is the analogue of the W_{ij} in the connectivity matrix in neuronal network models.

Ultimately we want to examine the dependence of the correlation structure and the effective connectivity among the observed group of neurons on the experimental conditions (current or recent stimulus, context, response, etc.) during which the recording was taken. If we analyze the neuronal spike trains in pairs, as outlined above, then even with the modest number of neurons that can presently be simultaneously observed in a multineuron experiment, combinatorial arithmetic will force the experimenter to examine and sort out literally thousands of cross-correlograms.

A recently developed analytical tool, at least in a screening strategy, allows avoidance of the combinatorial proliferation of cross-correlograms by treating the entire group of recorded neurons and spike trains as a single entity rather than as a large set of pairs (Gerstein & Aertsen, 1985; Gerstein, Perkel, & Dayhoff, 1985). The so-called gravity analysis transforms the N observed spike trains into an N-dimensional mathematical abstraction in which each neuron is represented by a charged particle. The charge is a low-pass filtered version of the spike train from the corresponding neuron. The charged particles exert force on each other, with like signs of charge attracting; as a consequence the particles move about. The largest force occurs when two particles have large charge at the same time, which, in turn, corresponds to near-coincident firing of the corresponding neurons. The end result is that those particles representing neurons that tend to have "excess" near-coincident firing will tend to aggregate. Thus the temporal analysis of a set of N observed spike trains has been transformed into a problem of cluster analysis in the abstract N-dimensional space.

The spatial clustering of points in the gravity representation is best examined in the full N space, where the shape of the aggregations can be interpreted in useful ways. However, for purposes of publication, since we can hardly make a picture of particles in an N space (with N greater than 3), we will use a projection from the N space to a two-dimensional plane. This, of course, is a procedure that can be deceptive, since points that cluster in the two-dimensional plane need not have done so in the full N-dimensional space. However, we will supplement the projection with a graph of the distances between all pairs of particles in the N space as the aggregation develops, so that validity of the information in the two-dimensional representation can be checked. The dynamics of the aggregation process may itself be of interest, and it is then appropriate to make a movie of the projection. For our purposes here, it will suffice to simply examine the aggregations attained as the available data reach an end. We assume, of course, a standard starting configuration of the particles for all calculations.

TIME SCALES

Almost all the measurements used on spike trains involve averaging over some time period, although this is not always explicitly stated. Thus cross-correlograms, for example, represent a measure of near-coincident firing as averaged over the piece of recording under study. In the same sense, the aggregations calculated in the gravity representations are the result of the temporal correlation structure of the observed spike trains, as averaged over the analyzed recording period. In other words, these analysis methods are not instantaneous measurements and imply a "reasonable" observation time.

If we want to compare the correlation structure among some observed spike trains in two different stimulus conditions, we must present the two stimuli alternately until a sufficient amount of recording for analysis in each condition has accumulated. This approach eliminates misinterpretation of slow physiological drifts, since these will apply equally to both stimulus conditions over the recording time. Before analysis the data are "cut and pasted" to produce material corresponding to a single stimulus. However, note that the stimulus alternation cycle is much shorter than the total analysis time: typical runs require 40 to 100 stimulus repetitions during the analysis time. Thus we are comparing the average correlation structure of the observed set of spike trains in each of two states that typically alternate on a time scale of 0.5 to 1 sec. Any observed differences between the correlation structures corresponding to the two stimuli will represent changes in the observed neuronal network that are on this time scale.

RESULTS: ASSEMBLY CORRELATION STRUCTURE

With multineuron recording, the analysis tools defined above, and an experimental design that presents several interleaved stimuli repeatedly, we now may examine the correlation structure exhibited by small groups of real neurons. The material shown in the figures is drawn from studies on auditory cortex of cat. Details of the experiments have previously been described (Bloom & Gerstein, 1986; Espinosa & Gerstein, 1988) and can be omitted for present purposes. The essential point is that we can compare the (average) correlation structure among the observed neurons under two (or more) different stimulus conditions by comparing the gravity condensations.

Figure 20.1 shows the distances between particle pairs for data containing eight cortical neurons under two different stimulus conditions. These gravity aggregations were run with appropriate compensation for the individual neuron

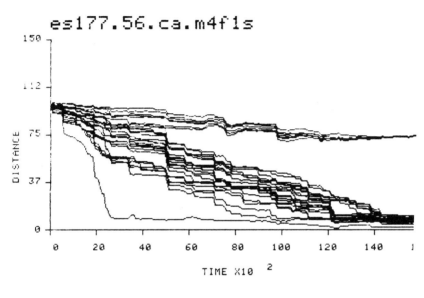

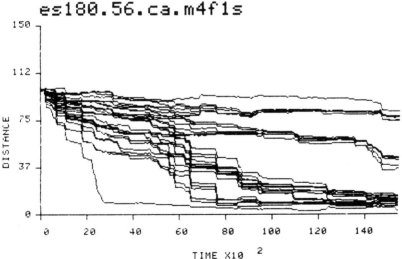

FIGURE 20.1.   Interparticle distances during gravity condensations for eight cortical neurons under two different stimulus conditions. Individual stimuli within each condition were presented every 550 msec. Each panel corresponds to one stimulus condition and shows all particle pair distances for the same eight observed cortical neurons.

firing rates, so that we are here examining the "excess" correlation that we earlier associated with "effective connectivity" and the W_{ij}. (For more detail on the compensation for individual neuron firing rates see Aertsen, Bonhoeffer, & Kruger, 1987; Gerstein & Aertsen, 1985.) It is apparent that the development of particle pair distances is different under the two stimulus conditions, and hence that the "excess" correlation structure of the spike trains was different in the two conditions.

Figure 20.2 shows the same data in the two-dimensional projection plane of the gravity representation. The starting arrangement is the same for each stimulus condition, as shown on the left; the final configurations on the right show that certain particles change their "allegiance." Again, this shows that the "excess" correlation structure was different in the two stimulus conditions.

Now it turns out that it is easy to find multineuron data that behave as shown in the figures. During the past year, we have obtained multineuron recordings from other laboratories which were recorded from a variety of creatures and brain structures. Many of these recordings demonstrate the same type of phenomenon seen in Figures 20.1 and 20.2: the correlation structure to some degree depends on the stimulus conditions.

As mentioned, the alternating stimulus cycle means that we force the change in correlation structure on a time scale of 0.5 to 1 sec, even though many repetitions of the cycle are needed to make the necessary measurements. Other measurements, which we have not described here, show that modulations of the correlation structure can take place on an even faster time scale of milliseconds (Aertsen et al., 1987; Aertsen et al., 1989).

Thus the results of experimental observation of small neuronal assemblies show that the correlation structure of firing is a dynamic, rapidly fluctuating quantity. This means that among real neurons, the effective connectivity (which corresponds to the W_{ij} of the modelers) behaves quite differently from the usual assumption of a slowly evolving constant.

INTERPRETATION AND POSSIBLE MECHANISMS

A dynamic correlation structure among a group of observed neurons can be explained by various known mechanisms that either operate at the level of synaptic properties or involve properties of the neuronal network. For example, the effective connectivity between two neurons could be rapidly modulated by a presynaptic input from another, unobserved neuron. Alternatively, the synaptic

FIGURE 20.2.   For the same data as in Figure 20.1, projections from the 8-space to a convenient plane. Top and bottom row represent, respectively, condensations during the two stimulus conditions. Left column are the (identical) projected initial particle configurations; right column are the projected final configurations. The straight lines in the right column join the initial and final projected positions of the particles; the actual projected trajectory is not shown.

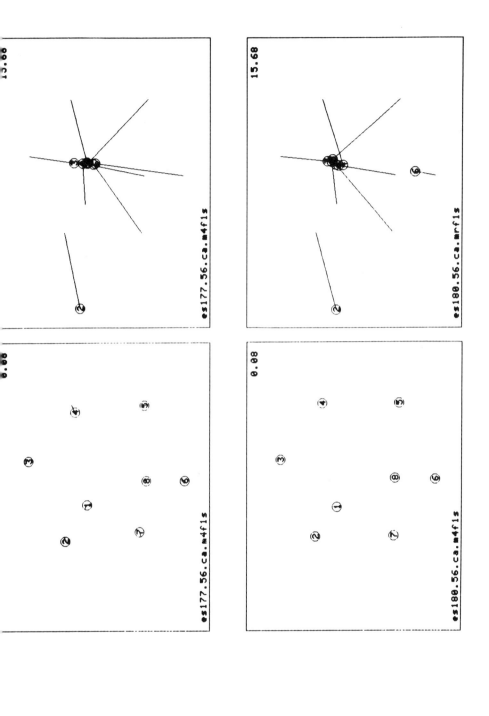

es177.56.ca.m4fls

es177.56.ca.m4fls

es180.56.ca.mrfls

es180.56.ca.m4fls

path between two neurons could go through an unobserved interneuron which itself has other input and hence modulates the effective connectivity between the two observed neurons.

At the network level, we may invoke the following type of explanation. Suppose we consider the observed neurons to be embedded in a large mass of interconnected neural tissue. Presumably stimuli that have different parametric values enter this large neural mass in different ways, probably at somewhat different locations. (This would correspond to the mapping of the sensory periphery onto the structure under study.) Thus each different stimulus sets up a disturbance that takes a somewhat different path through the neural mass and hence crosses the observed neurons in a somewhat different way, apparently causing the correlation structure of firing to vary.

Although all such explanations are plausible in a qualitative way, their quantitative applicability remains to be investigated, most simply by computer simulation methods. Such work is under way in several laboratories. An important (and largely unknown) parameter that is involved in such work is the amount of "spontaneous" (other) activity relative to the stimulus-related activity. In the limiting case of extremely small stimulus-related activity in a massive background of other network activity we would expect minimal modulation of the correlation structure by the stimulus. On the other hand, even in such a situation, modulation maybe imposed by other sources of input to the system. Since the time structure of such unknown input is not available, there is a serious measurement problem in that the usual averaging methods cannot be used.

SIGNIFICANCE FOR MODELING

As noted previously, most current models for networks of neurons do not explicitly contain W_{ij} with dynamic properties on the time scale demonstrated in the physiological measurements. The one exception is found in the work of von der Malsburg (1987), where Hebbian rules modulate synaptic efficacies on very short time scales and produce some useful consequences.

Is it important to adjust other network modeling so as to mimic the observed rapid modulation of effective connectivity? One possibility is that the rapid modulation is a stimulus-associated statistical variation that has no real physiological significance and is essentially a noiselike phenomenon. Another possibility is that the network explanation of the rapid modulation is adequate, and that models with essentially fixed W_{ij} nevertheless exhibit rapid stimulus-associated modulation of correlation structure. In both these cases, dealing with average W_{ij}, which vary only slowly, would seem to be justified, and development of network models can proceed along its current path. On the other hand, since real neuronal networks in the brain do show rapid modulation of correlation structure, it would perhaps be both safer and quite appropriate to see what changes occur in a given model if such properties are explicitly installed. The process of modeling always involves selection of the subset of real-world properties that are to be mimicked; it is important to make sure that such selection does not drastically affect the modeling results.

Acknowledgment

This work was supported by the System Development Foundation, SDF 0013, and by the Office of Naval Research, N00014-83-K-0387 and N00014-87-K-0766.

REFERENCES

Aertsen, A. M. H. J., Bonhoeffer, T., & Kruger, J. (1987). Coherent activity in neuronal populations: Analysis and interpretation. In E. R. Caianiello (Ed.), *Physics of cognitive processes* (pp. 1–34). Singapore: World Scientific Publishing.
Aertsen, A. M. H. J., Gerstein, G. L., Habib, M. K., & Palm, G. (1989). Dynamics of neuronal firing correlation: Modulation of "Effective Connectivity." *Journal of Neurophysiology, 61,* 900–917.
Bloom, M. J., & Gerstein, G. L. (1986). Dynamic changes in cortical connectivity during sound localization. *Society for Neuroscience Abstracts, 12,* 1274.
Espinosa, I. E., & Gerstein, G. L. (1985). Correlation among spike trains in cat's auditory cortex during presentation of three-tone sequences. *Society for Neuroscience Abstracts, 11,* 249.
Espinosa, I. E., & Gerstein, G. L. (1988). Cortical auditory neuron interactions during presentation of 3-tone sequences: Effective connectivity. *Brain Research, 450,* 39–50.
Farley, B. G. (1964). The use of computer technics in neural research. In R. F. Reiss (Ed.), *Neural theory and modeling* (pp. 43–72). Stanford, Calif.: Stanford University Press.
Farley, B. G., & Clarke, W. A. (1961). Activity in networks of neuronlike elements. In C. Cherry (Ed.), *Informaton theory (Fourth London Symposium).* London: Butterworth.
Gerstein, G. L., & Aertsen, A. M. H. J. (1985). Representation of cooperative firing activity among simultaneously recorded neurons. *Journal of Neurophysiology, 54,* 1513–1528.
Gerstein, G. L., Bloom, M., Espinosa, I., Evanczuk, S., Turner, M. (1983). Design of a laboratory for multi-neuron studies. *IEEE Transactions on Systems, Man and Cybernetics, SMC-13,* 668–676.
Gerstein, G. L., Perkel, D. H., & Dayhoff, J. E. (1985). Cooperative firing activity in simultaneously recorded populations of neurons: Detection and measurement. *Journal of Neuroscience, 5,* 881–889.
Glaser, E. M., & Ruchkin, D. S. (1976). *Principles of neurobiological signal analysis.* New York: Academic Press.
Hebb, D. O. (1949). *The organization of behavior.* New York: Wiley.
Kruger, J. (1983). Simultaneous individual recordings from many cerebral neurons: Techniques and results. *Review of Physiology, Biochemistry, and Pharmacology, 98,* 177–233.
Palm, G. (in press). Local rules for synaptic modification in neural networks. In E. Schwartz (Ed.), *Computational neuroscience.* Cambridge, Mass.: MIT Press.
Rochester, N., Holland, J. H., Haibt, L. H., & Duda, W. L. (1956). Tests on a cell assembly theory of the action of the brain, using a large digital computer. *IRE Transactions on Information Theory, IT-2,* 80–93.
von der Malsburg, C. (1987). Synaptic plasticity as basis of brain organization. In J. P. Changeux & M. Konishi (Eds.), *The neural and molecular bases of learning* (pp. 411–432). New York: Wiley.

21

Neural Networks and Networks of Neurons

GARY LYNCH
JOHN LARSON
DOMINIQUE MULLER
RICHARD GRANGER

Neural network models hold the promise of serving as a bridge, or translator, between the more familiar worlds of physiology and behavior. Behavior emerges from the collective activities of brain cells linked together in spatiotemporal patterns, and those activities are the result of the anatomical and physiological properties of individual neurons. Unfortunately, even a reasonably complete description of cellular neurobiology does not necessarily lead to precise predictions about the types of interactions that might occur between neurons in a particular brain region—let alone predictions about the coherent spatiotemporal patterns that presumably underlie visible behavior. It is easy to understand why this should be the case. Temporal interactions between any large group of objects are inherently difficult subjects for analysis; one need go no further than classical physics (e.g., celestial and statistical mechanics) to see this. Moreover, the influences that brain cells have over each other are by no means simple (i.e., synaptic responses are complex) and are transmitted via complicated architectures with any number of specialized and often subtle design features. In all, the objects of interest (neurons) are of several types, possess a host of relevant characteristics, and sense and exert a variety of influences over convoluted networks.

Obviously, a great deal of simplification is required if models of brain networks are to be developed. One of the successes of neural network modeling has been the demonstration that much can be learned about the aggregate activity of cells and its relationship to behavior using only very simple physiological rules and circuit designs. Moreover, in some cases the resulting models are tractable subjects for mathematical analysis, a point that is sometimes not appreciated by behavioral neuroscientists but that is of fundamental importance in efforts to develop theories of network behavior. By using mathematical techniques, it is possible to show that a given model will always achieve certain end points and thus that its behavior is not unique to a particular computer simulation (see Cohen & Grossberg, 1983; Hopfield, 1982; Kohonen, 1984; Rumelhart, Hinton, & Williams, 1986, for examples). Equally important, mathematical analyses can provide explanations and make predictions that are not likely to arise from experimental (in the present case, simulation) work (Kuhn, 1977).

Network models vary considerably, depending on the simplifying assumptions made and the goals of the enterprise. In some cases they are used to explore the consequences of hypotheses about the general operating principles of brain circuitries. Hopfield (1982), for example, investigates the possibility that the interactions between neurons converge to stable "states" (i.e., spatial or spatiotemporal patterns of cell activity) in much the way certain physical systems (e.g., gases, magnetic domains) do; these states would then form the representations of external objects. Gelperin and colleagues (Cook, Delaney, & Gelperin, 1985) found that a network of this type when used as a model of an invertebrate nervous system produces behaviors similar to those observed in experiments. Kohonen (1984; Chapter 16, this volume) notes that brain circuitry often resembles an input–output matrix and investigates the idea that such networks use a kind of matrix algebra to produce coherent activity and representations.

Another increasingly popular approach uses multilayered networks and a particular learning algorithm (backpropagation of error) to address a remarkable variety of behavioral problems (Rumelhart et al., 1986; Sejnowski & Tesauro, Chapter 17, this volume). Much of the appeal of this approach lies in the learning rule, since it can be shown mathematically to minimize errors (across trials) between the input cues to be encoded and the representations assigned to them (Widrow & Hoff, 1960). Of evident utility, this became more intriguing theoretically when it was understood (Sutton & Barto, 1981) that the algorithm corresponds to rules for classical conditioning defined by behavioral researchers (Rescorla & Wagner, 1972).

The success of neural networks in producing behaviors, and even complex behaviors, that resemble those exhibited by humans and other animals suggests that the models will ultimately provide some understanding of how aspects of psychology emerge from aspects of neurobiology. Clearly what is needed are experimentally testable predictions about neurons and about behavior. The models are concerned with spatiotemporal patterns in arrays of cells; unfortunately, using current technologies, these are extremely difficult to measure in brains. Indeed, our ignorance on just this point provides some of the impetus for modeling. In general the models do not yield detailed predictions about synaptic events, membrane properties, and the like, on the one hand, and acquisition rates, memory interference effects, and so forth, on the other. A bridge is being built but we must wait to see if and to what degree it connects the two worlds of behavioral neuroscience.

NEURONS IN NETWORKS

Another kind of modeling is concerned with the activities of individual (real) neurons and the question of how these arise from the brain networks within which the cells are found. Rather than beginning with hypotheses about the rules governing aggregate behavior of cells, this approach is concerned with finding local rules that produce effects observed in physiological experiments on single cells. Having identified such rules, one would hope that these will serve as the basis of more general theories of how cortex encodes experience. The emphasis in most models thus far has been on development, perhaps because many striking properties of cortical cells appear to be shaped in part by early experience.

Physiologists studying the visual system have provided a wealth of data on how experimental manipulations carried out during critical periods of development produce striking and detailed changes in the responses of cortical neurons to peripheral cues (see Singer, Chapter 10, this volume). Several groups are now building models with which to investigate various neuronal rules that could produce such effects (Cooper, Bear, Ebner, & Scofield, Chapter 15, this volume; Linsker, 1986, 1988; Singer, Chapter 10, this volume). Cooper and co-workers (Bear, Cooper, & Ebner, 1987) have had remarkable success in reproducing in simulations (and with mathematical treatments) some of the more prominent experimental effects observed in cat visual cortex; equally important, they used the model to make testable predictions, which in at least one case were confirmed. Their work also leads to unexpected but testable ideas about plasticity in neurons (e.g., the phi factor). In some senses then this work has achieved the two-way outlook of behavioral neuroscience mentioned earlier: it speaks to behavior (albeit at the level of behaviorally relevant activities of single cells) and to neurobiological properties. Linsker (1986) has also produced a model in which salient aspects of visual cortical physiology emerge using a development rule that is similar to those employed in certain of the neural network models mentioned earlier. The possibility that the hypothetical rules (back-propagation) used in neural networks might explain specific developmental effects observed at the single-cell level was explicitly tested by Zipser and Andersen (1988) with some success (see Andersen & Zipser, Chapter 13, this volume).

Yet another approach to exploring how various physiological rules in networks might produce effects observed in individual neurons and in the aggregate behavior of the network would be to start with physiologically defined rules. That is, rather than using hypothetical learning algorithms or deducing them from behavior or cellular end points, one could begin with experimental observations on synaptic plasticity, identify ways in which these are relevant to in situ events, and then ask what types of effects they produce when implemented in a network model. We have been carrying out a program of this type and the following sections briefly review some of our results.

LONG-TERM POTENTIATION AS A LEARNING RULE

Long-term potentiation (LTP) is in many ways an obvious candidate for the substrates of memory: it is an extremely persistent (Barnes, 1979; Bliss & Gardner-Medwin, 1973; Staubli & Lynch, 1987) synapse-specific (Andersen, Sundberg, Sveen, & Wigstrom 1977; Dunwiddie & Lynch, 1978; Lynch, Dunwiddie, & Gribkoff, 1977) increase in the size of excitatory postsynaptic responses elicited by brief episodes of high-frequency stimulation. Moreover, recent experiments demonstrate that drugs that block LTP also block certain forms of learning (Morris, Anderson, Lynch, & Baudry, 1986; Staubli, Baudry, & Lynch, 1984; Staubli, Faraday, & Lynch, 1985; Staubli, Larson, Baudry, Thibault, & Lynch, 1988). To use LTP as a learning rule we need to specify in some detail the relationship between physiological patterns occurring in situ and the induction of potentiation. Since LTP has been most fully characterized in hippocampus, this is a reasonable place to begin such an effort.

The hippocampal EEG assumes a characteristic 4- to 7-Hz rhythm known as theta whenever rats are engaged in exploratory behavior (Vanderwolf, 1969). The pyramidal cells in the structure fire in very short bursts of 3 to 5 spikes with the bursts often occurring during a particular phase of theta (Bland, Andersen, Ganes, & Sveen, 1980; Fox & Ranck, 1981; Ranck, 1973). The question then becomes one of whether a relationship exists between these characteristics (theta and bursting) and the induction of LTP. Our work indicates that this is the case. Short bursts (4 pulses at 100 Hz) delivered to the inputs to field CA1 elicit robust LTP when the bursts are spaced apart by 200 msec; intervals that are much shorter (< 100 msec) or longer than 200 msec produce progressively less LTP (Larson, Wong, & Lynch, 1986). It should be noted here that the potentiation induced in this fashion is extremely stable and can persist without evident decrement for weeks (Staubli & Lynch, 1987).

Convergence of different inputs on target cells is an essential feature of networks; therefore it is essential to know how convergence interacts with theta bursting and LTP. To answer this, we stimulated one collection of inputs to a target cell, waited 200 msec, and then activated a completely separate set of inputs to the same neuron. Five to ten such pairs were given with a delay of several seconds between each pair. The second, delayed input exhibited robust LTP, whereas the first was not detectably changed (Larson & Lynch, 1986). As a rule, then, we assume that activation of one afferent "primes" its target cells so that other inputs can change their synapses if stimulated about 200 msec later.

What about convergence within one phase of theta as opposed to convergence between waves? The experiments just described used synchronous stimulation of two large groups of axons because previous work (McNaughton, Douglas, & Goddard, 1978) indicated that LTP induction requires the cooperative action of many synapses. However, in situ the firing of different cells will not be so perfectly synchronized. To explore this issue, we carried out experiments in which three sets of afferents terminating in the same dendritic region were stimulated sequentially with their bursts only partially overlapping. Each input was first given a priming pulse; the three inputs then received a four-pulse burst (100 Hz) at a delay of 180 msec (first input), 200 msec (second input), and 220 msec (third input). Thus the burst to the second input overlapped that to both the first and third, while the first and third bursts did not overlap at all. The degree of LTP induced was greatest at synapses activated by the first burst, intermediate for the second, and least for the third (Larson & Lynch, 1989). It is interesting to note that this within-phase convergence rule is the opposite of the between-phase rule: with convergence during one phase the later arrival facilitates LTP in the early arrival, while across two phases the early arrival facilitates LTP in the later arriving input.

Having identified these LTP rules we can ask why they exist. This is a question of immediate importance to our understanding of the neurobiological factors that initiate synaptic change, but it is also of considerable significance for attempts to develop rules for networks. That is, a description of the physiological processes underlying the between- and within-phase effects is necessary for the development of rules that generalize beyond these particular activity patterns. Here we will only summarize the work on this issue; more complete descriptions can be found elsewhere (Larson & Lynch, 1986, 1988; Lynch & Larson, 1988; Lynch, Larson, Staubli, & Baudry, 1987).

The central feature of the "priming" effect that drives the between-phase rule appears to be a transient refractory period for feedforward IPSPs (Larson & Lynch, 1986; see also McCarren & Alger, 1985). Stimulated afferents in hippocampus initiate EPSPs in pyramidal cells but also trigger interneurons that produce IPSPs in the same cells (Alger & Nicoll, 1982). This IPSP lasts about 50 to 100 msec and then appears to become refractory (or suppressed) for about 200 to 500 msec. The theta interval (200 msec) defines a time after which the initial IPSP has dissipated and is difficult to reintroduce. EPSPs are considerably prolonged in the absence of the IPSP and summate within a burst to a much greater degree than is true for control conditions (Larson & Lynch, 1988). In essence, priming considerably amplifies the depolarization produced by a bursting input. Under some circumstances the amplified response is adequate to trigger an NMDA receptor–mediated response component as shown in experiments using selective antagonists of the receptor (Larson & Lynch, 1988). If this NMDA-related potential is blocked, LTP does not occur, a result that accords with previous findings (Collingridge, Kehl, & McLennan, 1983; Harris, Ganong, & Cotman, 1984; Morris et al., 1986). The NMDA receptor channel in its high-conductance state (i.e., under extreme depolarization) admits calcium into the target cell (MacDermott, Mayer, Westbrook, Smith, & Barker, 1986; Mayer & Westbrook, 1987) and calcium appears to be the trigger for LTP (Lynch, Larson, Kelso, Barrionuevo, & Schottler, 1983). The mechanisms whereby calcium produces LTP are controversial but are probably linked to the anatomical changes that correlate with LTP (see Lynch, Bodsch, & Baudry, 1988, for a discussion of intermediary mechanisms for LTP).

The refractoriness of the IPSP, temporal summation of responses during bursts, and the voltage threshold of the NMDA-mediated response are features that can be simulated and thereby provide some generality for a network rule.

Work on the causes of the within-phase rule is still in progress, but the causes appear to involve yet another peculiar feature of the NMDA receptor: its channel is slow to respond but once activated tends to remain open (Jahr & Stevens, 1987). Later depolarizing inputs then may serve to sustain NMDA-dependent events at synapses that were stimulated tens of milliseconds earlier (Larson & Lynch, 1989). Additional experiments should serve to specify the relevant events to a degree that is sufficient for incorporation into a plasticity rule for network simulations.

A NOTE ON THE SUBSTRATES OF LONG-TERM POTENTIATION

LTP can be modeled as a simple increase in synaptic strength; that is, activation of a given synapse produces a larger than normal voltage change in the target cell. Although this seems appropriate, it would be useful to know precisely what type of semipermanent change is in fact responsible for physiological potentiation.

Electron microscopic studies indicate that LTP is correlated with changes in the morphology of dendritic spines and a small increase in the numbers of certain types of contacts (Chang & Greenough, 1984; Lee, Oliver, Schottler, & Lynch, 1981; Lee, Schottler, Oliver, & Lynch, 1980; Wenzel & Matthies, 1985). The possibility exists that these effects are different degrees of a single process, that is, different degrees of spine transformation. It is reasonable to assume that the observed morphological correlates of LTP are responsible for synaptic facilitation, but there is no direct evidence on this point and secondary effects of structural reorganization may be involved. The recent discovery that LTP increases one component of postsynaptic response (that mediated by non-NMDA receptors) without affecting a second component (the NMDA-mediated component) considerably limits the possible locales for potentiation. This is all the more likely since paired-pulse facilitation (a very transient form of potentiation due to increased transmitter release) increases both components of the postsynaptic potential (Muller & Lynch, 1988). It is thus very unlikely that LTP is caused by a simple increase in transmitter release or a simple increase in synaptic contacts. More likely explanations are changes in the biophysics of the spine–dendrite coupling or an increased number of synapses that are impoverished in NMDA receptors.

IMPLEMENTING LONG-TERM POTENTIATION RULES
INTO A SIMPLE CORTICAL NETWORK

The hippocampus has proven extremely useful in developing an LTP-based learning rule, but it is not appropriate as a model for a simulation to test the consequences of that rule (see Lynch, Granger, Larson, & Baudry, 1988, for a discussion). Instead, we chose to use the superficial layers of the olfactory (piri-form-entorhinal) cortex for the purpose. This region is disynaptically connected to peripheral receptors for odors and thus can be assumed to play a primary role in virtually any olfactory-related behavior (see Lynch, 1986). Accordingly, it is not unreasonable to assume that events in the cortex will have detectable effects on behavior; this would greatly simplify the task of testing predictions from the simulation. Additionally, layers I and II of the cortex are comparatively simple and their anatomy has been defined in great detail, two essential features for a simulation (Lynch, 1986). The simulations we have carried out used 100 to 200 cells, local inhibitory interneurons, and sparse connectivity between the lateral olfactory tract (the extrinsic input to the cortex) and associational feedback systems with the target cells (Granger, Ambros-Ingerson, & Lynch, 1989; Lynch & Granger, in press). Physiological rules for the model included many of the LTP-related features described above as well as three forms of hyperpolarization: the feedforward IPSP, the late-hyperpolarizing potential (Alger, 1984), and a cell-specific after-hyperpolarization (Hotson & Prince, 1980). These are all promi-nent aspects of hippocampal physiology and have been identified in the piriform cortex as well (Haberly, 1985). Later versions of the simulation incorporated probabilistic transmission.

A particularly difficult problem for models of cortical networks is how to sim-ulate inputs that might occur during behavior. In the present case we would particularly like to know if the theta rhythm patterns used in the studies on hip-pocampus would constitute a "meaningful" signal to the olfactory cortex. There is reason to think that this might be the case since rats sniff at rates close to theta and indeed activity in hippocampus is correlated with the sniffs. Accordingly, a series of "electrical odor" experiments were conducted in which stimulation of the lateral olfactory tract (LOT) was used in place of natural odors in an olfac-tory discrimination task (Roman, Staubli, & Lynch, 1987). The animals were first trained on a series of discriminations using novel pairs of odors over several days. Then tests were made to determine if they could learn to discriminate an electrical odor from a natural odor or between two electrical odors (i.e., between stimulation at two sites in the LOT). Under these conditions, theta burst stim-ulation to the LOT was treated by the animals in a manner not obviously dif-ferent from real odors. Interestingly enough, stimulation used in the learning situation produced LTP in the LOT–piriform synapses but did not do so when used with naive rats (Roman et al., 1987). It might be noted that others have shown that induction of LTP in the perforant path–hippocampal system is dependent on the arousal state of rats (Jones Leonard, McNaughton, & Barnes, 1987).

In any event, LTP does appear in the piriform cortex during learning (at least of electrical odors) and theta bursting in the LOT is "interpretable" by the cortex as a meaningful input signal. Accordingly, the simulation receives as inputs short bursts of activity with the bursts separated by (simulated) 200 msec; each burst might be thought of as the input resulting from one of a series of "sniffs."

Interesting results emerged when the simulation was trained using LTP rules on a series of "odors" (an odor was represented as a specific 20% subgroup of the LOT lines) that overlapped or shared components among themselves (i.e., a given odor might share some percentage of its chemistry, and thus its input lines, with other members of a set of odors). After the model had learned several individual cues with such overlap, the spatial pattern (of activity) it generated on the first sniff became differentiated from the response pattern it emitted on later sniffs. Specifically, the first response was the same or nearly the same for all members of the odor group, whereas its later responses were specific to the cue being presented. In one experiment we presented the simulation with 22 separate cues; it produced 5 category (first sniff) patterns and 22 distinct third sniff responses. The network thus extracts information about similarity while at the same time emphasizing differences and then "reads out" this stored information by using successive sampling. Note also that the representations are stored hierarchically in that the category response always appears prior to the individuated response pattern. It is also important to emphasize that the LTP-based rules promote acuity; even cues that overlap by 90% generate network outputs after learning which have fewer than 50% of their cells in common.

These results indicate that empirically derived local (i.e., synaptic) rules for modifying contacts and global rhythmic rules do yield coherent aggregate behavior when implemented in a greatly simplified model of a cortical layer. The role that learning plays is somewhat different from that typically assigned to it but the phenomena we have observed are prominent in human recognition memory. People do partition their cue world into categories and do exhibit a hierarchical encoding (i.e., group–individual) not unlike that found in the simulation. A more critical evaluation of the simulation is being made by recording the activity of individual neurons in the olfactory cortex while rats are learning odor discriminations and then comparing the results with the predictions of the model. Several important features of the simulation have been confirmed. Coding appears to be very sparse in that only a small percentage of neurons react to any given odor and activity does seem to be time locked, probably due to the inhalation cycle and theta. We have also observed effects of learning on cell activity. A far more rigorous testing of the model will require large numbers of cues that can be subdivided into natural categories. Cue partitioning or categorization appears not to have been studied as such in rats. It is perhaps a measure of success of the simulation work that it emphasizes a form of learning that has received so little attention in animal psychology. Tests of the very specific predictions of the model (e.g., different patterns of activity arise with different sniffs) under these conditions will provide a rigorous evaluation of its validity as a description of how specific physiological characteristics produce aggregate effects in networks of neurons.

REFERENCES

Alger, B. E. (1984). Characteristics of a slow hyperpolarizing synaptic potential in rat hippocampal pyramidal cells *in vitro*. *Journal of Neurophysiology, 52,* 892–910.

Alger, B. E., & Nicoll, R. A. (1982). Feed-forward dendritic inhibition in rat hippocampal pyramidal neurones studied *in vitro. Journal of Physiology (London), 328,* 105–123.

Andersen, P., Sundberg, S. H., Sveen, O., & Wigstrom, H. (1977). Specific long-lasting potentiation of synaptic transmission in hippocampal slices. *Nature, 226,* 736–737.

Barnes, C. A. (1979). Memory deficits associated with senescence: A neurophysiological and behavioral study in the rat. *Journal of Comparative Physiology and Psychology, 93,* 74–104.

Bear, M., Cooper, L., & Ebner, F. (1987). The physiological basis for a theory of synapse modification. *Science, 237,* 42–48.

Bland, B. H., Andersen, P., Ganes, T., & Sveen, O. (1980). Automated analysis of rhythmicity of physiologically identified hippocampal formation neurons. *Experimental Brain Research, 38,* 205–219.

Bliss, T. V. P., & Gardner-Medwin, A. R. (1973). Long-lasting potentiation of synaptic transmission in the dentate area of the unanesthetized rabbit following stimulation of the perforant path. *Journal of Physiology (London), 232,* 357–374.

Chang, F. L. F., & Greenough, W. T. (1984). Transient and enduring morphological correlates of synaptic activity and efficacy change in the rat hippocampal slice. *Brain Research, 309,* 35–46.

Cohen, M. A., & Grossberg, S. (1983). Absolute stability of global pattern formation and parallel memory storage by competitive neural networks. *IEEE Transactions on Systems, Man, and Cybernetics, 13,* 815–825.

Collingridge, G. L., Kehl, S. J., & McLennan, H. (1983). Excitatory amino acids in synaptic transmission in the Schaffer collateral–commissural pathway of the rat hippocampus. *Journal of Physiology (London), 334,* 33–46.

Cooke, I., Delaney, K., & Gelperin, A. (1985). Complex computation in a small neural network. In N. M. Weinberger, J. L. McGaugh, & G. Lynch (Eds.), *Memory systems of the brain* (pp. 173–192) New York: Guilford.

Dunwiddie, T., & Lynch, G. (1978). Long-term potentiation and depression of synaptic responses in the rat hippocampus: Localization and frequency dependency. *Journal of Physiology (London), 276,* 353–367.

Fox, S. E., & Ranck, J. B., Jr. (1981). Electrophysiological characteristics of hippocampal complex-spike cells and theta cells. *Experimental Brain Research, 41,* 399–410.

Granger, R., Ambros-Ingerson, J., & Lynch, G. (1989). Derivation of encoding characteristics of layer II cerebral cortex. *Journal of Cognitive Neuroscience, 1,* 61–87.

Haberly, L. B. (1985). Neuronal circuitry in olfactory cortex: Anatomy and functional implications. *Chemical Senses, 10,* 219–238.

Harris, E. W., Ganong, A. H., & Cotman, C. W. (1984). Long-term potentiation in the hippocampus involves activation of N-methyl-D-aspartate receptors. *Brain Research, 323,* 132–137.

Hopfield, J. J. (1982). Neural networks and physical systems with emergent collective computational abilities. *Proceedings of the National Academy of Sciences USA, 79,* 2554–2558.

Hotson, J. R., & Prince, D. A. (1980). A Ca^{++}-activated hyperpolarization follows repetitive firing in hippocampal neurons. *Journal of Neurophysiology, 43,* 409–419.

Jahr, C. E., & Stevens, C. F. (1987). Glutamate activates multiple single channel conductances in hippocampal neurons. *Nature, 325,* 522–525.

Jones Leonard, B., McNaughton, B. L., & Barnes, C. A. (1987). Suppression of hippocampal synaptic plasticity during slow-wave sleep. *Brain Research, 425,* 174–177.

Kohonen, T. (1984). *Self-organization and associative memory.* Berlin: Springer-Verlag.

Kuhn, T. (1977). *The essential tension.* Chicago: University of Chicago Press.

Larson, J., & Lynch, G. (1986). Induction of synaptic potentiation in hippocampus by patterned stimulation involves two events. *Science, 232,* 985–988.

Larson, J., & Lynch, G. (1988). Role of N-methyl-D-aspartate receptors in the induction of synaptic potentiation by burst stimulation patterned after the hippocampal theta rhythm. *Brain Research, 441,* 111–118.

Larson, J., & Lynch, G. (1989). Theta pattern stimulation and the induction of LTP: The sequence in which synapses are stimulated determines the degree to which they potentiate. *Brain Research, 489,* 49–58.

Larson, J., Wong, D., & Lynch, G. (1986). Patterned stimulation at the theta frequency is optimal for induction of hippocampal long-term potentiation. *Brain Research, 368,* 347–350.

Lee, K., Oliver, M., Schottler, F., & Lynch, G. (1981). Electron microscopic studies of brain slices: The effects of high frequency stimulation on dendritic ultrastructure. In G. Kerkut & H. V. Wheal (Eds.), *Electrical activity in isolated mammalian C.N.S. preparations,* (pp. 189–212). New York: Academic Press.

Lee, K., Schottler, F., Oliver, M., & Lynch, G. (1980). Brief bursts of high-frequency stimulation produce two types of structural change in rat hippocampus. *Journal of Neurophysiology, 44,* 247–258.

Linsker, R. (1986). From basic network principles to neural architecture: Emergence of spatial-opponent cells. *Proceedings of the National Academy of Sciences USA, 83,* 7508–7512.

Linsker, R. (1988, March). Self-organization in a perceptual network. *IEEE Computer,* pp. 105–117.

Lynch, G. (1986). *Synapses, circuits, and the beginnings of memory.* Cambridge, Mass.: MIT Press.

Lynch, G., Bodsch, W., & Baudry, M. (1988). Cytoskeletal proteins and the regulation of synaptic structure. In R. J. Lasek & M. M. Black (Eds.), *Intrinsic determinants of neuronal form and function* (pp. 217–242). New York: Alan R. Liss.

Lynch, G. S., Dunwiddie, T. V., & Gribkoff, V. (1977). Heterosynaptic depression: A postsynaptic correlate of long-term potentiation. *Nature, 266,737–739.*

Lynch, G., & Granger, R. (in press). Simulation and analysis of a simple cortical network. *Psychology of Learning and Motivation.*

Lynch, G., Granger, R., Larson, J., & Baudry, M. (1988). Cortical encoding of memory: Hypotheses derived from analysis and simulation of physiological learning rules in anatomical structures. In L. Nadel, L. A. Cooper, P. Culicover, & R.M. Harnish (Eds.), *Neural connections and mental computation* (pp. 247–289). Cambridge, Mass.: Bradford Books/MIT Press.

Lynch, G., & Larson, J. (1988). Rhythmic activity, synaptic changes, and the "how and what" of memory storage in simple cortical networks. In J. L. Davis, R. W. Newburgh, & R. E. J. Wegman (Eds.), *Brain structure, learning, and memory* (pp.33–68). Boulder, Colo.: Westview Press.

Lynch, G., Larson, J., Kelso, S., Barrioneuvo, G., & Schottler, F. (1983). Intracellular injections of EGTA block the induction of hippocampal long-term potentiation. *Nature, 305,* 719–721.

Lynch, G., Larson, J., Staubli, U., & Baudry, M. (1987). New perspectives on the physiology, pharmacology, and chemistry of memory. *Drug Development Research, 10,* 295–315.

MacDermott, A. B., Mayer, M. L., Westbrook, G. L., Smith, S. J., & Barker, J. L. (1986). NMDA-receptor activation increases cytoplasmic calcium concentration in cultured spinal cord neurones. *Nature, 321,* 519–522.

Mayer, M. L., & Westbrook, G. L. (1987). Permeation and block of N-methyl-D-aspartic acid receptors channels by divalent cations in mouse cultured central neurones. *Journal of Physiology (London), 394,* 501–527.

McCarren, M., & Alger, B. E. (1985). Use-dependent depression of IPSPs in rat hippocampal pyramidal cells *in vitro. Journal of Neurophysiology, 53,* 557–571.

McNaughton, B. L., Douglas, R. M., & Goddard, G. V. (1978). Synaptic enhancement in fascia dentata: Cooperativity among coactive afferents. *Brain Research, 157,* 277–293.

Morris, R. G. M., Anderson, E., Lynch, G., & Baudry, M. (1986). Selective impairment of learning and blockade of long-term potentiation by an N-methyl-D-aspartate receptor antagonist, AP-5. *Nature, 319,* 774–776.

Muller, D., & Lynch, G. (1988). Long-term potentiation differentially affects two components of synaptic responses in hippocampus. *Proceedings of the National Academy of Sciences USA, 85,* 9346–9350.

Ranck, J. B., Jr. (1973). Studies on single neurons in dorsal hippocampal formation and septum in unrestrained rats. *Experimental Neurology, 41,* 462–531.

Rescorla, R., & Wagner, A. R. (1972). A Theory of Pavlovian conditioning: Variations in the effectiveness of reinforcement and nonreinforcement. In A. H. Black & W. F. Prokasy (Eds.), *Classical conditioning* (pp. 64–99). New York: Appleton-Century-Crofts.

Roman, F., Staubli, U., & Lynch, G. (1987). Evidence for synaptic potentiation in a cortical network during learning. *Brain Research, 418,* 221–226.

Rumelhart, D., Hinton, G., & Williams, R. (1986). Learning internal representations by error propagation. In D. Rumelhart & J. McClelland (Eds.), *Parallel distributed processing.* Cambridge, Mass.: MIT Press.

Staubli, U., Baudry, M., & Lynch, G. (1984). Leupeptin, a thiol proteinase inhibitor, causes a selective impairment of spatial maze performance in rats. *Behavioral and Neural Biology, 40,* 58–69.

Staubli, U., Faraday, R., & Lynch, G. (1985). Pharmacological dissociation of memory: Anisomycin, a protein synthesis inhibitor, and leupeptin, a protease inhibitor, block different learning tasks. *Behavioral and Neural Biology, 43,* 287–297.

Staubli, U., Larson, J., Baudry, M., Thibault, O., & Lynch, G. (1988). Chronic administration of a thiol-proteinase inhibitor blocks long-term potentiation of synaptic responses. *Brain Research, 444,* 153–158.

Staubli, U., & Lynch, G. (1987). Stable hippocampal long-term potentiation elecited by "theta" pattern stimulation. *Brain Research, 435,* 227–234.

Sutton, R. S., & Barto, A. G. (1981). Toward a modern theory of adaptive networks. Expectation and prediction. *Psychological Review, 38,* 135–171.

Vanderwolf, C. H. (1969). Hippocampal electrical activity and voluntary movement in the rat. *Electroencephalography and Clinical Neurophysiology, 26,* 407–418.

Wenzel, J. & Matthies, H. (1985). Morphological changes in the hippocampal formation accompanying memory formation and long-term potentiation. In N. Weinberger, J. McGaugh, & G. Lynch (Eds.), *Memory systems of the brain* (pp. 150–170). New York: Guilford.

Widrow, G. & Hoff, M. E. (1960). Adaptive switching circuits. *Institute of Radio Engineers, Western Electronic Show Convention Record (Part 4), 96–104.*

Zipser, D. & Andersen, R. A. (1988). A back-propagation programmed network that simulates response properties of a subset of posterior parietal neurons. *Nature, 331,* 679–684.

Index